# Healthcare in Private and Public from the Early Modern Period to 2000

A key volume on a central aspect of the history of medicine and its social relations, *Healthcare in Private and Public from the Early Modern Period to 2000* examines how the modernisation of healthcare resulted in a wide variety of changing social arrangements in both public and private spheres.

This book considers a comprehensive range of topics, from children's health, mental disorders and the influence of pharmaceutical companies to the systems of twentieth-century healthcare in Britain, Eastern Europe and South Africa. Covering a broad chronological, thematic and geographical scope, chapters discuss key themes such as how changing economies have influenced configurations of healthcare, how access has varied according to lifecycle, ethnicity and wealth, and how definitions of public and private have shifted over time.

Containing illustrations and a general introduction that outlines the key themes discussed in the volume, *Healthcare in Private and Public from the Early Modern Period to 2000* is essential reading for any student interested in the history of medicine.

**Paul Weindling** is Wellcome Trust Research Professor in the History of Medicine at Oxford Brookes University. His publications include *Victims and Survivors of Nazi Human Experiments: Science and Suffering in the Holocaust* (2014), *John W. Thompson, Psychiatrist in the Shadow of the Holocaust* (2010), *Nazi Medicine and the Nuremberg Trials: From Medical War Crimes to Informed Consent* (2004) and *Epidemics and Genocide in Eastern Europe, 1890–1945* (2000).

# Healthcare in Private and Public from the Early Modern Period to 2000

**Edited by
Paul Weindling**

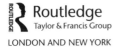

Routledge
Taylor & Francis Group

LONDON AND NEW YORK

First published 2015
by Routledge
2 Park Square, Milton Park, Abingdon, Oxon OX14 4RN

and by Routledge
711 Third Avenue, New York, NY 10017

*Routledge is an imprint of the Taylor & Francis Group, an informa business*

© 2015 Paul Weindling for the editorial material, and the authors for their individual chapters

The right of Paul Weindling to be identified as the author of the editorial material, and of the authors for their individual chapters, has been asserted in accordance with sections 77 and 78 of the Copyright, Designs and Patents Act 1988.

*British Library Cataloguing in Publication Data*
A catalogue record for this book is available from the British Library

*Library of Congress Cataloging-in-Publication Data*
Healthcare in private and public from the early modern period to 2000 / [edited by] Paul Weindling.
p. ; cm.
Includes bibliographical references and index.
I. Weindling, Paul, editor.
[DNLM: 1. Delivery of Health Care–history. 2. Private Sector. 3. Public Sector. 4. Health Care Reform–history. 5. History, Modern 1601–. W 84.1]
RA418
362.1–dc23
2014022952

ISBN: 978-0-415-72700-6 (hbk)
ISBN: 978-0-415-72703-7 (pbk)
ISBN: 978-1-315-73987-8 (ebk)

Typeset in Times New Roman
by Taylor & Francis Books

Printed and bound in the United States of America by
Edwards Brothers Malloy on sustainably sourced paper

To John Perkins for seeding the history of medicine at Oxford Brookes University

# Contents

# List of illustrations

# Acknowledgements

Work for this book was supported by a Wellcome Trust Strategic Award in Medical History [no. 082808/B/07/Z], which is gratefully acknowledged by the grant holders who have contributed chapters to the book. The award has funded an extensive programme of research since 2007 on 'Health care in public and private'. All contributors were initially based at Oxford Brookes University. We very much appreciate the supportive environment of Oxford Brookes for our research. We especially thank Dr Carol Beadle, Administrator of the Centre for Health, Medicine and Society: Past and Present for support during this grant, and for assistance with the preparation of the volume. Dr Beadle and Dr Aleksandra Loewenau co-ordinated the final preparation of the chapters, and skilfully carried out necessary textual editing.

# Abbreviations

| | |
|---|---|
| ANC | African National Congress |
| DPH | Department of Public Health |
| DSM | Diagnostic and Statistical Manual of Mental Disorders |
| FDA | Food and Drug Administration |
| ICI | Imperial Chemical Industries |
| ILO | International Labour Office/Organization |
| ICRC | International Committee of the Red Cross |
| LNHO | League of Nations Health Organization |
| MRC | Medical Research Council |
| NGO | Non-governmental Organization |
| NHI | National Health Insurance |
| NIH | National Institutes of Health |
| OSRD | Office for Scientific Research and Development |
| PAHO | Pan-American Health Organization |
| STS | Science and Technology Studies |
| UNAIDS | United Nations Programme on HIV/AIDS |
| WHO | World Health Organization |
| WMA | World Medical Association |

# List of contributors

**Dr Tom Crook** is Lecturer in Modern British History at Oxford Brookes University. Recent publications include (ed., with Glen O'Hara) *Statistics and the public sphere: Numbers and the people in modern Britain, c. 1800–2000* (Routledge, 2011) and (ed.) *Sanitary reform, class and the Victorian city* (Pickering and Chatto, 2013). He has also published single and co-authored articles in *Urban History* (2008), *Past and Present* (2011) and *Historical Research* (2015), and is currently completing a book entitled *Modern Governance and the Making of Public Health in England, c. 1830–1910*.

**Professor Anne Digby** is Emeritus Professor in History at Oxford Brookes University and her chief research interest is medical pluralism. She has published widely in the fields of British social policy and in the social history of medicine of both Britain and South Africa. Recent books have included *Diversity and Division in Medicine: Health care in South Africa from the 1800s* (Peter Lang, 2006) and a co-authored volume with Howard Philips, *At the Heart of Healing: Groote Schuur Hospital* (Jacana, 2008).

**Dr George Campbell Gosling** has held teaching and research positions at Oxford Brookes University, the University of Liverpool, King's College London and the University of Warwick. His work focuses on the history of medicine and charity in modern Britain and beyond. He co-edited (with Colin Rochester, Alison Penn and Meta Zimmeck) *Understanding the Roots of Voluntary Action: Historical Perspectives on Current Social Policy* (Sussex Academic Press, 2011) and his first monograph, exploring the limits of private healthcare in Britain before the NHS, will be published by Pickering and Chatto.

**Dr Elizabeth Hurren** is Reader in Medical Humanities in the School of Historical Studies at Leicester University. Her research expertise is on the history of poverty, welfare and medical research, featuring the public and private healthcare needs of the poorest in modern Europe. Recent books include: A. Gestrich, E. Hurren and S. King (eds), *Poverty and Sickness in Modern Europe: Narratives of the Sick Poor, 1780–1938* (Continuum, 2012) and *Dying for Victorian Medicine: English Anatomy and its Trade in* *the dead poor 1832–1929* (Palgrave, 2012). Currently, she is completing a Wellcome Trust-funded book on *Dissecting the Criminal Corpse: Post-mortem Punishment from the Murder Act (1752) until the Anatomy Act (1832) in England* (Palgrave, 2015).

**Professor Steven King** is Pro-Vice Chancellor and Head of the College of Social Science at the University of Leicester. For the last decade he has focused his research and publication on the intertwining questions of poverty, belonging and pauper agency. Recent publications include: A. Gestrich, E. Hurren and S. King (eds), *Poverty and Sickness in Modern Europe: Narratives of the Sick Poor, 1780–1938* (Continuum, 2012); S. King and A. Winter (eds), *Migration, Settlement and Belonging in Europe, 1500s–1930s* (Berghahn, 2013); and *Women, Welfare and Local Politics 1880–1920: "We Might be Trusted"* (Sussex University Press, 2010).

**Dr Alysa Levene** is Reader in History at Oxford Brookes University. Her research focuses on the history of childhood, welfare and the family from the eighteenth century to the twentieth century. She has published on the health and welfare of poor and abandoned children, illegitimacy, apprenticeship and hospitals, including *The Childhood of the Poor: Welfare in Eighteenth-century London* (Palgrave Macmillan, 2012), and the chapter on 'Childhood and adolescence' in Mark Jackson's *Oxford Handbook of the History of Medicine* (Oxford University Press, 2011). She is currently working on a project investigating family, welfare and community in nineteenth-century Britain.

**Dr Glen O'Hara** is Professor of Modern and Contemporary History at Oxford Brookes University. A former journalist, he is the author or editor of a number of books on twentieth-century British history, including (with Helen Parr), *The Modernisation of Britain? Harold Wilson and the Labour Governments of 1964–1970* (Routledge, 2006), *From Dreams to Disillusionment: Economic and Social Planning in 1960s Britain* (Palgrave Macmillan, 2007), and *Governing Post-war Britain: The Paradoxes of Progress, 1951–1973* (Palgrave Macmillan, 2012). He is currently writing a history of *The Politics of Water in Post-war Britain*, which will be published by Palgrave Macmillan in 2016.

**Dr Viviane Quirke** is Senior Lecturer in Modern History and History of Medicine at Oxford Brookes University. Her research focuses on the history of biomedical knowledge and practice, therapeutic innovation and the pharmaceutical industry. She is the author of *Collaboration in the Pharmaceutical Industry* (Routledge, 2008); co-editor with Jean-Paul Gaudillière of 'The era of biomedicine' (special issue of *Medical History*, vol. 52, 2008), identified as one of the highlights of the journal's past ten years; co-editor with Judy Slinn of *Perspectives on Twentieth-century Pharmaceuticals* (Peter Lang, 2010); and editor of 'Pharmaceutical styles of thinking and doing' (special issue of *Pharmacy in History*, vol. 52, 2010). Her current research areas are the history of pharmaceutical R&D,

focusing on the history of drug treatments for chronic diseases and the impact of drug safety regulation; the history of company-hospital relations and the development of clusters of innovation in Britain, France and the USA; and the history of cancer chemotherapy, studied from the perspective of both researchers and sufferers. Her next book, *Drugs, Disease and Industry: The Evolution of Pharmaceutical R&D at Imperial Chemical Industries*, is forthcoming with Oxford University Press.

**Dr Marius Turda** is Reader in Central and Eastern European Biomedicine at Oxford Brookes University. He is the author or editor of a number of books on the history of eugenics, race and biopolitics, including *Latin Eugenics in International Context* (Bloomsbury, 2014); *Eugenics and Nation in early Twentieth-century Hungary* (Palgrave Macmillan, 2014); and *Crafting Humans: From Genesis to Eugenics and Beyond* (Taiwan National University Press, 2013). He is currently compiling an anthology of eugenic texts and authors entitled *The History of Eugenics in East Central Europe, 1900–1945: Sources and Commentaries* (forthcoming, Bloomsbury, 2015).

**Dr Katherine D. Watson** is Senior Lecturer in the History of Medicine at Oxford Brookes University and a Fellow of the Royal Historical Society. Her research interests focus on areas where medicine, crime and the law intersect, including the history of infanticide and crimes against children, forensic medicine and science, and an unusual form of assault known as vitriol throwing. She is the author of *Poisoned Lives: English Poisoners and their Victims* (2004) and *Forensic Medicine in Western Society: A History* (2011), and has edited a collection of essays on the history of violence, *Assaulting the Past: Violence and Civilization in Historical Context* (2007). Her most recent publication, 'Women, violent crime and criminal justice in Georgian Wales', *Continuity and Change*, 28/2 (2013), arises from her current research on medico-legal practice in England and Wales 1700–1914, funded by the Wellcome Trust.

**Professor Paul Weindling** is Wellcome Trust Research Professor in the History of Medicine at Oxford Brookes University. His research interests cover the history of eugenics, public health organisations, and twentieth-century disease patterns. His current research focuses on social Darwinism and eugenics, international health in the twentieth century, and human experimentation post-1800, notably Nazi coerced experimentation. His publications include *Health, Race and German Politics Between National Unification and Nazism* (Cambridge University Press, 1989), *Epidemics and Genocide in Eastern Europe 1890–1945* (Oxford University Press, 2000), *Nazi Medicine and the Nuremberg Trials: From Medical War Crimes to Informed Consent* (Palgrave Macmillan, 2004), *John W. Thompson, Psychiatrist in the Shadow of the Holocaust* (Rochester University Press, 2010), and *Victims and Survivors of Nazi Human Experiments: Science and Suffering in the Holocaust* (Bloomsbury, 2014).

# 1 Introduction

## Public and private in the modernisation of medicine: Politics, professions, and practices

*Paul Weindling*

### Public and private: Polar opposites?

Medicine and healthcare provide penetrating insight into processes of modernisation, and the associated transformation of social structures and cultural values. The social and cultural implications of healthcare provision have been highly political as regards the state and voluntary sector, and in the developing of both the public and private spheres. Issues of national identity and personal identity are strongly defined and shaped by health. The repercussions appear across a wide variety of issues, ranging from healthcare as a political arena to the role of the professions with agendas affecting private interests and public service. Medical practices penetrate deeply into issues of privacy and the personal, as well as ranging across a wide terrain of institutional and professional structures. Epidemic crises and eugenic concerns with the quality of future generations are two cases in which the public has been paramount in intensely personal spheres.

Public and private can be taken as a long-running distinction with far-reaching repercussions for medicine in terms of individual and community health. The historian and campaigner for the socialisation of medicine, Henry Sigerist, addressed this in his pioneering analysis of the rise of modern medicine seen through the lens of 'the social history of medicine', a term that he introduced in 1940.[1] Yet for Sigerist, the more medicine was socialised, the more optimistic he was about its benefits. He was naïve about gender and how medical knowledge could be coercive and dehumanising.[2]

The politics of how best to deliver healthcare has often been contentious since the sixteenth century, when guilds of physicians, barber surgeons and apothecaries protested against competition from 'irregular' healers. Iconoclastic and radical Paracelsian practitioners had visions of chemical medicine for the poor, as opposed to costly medicine for the rich.[3] In the course of the seventeenth century, new types of policlinics and dispensaries, and public hospital provision all sought to provide a medicine for the people. The French Paracelsian Théophraste Renaudot opened a pioneering public clinic in 1630. The emergent professional organisations and associated institutions deepened the idea of the public sphere as being essentially communicative.[4] What sharpened was the clash between the private professional interests and schemes for making medicine accessible to wider publics. These arising disputes can be seen in the context of sexually transmitted diseases and tuberculosis when the public interest was for the afflicted to be treated. Public and private have been engaged in a protracted conflict, as professional interests seek to protect their autonomy from socialised schemes of medical provision. At other times, there has been complementarity and symbiosis between public and private as reflected in ideas of health, experiences of sickness, and in various forms of medical knowledge and provision. Certainly, the multifarious meanings of public and private in medicine require elaboration, explanation and exemplification as complex and fluid categories.[5]

The cultural upheavals generated by Renaissance and Reformation science-based medicine had a profound impact on the sensibilities surrounding the emergence of ideas on modern life from conception to death. On the one hand, medicine generally, and science-based medicine especially, offer the historian penetrating insights into privacy and intimacy (as with sexual and reproductive issues), everyday customs surrounding well-being, and the coping with stress (itself a medically defined category). On the other hand, medicine has been highly public, with spectacles (such as public anatomical dissections since the sixteenth century), practices such as the mediaeval traditions of healing by touch, and the idea that the physician should act in the public interest in matters of sanitation and reproduction. The physician/healer was both a public figure and yet detached because of specialist esoteric knowledge and powers. The Norwegian dramatist Ibsen in his 1882 play *An Enemy of the People* showed the reforming physician as being at loggerheads with vested commercial interests. The boundaries between public and private have been shifting, often socially contested, but sometimes complementary to each other. The issues that have arisen in turn provide insight into social norms and structures, so that the history of medicine contributes to mainstream history. Beyond this, historians have an important role to play in providing accountability by assessing past medical conduct, and taking a forward look at socio-medical problems by contributing to policy.

This volume seeks to analyse key aspects and episodes in the history of medicalisation and professionalisation in ways that are thematically cohesive and historically contextualised. Chapters examine issues broadly, contextualising, comparing, and identifying the interactions of interest groups and states. We take a thematic approach rather than one restricted to any short period and particular location. Our common concern is the crucial polarity of public and private. Our studies explore the time- and region-specific character of the mixed economy of healthcare, and the nature of patient and professional experiences of such systems. Of particular interest is how these issues reflected a complex interplay between public (the state, national and local), private (from the professional entrepreneur to family and self-help), and philanthropic bodies, which range from corporate to mass public donor medical charities. Our diverse investigations have focused on the financing of health services, the character and meaning of institutional provision, differential patient access to treatment, professional careers, and the geographical reach of the medical market. It has become ever clearer that there was an indistinct, porous and fluctuating frontier between the different sectors. The relative importance of each sector and the nature of the borderlands between them have been shaped by exogenous influences such as economic, political or socio-structural conditions, shifts in the perceived role of the state, a changed understanding of diseases, the development of information networks, and economic imperatives. While these are all factors operating in general, and indeed in global, history, there are also factors more specific to medicine, such as the balance of professional and patient power, patient choices, and medical innovation and the prevailing knowledge systems, which are important influences in a story characterised by fluidity and diversity of types of healthcare provision.

The powerful processes shaping medical provision since the Renaissance, notably professionalisation and the expansive embracing of diverse personal and public sectors referred to as 'medicalisation' have been characterised in conflicting terms. The French philosopher Michel Foucault and the critic of modern institutions Ivan Illich castigated medicine in terms of 'medicalisation' as a repressive, menacingly destructive process.[6] There have been highly uneven and indeed contested processes of social change and conflict involving medical provision and impacting on the health of populations. We find varieties of therapy, different arrangements in medical provision, and changing public expectations. The impacts were uneven, and occurred at differing times and with varying intensity in different locations.

Our chapters build on and carry forward these new historiographical perspectives. Chapters explore what has come to be known as 'the mixed economy of healthcare' across a large chronological (1650–2000) and geographical (encompassing Britain, Europe, the United States and Africa) range, and engage with the histories of a wide spectrum of social, professional and life-cycle groups. In so doing, they form the foundation for a synthetic and analytical overview of the interplay of the public, private and philanthropic in the provision of healthcare in the modern world.

Our studies are organised around the twin themes of public and private provision of healthcare. Debates over current healthcare policy centre on the ambiguous dichotomy of public and private. These include the desirable balance between the public and private work of practitioners; the rights of patients and the duties of institutions and professionals; the rights of the state to intrude (in health terms) into the private domains of the person and the family; and the balance between the private imperative involved in genetic intervention and the interests of science as a state-monitored and protected 'public good'. The chapters explore aspects of the roots of these historical and modern policy issues with wide thematic and comparative coverage.

## State and community

The emergence of medicine in the public sphere is intertwined with state and community formation. Tensions arise between community and state schemes. Beyond the nation state, there was the emergence of a new and equally contested international sphere. Administrative arrangements varied in terms vividly explored by Tom Crook for the nineteenth century, and Glen O'Hara and George Gosling for the second half of the twentieth century. Sanitation, housing, and even the processes of dying and disposal of the dead evoke these discordant discourses.

The German case is of special interest for establishing the modern pattern. Germany provided the modern model of the scientifically trained physician. On the one hand, any 'Herr Doktor' would have completed an MD dissertation; on the other, he (women were admitted to the profession only in the early twentieth century in Germany) would have passed state medical examinations. Clinical appointments at universities were full time salaried appointments. The German case became internationalised with the Flexner Report for the Carnegie Foundation in 1912. This set the pattern for the German system becoming the norm at American medical schools. The state-regulated insurance system in Imperial Germany expanded the market for medical care immensely.[7] This created a tension between the public and private spheres, as the profession doggedly defended a free market in terms of patient choice. Yet the slogan of patient choice in reality reflected the collective interests of physicians, as obstructing any form of socialisation of medical provision. These structural tensions have continued to surround modern medicine in many countries and contexts until today, as well shown by controversies surrounding 'Obamacare' in the United States.

One might see the process of medicalisation as symptomatic of the wider transformations of modernisation. This involves how the provision of systems of medical care such as those under the poor laws became universalised, science-based professions and industrial systems of production of pharmaceuticals. One can, however, see a persistence of other forms of practice, healing and medicaments, shown by numerous forms of alternative healing and nature therapy. The public constituted an expanding market for medical care, even though both the state and profession sought to regulate this market. Charles Webster introduced a market-based perspective to reveal a diversity of practitioners in the early modern period. The early modern period was characterised by physicians making unrealistic claims of a monopoly, when the actual situation was of a plurality of healers. This situation finds a parallel in the African case analysed by Anne Digby: here traditional healers retained a position until modern times.

Medicine became increasingly interventive in the private sphere, as it came to pervade domestic arrangements and the family. Alysa Levene (following the German philosopher Jürgen Habermas) views the family as 'the intimate sphere', providing a range of details concerning medical aspects of domesticity and personal relations. Hygiene governed domestic space, the space between individuals, and the definition of sexuality. Norbert Elias analysed the civilising process in terms of the sociology of knowledge. Elias developed notions of individual autonomy, privacy and intimacy. These were tempered by Elias's experience as a medical student, so that the 'trickle down' process of the regulation of codes of behaviour included an increasingly hygienic lifestyle.[8]

The pace and intensity of these processes have given rise to sharply divergent interpretations. One is of a 'scientific revolution' impacting on medicine and replacing traditional healers. Another is of gradual processes dependent on the market and consumption patterns. Wider questions arise as to the significance and impact of laboratory medicine. Thomas McKeown argued in the early 1970s that science-based therapies were of little consequence, and were implemented after declines in mortality from TB and other major infections; he considered improvements in diet and housing to have had a major effect in reducing mortality from infectious diseases.[9] The historical focus on innovation rather than implementation has meant that these issues remain open and unresolved.

Wider theories of modernisation involve the rationalising of reproductive behaviour. Theories of the 'demographic transition' (a term coined by Frank W. Notestein around 1945) and 'epidemiological transition' (a term coined by Abdel Omran) have provided a dynamic context for framing medicine.[10] The demographic changes had profound implications for the health of children, as shown by Alysa Levene. Rates of maternal mortality remained persistently high.

Eugenicists were pioneers in detecting both the shift to smaller families and the shift from infectious to chronic diseases.[11] While correctly diagnosing these trends, they denounced them as pathological in terms of subverting population health and fertility. Eugenicists were critical of women entering the labour market. To act as a corrective, eugenicists demanded a shift from the physician acting in the interests of the individual patient, thereby threatening national health by maintaining the lives of the hereditarily unfit, to a role of professionals acting in the service of the state.

For a long time historians of medicine equated state-funded medical provision with improvements in health. A classic expression of this can be found in the works of the American historian of public health, George Rosen, and Henry Sigerist, who revolutionised the history of medicine by rejecting the narrowness of the textual exposition of physicians' writings.[12] More critical views began to be voiced from the 1980s with a renewed emphasis on the patient.[13] The history of eugenics showed the darkly destructive side of medical power entrenched in new administrative structures: Jane Lewis critically analysed Ministry of Health policies in the 1920s for defective provision for female health in the UK.[14] Yet above all it is the case of German eugenics that most vividly shows the destructive potential of any state system in terms of genocidal policies of forced abortion and sterilisation, and murder of unwanted populations of the mentally ill, the disabled, and Jews and gypsies, among numerous other targets, on medical and racial grounds.[15] The Dutch sociologist Abram de Swaan has examined implications of the shift from the local to the national with the extension of state power in healthcare provision on a collective and compulsory basis, administered and enforced by the state.[16] Yet de Swaan's view is open to question. O'Hara and Gosling see the private within the public in the case of the central state-administered NHS. Looking more widely at developments concerning the costs of insurance provision, we find a sphere that is non-state but not private. Structurally, the Bismarckian social and medical insurance of the early 1880s involved a multiplicity of organisations with decentralised administration. The total socialisation of medicine emerges as utopian in its terms of actual realisation. The pragmatic view is that of a 'mixed economy of healthcare', yet varied forms of socialised not-for-profit provision range between public and private.

The seventeenth century saw the first policlinics and dispensaries for a wider public. The dispensary movement and infirmaries expanded in eighteenth-century England as forms of patriarchal charity – a sick person needed a ticket from a donor to be seen. The extension of state provision was accompanied by ideas of a right to healthcare. While the French Revolution left a legacy of ideas of social medicine, the idea of a right to democratically accountable healthcare had to wait for the revolutions of 1848. The Berlin poor law doctor and medical statistician Saloman Neumann demanded healthcare as a democratic right. The liberal pathologist Rudolf Virchow forthrightly called for a free profession. Here we find a paradigmatic clash between the idea of healthcare as both an entitlement and politically accountable to its clients, and the notion that the quality of healthcare depends on freedom. While ideas of a free profession have been associated with the idea of a duty of care to the individual patient, the realisation has been highly variable. The issues of public accountability of medicine and a free profession based on medical research have remained contested. In Britain the reforming Anatomy Act of 1832 (a year also of political reform) boosted the idea of a science-based professional education.[17] While the 1930s saw a movement for science-based medicine as part of a planned society, the Cold War saw a reversal of values, with the idea of the freedom of science as an individual pursuit, funded by the state but not subject to public accountability, gaining prominence. Set against this were notions of consent as a reaction to the Nazi experiments. Researchers have a strong sense that research requires autonomy, while there is an evident need for public accountability and public understanding of science. Michel Foucault's view of an authoritarian and exploitative medical gaze represents an extreme view of medicine as manipulative and coercive.

The state takeover of poor relief from community-based provision led to deep controversies over welfare and entitlement. Even though there was a shift from local propertied classes to bureaucrats, Abram de Swaan has argued that the primary beneficiaries of welfare systems are the propertied classes. The chapter on international health in this volume shows how welfare

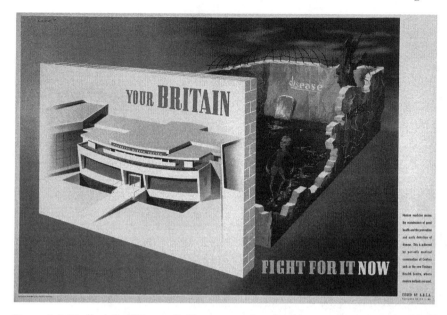

*Figure 1.1* Medical facilities available at a modern health centre contrasted with ill
health in old-fashioned housing, 1942. © The Wellcome Library, London.

state provision has benefitted the entitled but simultaneously deprived the
poor, sick and starving of the ability to escape threats by migration. From
the late nineteenth century, ideas of racial and ethnic cohesion intensified,
precipitating a shift to more complex forms of the state. As the chapter by
Marius Turda shows, the interwar Central European states well illustrate the
emergence of new state formations. Whereas in Imperial Germany welfare
was deemed a private charitable matter, the new Weimar constitution of 1920
made welfare a state responsibility. Health and welfare ceased to be a private
matter, and became a concern of the state: ironically, democratisation opened
the door to professional power in the shape of eugenics and ultimately the
coercive racial policies unleashed from 1933 under the Nazis.

After the devastation of the Second World War came a new human rights
revolution to protect populations from coercive injustice. The 'Constitution
of the World Health Organization' reaffirmed health – and by extension
healthcare – as an international civic right in 1946. But the World Health
Organization was cautious as regards the implementation of universal medical entitlement at a time of physician opposition to state health systems.

## Problems and controversies

The question of what is private and what is public becomes a major set
of controversies. Issues concerning the costs of healthcare and its public
provision remain at the core of what this book shows are long-running and

wide-ranging controversies. We address different combinations of the following key questions:

- How and why have political, patient and professional perceptions and
  expectations of publicly versus privately funded healthcare developed?
- In particular, how have definitions of 'public' and 'private' responsibilities
  varied over time and place?
- How have the changing economics of health influenced perceptions,
  experiences and configurations of healthcare?
- For patients, how did the constellation of healthcare (and the respective
  locations of public and private), rights to treatment and health outcomes
  vary according to life-cycle stage, ethnicity or wealth?
- How has the role of philanthropy influenced the development and patient
  experience of the mixed economy of healthcare?
- How were the indistinct and porous boundaries between public, private
  and philanthropic healthcare experienced and negotiated by patients and
  practitioners in the past?
- What sorts of professionals and patients have populated the borderlands
  between the sectors in the past?
- What are the relationships between a particular configuration of public
  and private resources and the mainstreaming or marginalisation of
  groups of patients (e.g. British paupers or black South Africans)?
- How have patients and professionals thought about their rights and
  duties in differently configured mixed economies of healthcare? How, in
  particular, could patients seek to establish rights to health resources?
- How and why have public, private and philanthropic institutions developed and what have their roles been in differently configured systems?
- How has the transfer of theory and practice across sectoral boundaries
  influenced the experiences, perceptions and expectations of publicly,
  privately and philanthropically funded healthcare?
- How have public healthcare systems participated in knowledge creation,
  testing and innovation with private companies?
- How did public, private and philanthropic medicine come to be shaped
  by scientific ideologies such as eugenics, and how did eugenics fare under
  radically antagonistic political systems?

## Contents and concepts

The various studies here outline and analyse crucial aspects of the polarities
between public and private in their diverse and intersecting forms. To set the
scene, it should be noted that between 1500 and 1700 an individual's health
was mainly a private matter. The historian Tim McHugh has argued that the
Reformation changed ideas of health concerning the body, and obligations of
charity. In England William Petty, a scientist and economist, planned a new
type of public hospital. By the eighteenth century philanthropically funded but

secular infirmaries contrasted to Church-provided hospitals in Europe. A contrast can be drawn between healthcare as a secular responsibility in England, and the French Catholic Church as a provider of medical charity. In Austria Enlightened Catholicism prioritised an active charitable love of one's neighbour, and an active healing role of Church institutions and parish priests.

Mercantilist economic theorists from the seventeenth century onwards emphasised the importance of the health of the population to the strength of a state. States began to co-ordinate and intervene when faced with epidemics and famine. The eighteenth century saw the first steps toward protecting the population's health through environmental improvements.[18]

The healthcare of the poor became a major focus for emerging states as well as for localities. Steven King has argued that the healthcare needs of the poorest sections of British, American and European society were met with a complex medical economy of makeshifts. From the 1650s, systematic contracting of doctors to institutions began, and charities and parishes in Britain and Europe became active organisers of healthcare provision. The chapter by Elizabeth Hurren and King examines the changing balance of public, private and philanthropic healthcare from the perspective of the poor. They delineate different experiences of health systems in Europe and North America, and draw attention to the power and influence of poor patients as having in the past arguably been more significant than in the present.

Alysa Levene examines how the key dependent group of children were a focus of public and private care. Her work on foundlings addresses the interaction between private practitioners, families as healthcare providers, charities and public concerns over child health. Importantly, public bodies such as charities and the state intruded into the private life of the family. She sees children as 'the most private aspect of the private sphere', protected by their living space and by their parents. Here a tension arose: children had long been seen as the private assets of their parents, but added to this was a growing sense that they were also the resources of the state. States exercised increasing powers over hitherto private matters of schooling, employment, nutrition, childcare and health.

Katherine Watson explores forensic science as offering key insights into medical responses to crime and social deviance. She considers the role played by psychiatry in criminal trials for homicide and illicit sexual activity since the late eighteenth century. In France and Germany, where forensic medicine developed comparatively early, and then in England and Wales, and the United States, forensic psychiatrists established themselves as authorities on the links between criminality, mental disorder and dangerousness, thus helping to shape public perceptions of crime and criminals. Throughout, the figure of the medical expert functioned as a bridge between medicine and the law, balancing the needs and rights of mentally ill offenders with the safety of the community.

The nineteenth century became an era of inspection: factories, schools and homes all became subject to surveillance. A complex and fraught borderline arose between protection and intrusion. Here it is interesting to compare the extent of intrusion. By the early twentieth century there was greater readiness to intrude in the home and (with coercive sterilisation) bodies than in the productive process in the economy.

Tom Crook delineates how the imperative of health has transformed the design and practice of public and private space in the transition to becoming a modern, urbanised society. The history of public and private space is a complex and manifold one, and health is not the only imperative that deserves consideration: so too do the imperatives of civilisation (Elias), discipline (Foucault), and private selfhood (Taylor). Crook discerns how reforming public and private space allows for a productive consideration of the ways healthcare has shaped our bodily conduct and reconfigured the way we relate to ourselves and to others, morally just as much as physically. More simply, it helps to illuminate the multiple ways caring for health has remade the architecture of 'public' and 'private' life, and the experience of the everyday.

The 'medicalisation' of space comprised linked processes: the de-congestion of urban space and the building of healthier, more open public spaces (streets, squares and parks); the 'cellularisation' of space in disciplinary institutions (hospitals, prisons, asylums and workhouses), premised on according the inmate an observable, hygienic space; and, finally, the provision of various cubical spaces, such as those containing baths, beds and toilets, designed to secure for the subject a private sanitary space of his or her own. Crook concludes by looking at complexities of use and appropriation, and the limitations of space as a tool of government. He examines the need for ongoing maintenance and cleanliness, and the importance of class – especially in the British context – as a means of understanding the differential provision of public and private space.

George Gosling and Glen O'Hara place the developing National Health Service (NHS) within a wider international context. The NHS is notable as a central state system financed from general taxation, if not unique then a relatively rare example of public medicine that contrasts to insurance-based provision. Yet there are a number of decentralising forces: a continuing status of members of the medical profession as free contractors, and the lack of fully comprehensive coverage, as shown by dental care. The chapter here highlights privatisation within the system. The NHS stands as an example of an idea of national citizenship and nation-building in the second half of the twentieth century. Rather than an example of wholesale nationalisation of healthcare provision, Britain's NHS evolved into an uneasy compromise. It was less a fully-integrated and well-funded universal system along Nordic lines, or a contractual social insurance system as in the rest of Western Europe, or even an individualistic and pay-as-you-go arrangement akin to those accepted in Australia and the United States. Instead, the NHS took over and adapted elements from the old Poor Law system – a role for local government in the delivery of health-related social services, for instance, and a divide between prestigious (and often London-based) teaching hospitals and humbler, less well-funded local institutions. This eventually gave rise, during the 1970s and 1980s, to the idea that the Service should be 'reorganised', with the entire structure brought together in a single system of top-down management – a complicated and heavily bureaucratic process that eventually left the NHS seemingly unable to respond to patients' and families' needs and concerns. The scene was set for an even more fundamental series of changes, beginning in the late 1980s and picking up speed in the early twenty-first century: the creation of heavily-regulated quasi-markets that to some extent returned to the 'mixed economy of healthcare' that had prevailed before the NHS was created. The authors show how the British healthcare system had therefore come full circle, while remaining unlike almost any other in the world: an example of the role of governments in structuring the public sphere, but also a unique scheme that helps to highlight and give shape to our understanding of others.

Marius Turda discusses various traditions of private and public health-care characterising Central and south-eastern Europe from the nineteenth to the (mid-) twentieth centuries. The region offers an epidemiological and demographic contrast to Western Europe. He delineates how it is a very diverse region, not only in terms of its geography, but also in terms of culture and religion. The region shows an inherent fluidity and instability in terms of the transition from four empires (Ottoman, Austro-Hungarian, Russian and German) to states defined on the basis of ethnic self-determination. The chapter shows how the newly constituted national governments attempted to re-inforce the importance of a healthy population to their nation-building ambitions. In collaboration with foreign institutions, the Central and south-eastern European states provided financial support for the establishment of health institutions and infrastructure. These public approaches were developed in tension with private professionalising interests. To an extent the tensions were bridged by the transformation of physicians into devoted supporters of the national community. The Nazi occupation and the Holocaust tore apart the cohesion of state systems and professional elites. After a brief period of fluidity after the war, the imposition of a Soviet-style socialised system meant the predominance of a public framework. Within this, as a survey by Michael Kaser shows, private interests – professional, insurance-based, and confessionally based medical provision – continued to flourish.[19]

The impact of Western medicine on the wider world is analysed in the chapter on South Africa. Anne Digby takes an innovative patient-oriented approach by addressing the patient pluralism practised by different ethnic groups, exploring choices made across private and public health provision. South Africa is placed comparatively within the context of Southern and Central Africa, and beyond this in relation to developments on the continent of Africa, where there has been a huge burden of disease on usually poorly resourced public and private healthcare. The analysis is of wider global significance in terms of the immense burdens of disease and limited therapeutic resources.

The chapter shows how South Africa is unusual in being both a developed and a developing country, and this has influenced its mixed economy of healthcare. The nation's varied ethnic composition and the policies that addressed (or too often neglected) this diversity imposed further burdens on the sick and the impoverished. In focusing on the financing of healthcare this chapter maps structures and policies onto this complex and changing foundation. Digby addresses the changing dimensions of public and private healthcare by analysing the structures underpinning inequitable access. Responsibility for public healthcare was fragmented between central government (in charge of public health), four provincial authorities (directing hospitals) and many local authorities (responsible for environmental health and infectious diseases). She outlines how a significant but abortive attempt to create a national health system in the 1940s was cut short by the Nationalist government of 1948 and its apartheid policies, but was revived after the democratic transition in 1994. A major divide is that of urban-centred healthcare while the majority of the population lived in rural areas. The chapter discusses a health policy that began after the democratic transition of 1994 to address the overwhelming strength of funding in urban tertiary institutions together with the concentration of medical – and to a lesser extent nursing – personnel in urban areas by giving priority to primary healthcare, building a network of rural clinics, and requiring community service from recent healthcare graduates. Finally, the chapter briefly looks at the huge impact of the HIV/AIDS pandemic on this.

Viviane Quirke draws threads of themes of manufacturing and commercial interests, state regulation and market-based consumption by examining the global significance of pharmaceutical innovation and manufacturing. She examines the interaction between the public and private spheres that has underpinned pharmaceutical innovation and has in turn been shaped by it. The public–private interactions involved in pharmaceutical innovation, marketing and consumption have been considerable. On the consumption side, private marketing has been highly regulated by public bodies, with professional experts playing a key role on both sides. Indeed, the dual nature of expertise has far-reaching implications.

Paul Weindling's international analysis is premised on the spread of sickness insurance in the areas of family health and welfare, as well as of the new socialised systems of emergent welfare states. The chapter is innovative both in its century-long time span and in considering the effects of the Holocaust on post-Second World War developments. The frame of reference is international, and international organisations are the main focus. International health organisations have regulated medical matters between states, across whole regions, and on a global basis, and provided relief to the diseased, famished and oppressed. They functioned as multilateral organisations through the League of Nations and then the United Nations. Others were empowered by a sense that the humanitarian issues were best dealt with by organisations acting beyond the state and the multilateral framework. At their most limited, international health agencies continued the sanitary controls of the nineteenth century, imposing quarantine and closing borders to exclude disease carriers. At its most interventive, public health offered total sanitary surveillance of whole communities. There was a shift from the limited liberal state in which most health-related matters were essentially in the private sphere to transnational organisational forms complementing new comprehensive welfare states. This chapter concludes with the emergence of diverse models of public and private medicine at the new international level, and their responses to mass migration, socio-economic upheavals, two world wars and the Cold War.

## Historical perspectives

What emerges is that although medicalisation and professionalisation were key features of the modernising process, these processes and their outcomes were diverse. Between the private and the public, strengthening professional interests exercise a powerful force. Modern societies are in many ways professionalised and knowledge-based, and medicine well illustrates this.[20] The rubric of public and private captures the resulting diversity and pluralism. Yet the boundaries between the public and private, although contested, show considerable overlaps. Interpretations of topics such as social medicine are highly coloured by the political perspective on the issue of welfare provision. One role for historians is to look beyond the polemics at the actual functioning of institutions and interests.

The relationship between public and private has varied between an informal complementarity and forceful intrusion. The Nazi denial of rights to reproduce and penetration (in terms of state powers) into the reproductive organs well shows this: the unfit and undesirable were castrated and sterilised. Here there was a strong alliance between the medical profession, keen to extend its powers, and the state. As the SS marital regulations showed, the fit elite of the German nation were subjected to screening and regulation. State population policies were a prominent feature of the twentieth century, with regulation, intrusion and transplantation of whole population groups.

Systems of human rights have been necessary to offer protection against violations and the undermining of freedoms in the name of medicine and health regarding behaviour and sexuality. There continue to be fierce clashes over issues that in the West are regarded as elemental human rights, not least abortion as a woman's right and the person's body as a sovereign inviolable sphere. Broadly speaking, one can see the informal and 'private' dissemination of values and patterns of behaviour as contrasting to publicly regulated systems. Professional- and expert-based delivery of healthcare cuts across the public-private dichotomy, opening up rich fields for historical analysis. More widely, but more elusively, one hopes that the history of this essential public–private dichotomy will lead to best practice, prudent policy and above all to insightful understanding of complex and intricate processes, medical provision, and qualitatively improved health outcomes.

# Notes

1 Henry Ernst Sigerist, 'The Social History of Medicine', *The Western Journal* of *Surgery, Obstetrics and Gynaecology*, 48 (1940): 715–22.
2 Dorothy Porter, 'The Mission of Social History of Medicine: An Historical View', *Social History of Medicine*, 8 (1995): 345–59.
3 Charles Webster, *Paracelsus: Medicine, Magic, and Mission at the End of Time* (New Haven: Yale University Press, 2008); Charles Webster, *Health, Medicine, and Mortality in the Sixteenth Century* (Cambridge: Cambridge University Press, 1979).
4 Steve Sturdy (ed.), *Medicine, Health and the Public Sphere in Britain, 1600–2000* (London: Routledge, 2002).
5 Jeff A. Weintraub and Krishan Kumar (eds), *Public and Private in Thought and Practice: Perspectives on a Grand Dichotomy* (Chicago: Chicago University Press, 1997).
6 Ivan Illich, *Medical Nemesis* (London: Calder & Boyars, 1974); Michel Foucault, *Naissance de la clinique – une archéologie du regard médical* (Paris: PUF, 1963); Michel Foucault, *Madness and Civilization: A History of Insanity in the Age of Reason* (London: Tavistock, 1965).
7 Reinhard Spree, *Health and Social Class in Imperial Germany: A Social History of Mortality, Morbidity and Inequality* (Oxford: Berg, 1988).
8 Norbert Elias, *The Civilizing Process, Vol. 1: The History of Manners* (Oxford: Blackwell, 1969), and *The Civilizing Process, Vol. 2: State Formation and Civilization* (Oxford: Blackwell, 1982).
9 Thomas McKeown, *The Modern Rise of Population* (London: Edward Arnold, 1976); Thomas McKeown, *The Role of Medicine: Dream, Mirage or Nemesis?* (London: Nuffield Trust, 1976). www.nuffieldtrust.org.uk/sites/files/nuffield/publication/The_ Role_of_ Medicine.pdfI (accessed 10 May 2014).
10 Abdel R. Omran, 'The Epidemiologic Transition: A Theory of the Epidemiology of Population Change', *Milbank Memorial Fund Quarterly*, 49 (1971): 1, 1–42. For background see George Weisz, *Chronic Disease in the Twentieth Century* (Baltimore: The Johns Hopkins University Press, 2014).
11 Paul Weindling, 'From Infectious to Chronic Diseases: Changing Patterns of Sickness in the Nineteenth and Twentieth Centuries', in Andrew Wear (ed.), *Medicine in Society* (Cambridge: Cambridge University Press 1992, reprinted 1994), 303–16.
12 George Rosen, *A History of Public Health* (Baltimore: The Johns Hopkins University Press, 1993); Milton Roemer (ed.), *Henry E. Sigerist on the Sociology of Medicine* (New York: MD Publications, 1960).
13 Roy and Dorothy Porter, *Patient's Progress: Doctors and Doctoring in Eighteenth-Century England* (Cambridge: Polity Press, 1989).
14 Jane Lewis, *The Politics of Motherhood: Child and Maternal Welfare in England, 1900–1939* (Beckenham: Croom Helm, 1980).
15 Dorothy Porter, *Health, Civilization and the State: A History of Public Health from Ancient to Modern Times* (London and New York: Routledge, 1999); Paul Weindling, *Health, Race and German Politics between National Unification and Nazism* (Cambridge: Cambridge University Press, 1989).
16 Abram de Swaan, *In Care of the State: Health Care, Education and Welfare in Europe and the USA in the Modern Era* (Cambridge: Polity Press, 1988).
17 Ruth Richardson, *Death, Dissection and the Destitute* (London: Routledge, 1988).
18 I wish to acknowledge and thank Tim McHugh for his views on this topic.
19 Michael Kaser, *Health Care in the Soviet Union and Eastern Europe* (Beckenham: Croom Helm, 1976).
20 Alfons Labisch and Shizu Sakai, *Transaction in Medicine and Heteronomous Modernization: Germany, Japan, Korea and Taiwan* (Tokyo: University of Tokyo Center for Philosophy, 2009).

# 2 Public and private healthcare for the poor, 1650s to 1960s

*Elizabeth Hurren and Steven King*

## Introduction

The supply of medical services (the 'medical marketplace') between the seventeenth and twentieth centuries was, as Paul Weindling points out in his introduction, underpinned by a complex and fluid amalgam of public, private and charitable/mutual provision. At any chronological point, the constellation of such provision reflected the outcome of debates about a number of key questions that we have come to think of as essentially 'modern' but that in fact have a ringing echo across the period considered in this chapter. Such questions include: Who should fund healthcare and what balance should there be between private individuals (via savings and insurance) and local and national governments via taxation? Who should regulate healthcare? What should the balance be between the rights of patients and the duties of doctors? Should state-funded healthcare systems be residual (as in America until recently) or comprehensive, as in Britain? What should countries do with those – chiefly for instance in-migrants or immigrants – who have not made accumulated contributions to the societies on which their healthcare needs are imposed? How much should private provision be allowed to entwine with public healthcare systems? What role is there for mutual organisations in the provision of medical services? And what should be the balance between provisions in institutions like hospitals versus care in the community or the homes of the sick? National and local debate about these matters was as vibrant in seventeenth-century France as in twenty-first-century America. The issues will increasingly manifest themselves in the emerging economies of Asia and South America as the state's capacity to pay for healthcare collides with the willingness to do so.

Within this broad context – and notwithstanding the assertions of modern politicians who essentially see it as a recent phenomenon – choice (of provider, treatment, location) has been one of the most consistent leitmotifs in the history of healthcare. For the middle classes (or 'the middling orders and sorts', to adopt pre-twentieth-century nomenclature) such choices have always been real. The American middling orders of the later eighteenth and early nineteenth centuries who sought healthcare from multiple doctors, treated themselves, used astrologers and herbalists and took the waters at medicinal springs are not so different from their counterparts in the twenty-first century who might use the multiple private and state providers, treat themselves, take spa breaks and seek out astrologers, card readers and herbal supplements.[1] Middling people, with or without money but always with a voice, rapidly learnt to navigate the different constellations of public and private healthcare provision across history. It is less clear that the poor[2] and groups such as recent migrants have had the same navigational abilities and tools and the same attendant choices. Indeed, for some of the period considered here medicine has explicitly or implicitly been something that was 'done to' the poor. Against this backdrop modern politicians have tended to put choice and quality of service for the poor – whether this be the imposition of service targets on the British NHS or the development of 'Obamacare' in America – at the heart of their attempts to balance private, public and alternative provision of healthcare services. Reflecting this simple but important observation, our chapter is underpinned by a basic philosophical contention: to understand the structure, balance and nature of healthcare services across Britain, Europe and America, the key yardstick is how such services were and are experienced by the very poorest.

Using this group as a prism, the rest of our chapter takes up three key themes: First, the changing constellation of public, private and philanthropic/ mutual healthcare in Britain, Europe and America. Our synthesis runs from the 1650s (when we first see *systematic* contracting of doctors to institutions, charities and communities providing medical services to the poor in Britain and Europe), through the later nineteenth century when America and Europe engaged in very different internal conversations about the nature and purpose of medical care for the poorest, and to the rise of the voluntary and municipal hospital movements of the nineteenth and twentieth centuries. The synthesis ends at the point in the 1960s when the Swiss and Dutch welfare states and related healthcare systems were finally codified at national level.[3] Second, we focus on how patients experienced these different amalgams of state, private and philanthropic provision. Acknowledging that experience varies according to gender, the age of individual patients, the amount of money or patronage available to the sick person and one's physical location within any country, we nonetheless focus on the experiences of the poor and associated groups such as migrants as the prism through which to understand what health systems 'meant' to those who tried to navigate them. Finally, we turn to the question of how patients, doctors and state/philanthropic healthcare providers conceptualised their respective rights and duties across the period considered in the chapter. Our focus once again turns away from the middling orders and classes, who have traditionally had the rhetorical, legal and economic power to create rights for themselves and duties for the state, towards the poor and other 'outsider' groups who have not. Clearly, given the constraints of a single chapter our approach will be broad-brush, but some of the shared experiences across time and space will be striking. Throughout the text we explicitly link healthcare and the wider welfare systems of the countries considered here, both because the latter often grew out of the former and because for the very poorest health and welfare dependence are, and have always been, entwined in a lethal circle.

## The constellation of healthcare

Historians differ strongly over the relative trajectory, purpose and reach of European and American welfare systems.[4] A consideration of national surveys and (particularly for the essentially federalised Swiss Cantons, America and the Italian city states) smaller-scale community studies would, however, suggest an increase in local or national state spending on both welfare and the healthcare needs of the poor from the later eighteenth or early nineteenth centuries.[5] The experience was of course not uniform. Scotland and Ireland had little by way of state-funded welfare until well into the nineteenth century, especially as compared to England and Wales. Healthcare provision at the municipal level for the Dutch was immeasurably better in the early nineteenth century than was the case for America. Nonetheless, it is possible to see an uptick in welfare spending across the regions considered in this chapter. This observation sits neatly with a grand meta-narrative that might see a transition over time and country between healthcare as essentially a private good to be addressed with private and philanthropic resources, to healthcare as a public and national good to be addressed initially with a mix of philanthropic and state funding and then (from the twentieth century) increasingly by a partnership between state and individual mediated by the tax or insurance systems.

While convenient, this sort of narrative does no justice to the diverse ideological, organisational, economic, political and institutional frameworks shaping healthcare provision either in the past or now. In the rest of this section we thus attempt a synthesis of the spectrum of experience in Europe and America, set against the emergence of common threads in the ideology, organisation and financing of healthcare provision. This work must be read with two broad caveats borne in mind. First, the boundaries between state, philanthropic and private healthcare provision were often impermeable. Nowhere is this clearer than in the provision of tax-based state subsidies for religious organisations, essentially philanthropic entities, to provide medical services to the general population, or more specifically to the poor, between the seventeenth and twenty-first centuries.[6] Second, whatever the particular constellation of providers at any chronological point, states tend to get involved directly in healthcare at the local or national level at times of demographic or other crisis. The plagues of the seventeenth century, cholera in the nineteenth century, polio in the twentieth century and bird flu in the twenty-first century have created national panics and demanded that the state superimpose itself on existing healthcare services, even if it uses the same structures as a delivery mechanism. It is for these reasons that one must talk about state, philanthropic and private provision in only the loosest of senses.

Against this backdrop, seventeenth-century Britain and Europe exhibited a complex mix of provisions for the poor. At its core was self-help within the context of a model of health that placed great emphasis on the inevitability of suffering.[7] This area included herbals, wise people, astrology, medicinal springs and only the occasional doctor. Self-help was also the first and often the last port of call for the middling orders of most European states. Such essentially 'private' provision was supplemented with residual post-Reformation religious charity in Britain and a much more forceful and dynamic system of religious nursing and domiciliary care in both Protestant and Catholic Europe.[8] While this area of healthcare, broadly philanthropic in nature, declined in relatively linear fashion in England and Wales, across Europe it experienced many revivals into the twentieth century. Other forms of medically orientated charitable provision varied significantly in scope and trajectory across the countries encompassed by this chapter, weakening in England and Wales, low but persistent in Scotland, and high and rising in much of the rest of Europe. Nowhere is the latter trend clearer than in France where we see the foundation of a network of (usually urban) charitable hospitals.[9] Across most of Europe, however, the later seventeenth century witnessed an upsurge in organised, institutionalised and personalised philanthropic provision for the poor. The position of the state in this picture is complex, and made more so by periodic attempts (usually ineffective) to hypothecate some forms of tax revenue to support philanthropic endeavour. In England and Wales, the 'Old Poor Law' of 1601 provided a national, tax-based framework for the delivery of welfare and healthcare, though for much of the seventeenth century this 'state' system played second fiddle to philanthropic resources. The Swiss federation and the Netherlands never achieved the same robust national framework, but both sought to create and control larger-scale healthcare structures at an early date. In the rest of Europe the state constituted at best a minor and often unwilling partner in the constellation of healthcare except in areas where failing to respond might cause social unrest – such as the need to provide medical and welfare aid to ex-soldiers or to construct sanitary cordons at times of epidemics. For the seventeenth century, then, it is possible to point to a constellation of healthcare for the poor revolving very firmly around self-help, organised and endowed charity and informal charitable initiatives by individuals and groups such as landlords, clerics, doctors and guilds.[10]

The eighteenth century was to see this constellation disrupted. In England and Wales the Old Poor Law of 1601 established itself and became a truly national system of welfare. While historians differ on the generosity and scope of welfare spending, it seems clear that health-related spending from local taxes on property became a mainstay of welfare provision. In particular, the patchy seventeenth-century practice of doctors being contracted to communities to provide medical care to the poor gained purchase nationally from the 1730s before developing into a comprehensive system by the early nineteenth century. A nascent hospital system funded by philanthropic donations and endowments complemented the parochially based Poor Law, but it is clear that for England and Wales there was a decisive shift in healthcare provision towards the state. England and Wales were of course not alone in having or gaining state or state-influenced welfare systems in the eighteenth century. Flanders, the Netherlands (at least at the municipal level), and some of the Swiss Cantons or Austrian regions could all boast recognisable 'poor laws'. Only in America, however, did state involvement translate to long-term contract-based provision of medical care by doctors along the lines of that developed in England and Wales.[11] Elsewhere, the state remained particularly likely to get involved in the medical welfare of particular population groups – for example, the aged, foundlings, soldiers – and played an increasingly important role in responding to national crises. Venereal disease also exercised political leaders and state institutions in the form of 'lock hospitals', many with powers of incarceration, which were common in both Europe and North America.[12] Such involvement makes it possible to talk more confidently about the emergence of a mixed economy of healthcare, involving the systematic fusion of state, philanthropic and private healthcare solutions. This said, welfare in general and medical care in particular remained for most European states firmly entrenched within the remit of localities or municipalities and the institutional, guild and informal charitable networks that had long been in place. A resurgence in philanthropic giving for the purpose of building hospitals, nursing homes, specialist medical institutions, and foundling hospitals emphasised this localism at the same time as it laid the foundations for the emergence of national institutional networks in Europe and America in the nineteenth century. This is especially clear in France, where localities fiercely defended their autonomy from the state in these terms well into the twentieth century.[13] The result was a complex patchwork of medical provision across the European and American space that stands in contradistinction to the much more uniform structures to be found in England and Wales for this period.

Napoleon's conquest of Europe in the 1790s and early 1800s prompted the seizing of charitable endowments, particularly from religious institutions, and their deployment in a recognisably French system of relief for the poor and the sick. For some countries, such as Prussia or the Netherlands, his eventual defeat left few legacies. Philanthropic funds were returned to their original 'owners' or were re-purposed under municipal control.[14] Elsewhere, the marks of Napoleonic reform, particularly in the sense of ongoing institutional provision for the sick poor where little had previously been available, were stronger. War/militarisation more generally changed the perspective of politicians on the proper role of the state in healthcare. Persistent problems of recruiting healthy men for armies on the one hand, and the need to cope with significant numbers of injured and disabled soldiers on the other, drove an impetus for systematic networks of care. Nowhere was this impetus greater than in America. Across the Atlantic the implementation of the English and Welsh New Poor Law in 1834 systematically introduced workhouses as a vehicle for welfare. While their impact on relief practice has been overstated, it is clear that by the 1850s such workhouses had become sites of care of the aged and diagnostic and treatment spaces.[15] Elsewhere in nineteenth-century European and American cities, state-funded workhouse-type systems developed rapidly, many of them with carceral powers, but they too increasingly played a central role in healthcare for the poor. Sweden and other Scandinavian countries led the way with powerful networks of institutions seeking to treat and control the spread of venereal disease, and across Europe and (particularly) America state asylums increasingly mopped up the 'lunatic' poor who might otherwise have resided in workhouses, domestic situations or private asylums.[16]

Of course, increased state involvement in healthcare for the poorest was not always clean and concerted. Often (as in France) mistrust between the centre and localities hampered the expansion of formal state provision. Nor was it uncontested or unaccompanied. Even in England the nineteenth century witnessed a sustained upsurge in philanthropic giving for medical institutions and charities, adding thousands of beds in voluntary hospitals and specialist institutions for the impaired to the landscape of the mixed economy of healthcare. Nowhere was this philanthropic impulse more keenly directed than in America, which by the early twentieth century had easily surpassed European figures for hospital beds per capita.[17] Nor should we forget that the nineteenth century witnessed a remarkable upsurge in self-help activity in the form of friendly societies, sickness clubs and union- or guild-organised medical care, as well as a reinvention of the possibilities of self-treatment arising out of the independent pharmacy movement. In short, the sick poor of Europe and America were enmeshed in an increasingly dense and vibrant medical economy by the later nineteenth century and were likely to spend more of the time that they were sick in institutions or otherwise under formally organised medical supervision. Indeed, a fusion between state and philanthropic activity gave certain groups of the poor – the aged in particular – a much greater choice of healthcare than they had experienced in the past. Within this broad framework, however, the nineteenth century witnessed a discernible shift towards state, state-inspired or state-sponsored provision. The European nation-building of the 1840–1870s period enhanced the sense that it was right for the state to be firmly involved in the finance, organisation and delivery of healthcare. With this altered ideological perspective came a dilution of a lingering sense that the poor were themselves responsible for much ill health and thus poverty because of their own moral choices. Poverty thus became remediable rather than natural and across Europe and America the institutionalised sick became a particular focus for this remediation process.

It would be a mistake, however, to regard the nineteenth century as a unified period. From the 1870s an increasing interchange of administrators, ideas, structures and ideologies between European states and between Europe and America created a framework for the convergence of ideas on welfare and healthcare.[18] We witness parallel and overlapping conversations about rights to welfare (chiefly the pension) and the need for the state to protect certain groups (children, the disabled, etc.). Even more powerfully, it is

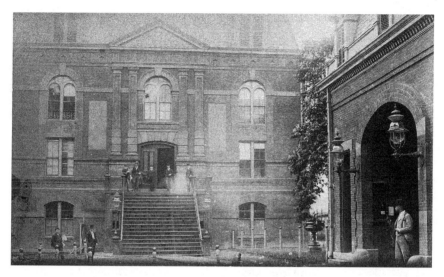

*Figure 2.1* Bellevue Hospital, New York City, 1885–1898. © The Wellcome Library, London.

possible to trace a shared public and political discourse over the models that might be used to fund increasing state-sponsored provision of healthcare services, ranging along a spectrum from schemes that drew on general taxation (albeit with a notional hypothecation of certain taxation streams and a narrative about accumulated individual contribution) through to insurance schemes where the entire burden would fall on the individual or their employer with or without the state funding a residual system. American and Dutch discourses in this area were particularly acute, though the convergence of German and British conversations has attracted most historiographical attention.[19] In the midst of these developments, extensive migration between European states and between Europe and America increasingly highlighted welfare and healthcare anomalies. Restrictions on the welfare rights of migrants put them at a substantial disadvantage compared to native populations and it is unsurprising to see states such as France, Germany, Italy and Switzerland entering into bilateral agreements for the mutual welfare and health support of immigrants. In effect such agreements set minimum standards of welfare and healthcare for both migrants and natives where none had previously existed. They also directly underpin the increasing activity in the twentieth century of the International Labour Organization, World Health Organization, the Rockefeller Foundation and other non-governmental organisations in pushing for international responses to common healthcare problems in both the developed and developing world.[20]

The shared conversations of the 1870s and 1880s took some time to come to fruition. They were set against the backdrop of the increasingly formal organisation of the European and American medical profession, the rapidly rising costs of care as medical regimes moved from a largely palliative to a significantly curative basis, and the increasing sophistication and commercialisation of medicine that, for much of the twentieth century, sucked knowledge and practice beyond the control of the individual and thus made self-dosing more and more of an ancillary activity. These are themes partly picked up in Viviane Quirke's contribution to this volume. The shared conversations were also concerned with the dual threats of moral hazard and the free rider problem, two issues that remain central to the debate about the cost and scope of modern healthcare systems. By the early twentieth century, however, the foundations of the trio of healthcare models that would dominate the twentieth century were decisively set. In Britain, the long-established link between welfare, healthcare and general/local taxation was played out in a series of measures that gave welfare and de facto healthcare rights to narrowly defined sections of the population, including for instance pensions for those over 70 who had met a raft of qualifying criteria. This policy change coincided with a decline in both philanthropic giving for medical projects and institutions and, notably, self-help and mutual healthcare solutions. By the 1930s, and even more so after the foundation of the National Health Service – an entity initially funded through general taxation and free at the point of use – the medical economy of makeshifts for the poor became increasingly narrow and state focused.[21] In other European states an amalgam of philanthropic, religious, municipal, state and mutual provision perhaps persisted for longer than in Britain. The French and Dutch welfare systems stand out particularly in this respect. Nonetheless, by the early twentieth century a clear path towards the insurance-based schemes and state safety net systems that were to dominate European welfare and healthcare had been established.[22] Unsurprisingly, America represents a third core model. Here, philanthropic provision, mutuality, self-help/organisation and work-based medical welfare generated a complex, often regionally specific, medical economy of makeshifts for the poor or potentially poor to the 1960s and beyond. Individual private insurance schemes were increasingly superimposed on this healthcare landscape, in effect creating a class of the very poorest for whom access to healthcare in anything other than residual form was a luxury rather than a right.[23]

Many of these twentieth century themes are taken further by others in this volume. Looking backwards, it is clear that the American and European sick poor were obliged to navigate an extremely complex mixed economy of healthcare across the period covered by this chapter. While the end point – an increasingly state-dominated system in Europe and a much more complex medical economy in America – is clear, the journey from 1650 was by no means linear. There were (and remain) distinct ideological, structural and organisational differences between European states in their approach to healthcare, epitomised by the British Old and New Poor Laws at one end of the spectrum and intense French localism on the other. Within individual states there were also stark differences in the constellation of private, philanthropic and public health services according to region or place. Such differences were most acute in America, but even in Britain the difference between England and Wales, with an increasingly expensive national welfare system with issues of healthcare at its core, and Scotland, with no formal welfare or healthcare provision before the 1840s, is compelling. We move now to consider the process by which the sick poor made sense of the differential rules and expectations of these systems and how they experienced healthcare structures.[24]

## Patient experiences of the healthcare system

It will be clear from the changing constellation of public, private and philanthropic healthcare identified above that the general experience across the period and countries covered here was for patients to spend progressively more of their medical lives under the care of doctors and in state-funded or state-controlled institutions. Rights to healthcare had also, by the twentieth century, superseded the discretionary systems of earlier centuries. In the case of the very poorest sections of society, however, a consideration of records from philanthropic hospitals, the case notes of doctors or the records of state institutions such as workhouses suggests that this engagement lacked consistency. Nineteenth-century patient case records from Europe and America convincingly demonstrate that the poor engaged with medical institutions *in extremis* and often towards the end of an illness that would prove fatal. By contrast, this group was much more likely to seek the charitable assistance of individual doctors or to try and access medical charity. A phenomenon that politicians and doctors have come to think of as essentially 'modern' has striking consistency over several centuries. We must thus beware of assuming an indelible link between the presence and notional availability of medical institutions – whether philanthropic, private or public – and improved health outcomes for the poorest sections of European and American society. As in the twenty-first century, such health services provided an explicit subsidy to the middling orders and the respectable labouring classes rather than inevitably improving the lot of the poor.

Such observations raise important questions about how this group navigated the state, private and philanthropic sectors and responded to changes in their constellation. Some sense of this issue can be garnered from the words of the poor themselves. Those who were 'out of their place' when they fell into poverty had simply to make do, return to the place where they had a legal or moral right to apply for welfare or healthcare, or write to that place asking to be relieved in their own homes. The majority wrote or got others to write on their behalf to their 'home' communities. Recent research on Britain, Europe and America has revealed tens of thousands of these 'pauper narratives' and further indirect references that indicate that many hundreds of thousands were sent but have not survived. In chronological terms they run from the mid-eighteenth century (the point at which postal and money transmission services were sufficiently well developed in many countries to make writing easy and potentially fruitful) to the 1930s.[25] Their contents range from the formulaic and formal to the rambling and orthographic, but collectively they provide an important window onto the way that the sick poor experienced the welfare and healthcare systems.

These letters tell us that at the core of the issue of how poor people experienced differently constituted healthcare systems were three intertwining considerations that span the period considered here. The first relates to accessibility and eligibility. Travelling for healthcare had both direct (financial) and opportunity (childcare, work foregone) costs. It is thus unsurprising that where we have their words, these indicate that the very poorest of Britain, Europe and America preferred local solutions – the charity of local doctors, institutions located in their own towns and receipt of cash allowances that would allow them to purchase their own local healthcare solutions – to potentially more 'modern' institutions run on behalf of the state or subscribers at a greater distance. Changes to the constellation of healthcare systems that resulted in provision at greater distance reduced the engagement of the poorest with those systems and pushed them to seek medical aid much later in the illness cycle than had been the case previously. This was the case with the English and Welsh New Poor Law, for instance, and even more forcefully with many Prussian and later German workhouses and care institutions that tended to be run at the regional rather than the local level.[26] Even under the state-sponsored healthcare systems of the twentieth century, localism has become a cherished characteristic of patient groups. The exception to this rule seems to be healthcare or institutions funded through the mutual or self-help model, for which the poor of Europe and America appear to have been willing to travel some distance. These places offered care as of right rather than an act of charity. British and American letter writers had a keen appreciation that nineteenth and twentieth century philanthropically funded hospitals would not treat certain categories of illness, required a letter of support from a subscriber in order to admit the poor, sometimes demanded that patients come with appropriate clothes and cash for washing, and always imposed strict rules in terms of behaviour, morals and visiting. By the later nineteenth century many American hospitals were requiring guarantees of patient removal after treatment was completed and insisted that all patients submit to an assessment of means.[27] Few of the very poorest could or would try to meet these sorts of eligibility criteria and it is unsurprising to find that workhouses and state hospitals and asylums formed a residual pool of support for these groups. Even here, however, there were implicit eligibility criteria based on skin colour (black people in Britain were rarely turned down when applying for welfare), origin (the Irish found it particularly difficult to obtain treatment in the English healthcare system prior to the NHS) and financial means. Indeed, the absence of the very poorest in some of the healthcare institutions of Europe and America in the nineteenth and early twentieth centuries is striking. Their letters confirm that some of the changing constellations of healthcare provision traced in the last section simply slipped by the notice of the poor.

A second consideration influencing the way that the poor experienced healthcare is that of continuity and predictability. While the links between citizenship and healthcare across the period covered by this chapter are complex, little or no provision was underpinned either by formal rights or associated minimum standards. In situations as varied as seventeenth-century England, nineteenth-century America and early twentieth-century France, the poor simply could not predict how the local state (parishes, municipalities, communities) would react to a plea for medical welfare funded either by local taxes or a combination of taxes and co-ordinated/directed charitable resources. Indeed, prior to the twentieth century it was quite usual for the character, duration and scope of healthcare to vary radically from one place to another, even if they were contiguous. Paupers often complained of the care/resources offered by their 'home' communities and the situation in their host communities. Where healthcare for the poor also became a political or moral tool – as it did for instance at Lyon in early twentieth-century France[28] – these issues of continuity and predictability were magnified. Voluntary or state hospitals had more predictable, if more discriminatory, admissions criteria for discrete episodes of illness but pauper letter writers did not regard their time in them as any more than a brief sojourn. Letters show clearly that the very poor could not depend on a repeat admission where a condition returned. Moreover, hospitals had various exit points for patients, ranging from incurable through 'relieved' to 'cured'. Institutions with limited budgets inevitably viewed extended stays and a failure of conditions to respond to initial treatment with concern and, while some paupers complained that they had been kept too long, many more were discharged either with the conditions that had prompted their admission in the first place or with something worse that they had caught in the hospital itself. Private insurance-based institutions or those funded by the state through general taxation often offered continuity of treatment, but they were by no means immune from the calls of economy as duration of stay increased or tax and insurance revenues fell. At the opposite end of the spectrum, workhouses were very predictable, even if (at least according to much of the older historiography) not very palatable. As they became increasingly medicalised across the nineteenth century they constituted a collection point for the very worst illnesses. Indeed, it has been argued that in both Britain and America such institutions improved the general health of the population by removing the most infectious and ingrained medical cases from the wider community and (by inertia or law) keeping them confined.[29] It is perhaps for this reason that European historians in particular have begun to see the workhouse in a more positive light, as part of the medical economy of makeshifts available to the very poorest.

For pauper writers, continuity of care and resource were a flashpoint in their engagement with officials and they actively sought to navigate the public, private, philanthropic and self-help matrices available so as to garner certainty. For example, across the period, and bridging the Atlantic, in both Europe and America, paupers actively sought the nursing and medical care provided by religious organisations. These bodies were both more local and provided continuity of care where illnesses were of a chronic or long-term nature. Letter writers also appear to have valued the philanthropic efforts of doctors in private practice. While it is easy to see such activities as begrudgingly given (as it was for instance by Arthur Conan Doyle when he was practising medicine in Portsmouth, England) and purely instrumental, it is clear that, once started, doctors found it almost impossible to step back from the implicit contract with their communities created by offering free attendance to the poor. Moreover, we are struck when reading European and American pauper narratives by just how frequently doctors went to considerable, expensive and elongated efforts to cure the dependent poor even when they had absolutely no hope of recovering their costs. The sick poor also relied, of course, on their family, friends and neighbours for the delivery of nursing and healthcare on a predictable basis. Even under the national state-funded welfare and healthcare system in Britain between 1601 and 1929 there was a clear preference among pauper writers to seek private rather than philanthropic or state-provided medical care. Most of those who wrote in this period, for instance, requested cash with which to navigate the private medical marketplace rather than the attendance of the parish or union doctor.

A final consideration shaping the way that the poor experienced healthcare is that of navigability and contestability. Whether in Germany, France, England or America, pauper narratives demonstrate persuasively that the sick poor were keenly aware of law, convention and customary practice. They pooled knowledge and were remarkably persistent in their attempts to secure healthcare or the resources to commission it. Moreover, their letters were often differently structured and rhetorically presented according to whether they were addressed to those in charge of philanthropic institutions, the various arms of state or those providing private charity. And we obtain a real sense that those in liminal positions – the Irish in England, Italians in France, those of colour in most countries – understood that their eligibility demanded a certain set of reference points coded in accepted ways. Thus, in letters seeking healthcare, black letter writers in England usually emphasised their service – to employers, the country or their communities – and their friendlessness, rhetorical and strategic devices rarely deployed by the native white population. Yet the ability of individuals to navigate differently constellated healthcare systems was crucially dependent on the locus of power. Where authority to make decisions on individual cases was placed in the hands of paid officials (for instance, professional almoners in American and British hospitals[30]) or those at the centre of national and regional administrative systems, or where accessing one aspect of healthcare became dependent on prior access to another form of healthcare, necessitating multiple letters to different audiences, so the sick poor appear to have lost their ability to navigate the system in which they were enmeshed. In the increasingly complex

American healthcare system of the late nineteenth and early twentieth centuries, the pauper response was simply to stop writing and to draw on the voices and authority of epistolary advocates such as employers, landlords or the clergy. Similar considerations apply to the contestability of healthcare systems and decision making. Paupers across Europe and America were remarkably adept at contesting both their eligibility for state-sponsored medical care and the form this took. In some regions they demonstrated an intimate knowledge of medical conditions, appropriating the language of doctors and other officials to describe their symptoms and contest their treatment.[31] There is much less evidence of the sick poor negotiating their treatment in philanthropic institutions and almost no evidence of their contesting the care available via self-help networks, sick clubs, mutual organisations and other arenas where they perceived themselves to have absolute rights to a particular level of care. In turn, however, the centralisation and regionalisation of state-organised healthcare administration in the later nineteenth and early twentieth centuries, accompanied as it was by a decline of philanthropic provision and the rise of entitlement systems of welfare and healthcare, reduced the volume of letter writing by the sick poor. Rule-based systems, themselves deeply inscribed in complex administrative structures, reduced the ability of the poor to publically contest the character and duration of their healthcare.

The evidence from the pens of paupers themselves or from their epistolary advocates clearly points to a disjuncture between the changing constellations of public, private and philanthropic healthcare and the underlying medical welfare experiences of the sick poor. This group actively sought to navigate and negotiate healthcare provision so as to ensure localism, prioritise rights-based treatment and focus on individual philanthropy. Moreover, they actively sought resources from the local state in a form that would allow them to participate in the private medical marketplace rather than asking for direct medical care. The fundamental transition to state-based or state-sponsored welfare and healthcare solutions in Europe in the late nineteenth and early twentieth centuries changed this dynamic, resulting in a healthcare system to which the sick poor were subject, rather than them retaining their role as active participants. Exactly the opposite was the case in America in the same period, where a complex mixed economy of healthcare and a relative absence of state solutions left the sick poor notionally with more power but also a more difficult job of navigation.

## Rights and duties

One of the purposes of pauper letters and other forms of engagement between the sick poor and medical and welfare officials was to try to establish de facto rights where none existed and state and medical duties where none could be enforced. With very few exceptions, neither welfare systems nor the healthcare structures that grew out of them offered a legal guarantee of support. At best, as in England and Wales, the sick poor had an enforceable right to apply for medical aid and a right to appeal where it was not granted. This does not, however, amount to a right even if custom and the actions of pauper letter writers and their advocates created 'rights' that made failing to treat certain groups of sick paupers – the aged, for instance – a matter of dispute. Indeed, it would be no exaggeration to say that many more people in Europe in the seventeenth and eighteenth centuries were subject to forced treatment – notably for lepers, smallpox victims and venereal patients – than had anything resembling a right to healthcare. Looked at from the perspective of the early twenty-first century we might see a fairly simple journey from this situation to one in which patients had guaranteed rights to care inscribed firmly within a framework of state and professional duties. Setting aside the question of whether one can point to such a system in America or Europe even in 2014, there is a sense in which this journey was surprisingly patchy, non-linear and incomplete even by the end of the period covered in this chapter. It is striking, for instance, that much of the twentieth-century legislation establishing healthcare systems was not about giving rights. Indeed, one might argue that such legislation was, in tone and intent, about limiting and curtailing such rights. This was particularly true of British and European legislation up to the 1930s. Moreover, some patients – poor patients in particular – started the period with no rights and had not markedly improved their position by its end even as the balance between public, private and philanthropic healthcare systems shifted. Those with venereal disease constitute one such group, but by far the largest was composed of the mentally ill poor who often lacked advocates, their own voice and the economic or social power to navigate the health systems to which they were subject. The great decanting of this group from asylums to communities in the later twentieth century is a direct response to this situation. Even where rights were granted, they might be structured and graded; in Switzerland, for instance, multiple levels/grades of citizenship were associated, for much of the twentieth century, with multiple baskets of rights to heath care and welfare payments.[32]

Accepting that the journey to rights for the sick poor and duties for doctors and the state was not as smooth or comprehensive as we might imagine, two staging posts for that journey are extremely important and have striking modern resonance.[33] The first is a growing nineteenth-century culture of challenge to medical neglect in institutions. While the middle classes had always been able to challenge poor care and to substitute one form of care for another, this was less of an option for the European and American poor. By the nineteenth century, however, a century-old tradition of paupers writing to officials coincided with an explosion of investigative journalism on both sides of the Atlantic and made it immeasurably easier for the sick to complain about their treatment. The explosion of complaints by paupers or their families and friends about medical and other neglect in state-funded or state-sponsored institutions from the 1840s is both remarkable and uniform across European and American welfare systems. Directed at both local authorities and (increasingly) centralised administrations, some of these complaints were

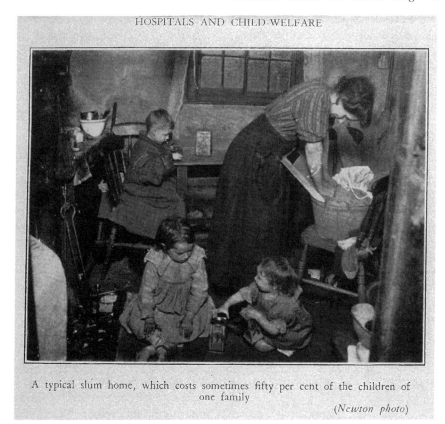

HOSPITALS AND CHILD-WELFARE

A typical slum home, which costs sometimes fifty per cent of the children of
one family

(*Newton photo*)

*Figure 2.2* A mother and three children in a slum dwelling, 1920. © The Wellcome
Library, London.

used for political ends. They also had a much wider impact, and nowhere
more so than in Britain. Here, as Kim Price has shown, complaints about
medical neglect focused on a wide spectrum of medical practice in institutions: attendance, dosing, sexual misbehaviour with patients, experimenting
on the poor, inadequate attention to dressings, cruelty and bad nursing.[34]
This litany re-inforces the idea that the sick poor and their advocates had
the knowledge and the means to dissect the medical care they were offered.
In turn such complaints were rapidly picked up by local and national
newspapers. Whether proven or not, complaints always prompted extensive
investigation and recommendations for future conduct at the individual or
corporate level. Sometimes these investigations resulted in criminal prosecu-
tions. Outcomes were invariably publicised in local government circulars and
guidance but they were also, and much more importantly, subject to scrutiny
by local and regional committees of doctors and at annual conferences of
poor law medical officers and welfare officials. In short, complaints created a
weight of precedent and guidance that shaped behaviour and imposed rights

to certain minimum standards of care and duties to provide it, even in the absence of formal legislation. This is an important observation when combined with the suggestion above that the constellation of healthcare began to move sharply towards state-orientated solutions in the nineteenth century.

In another area of the medical economy – the voluntary hospital – formal neglect cases are more difficult to pin down in either Europe or America. Indeed, the annual reports of these institutions were usually replete with testimony from grateful patients. Yet even a cursory glance at newspapers from the 1840s and 1850s dispels the illusion established by annual reports. To be sure, the medical neglect cases reported for most voluntary hospitals were less stark than those in state institutions, but they were persistent. Their impact was also instant. Such institutions depended largely on the continued support of subscribers and while American institutions in particular sought over the nineteenth century to diversify their subscriber list so as to generate mass financial support, in most places the influence of a few large and wealthy donors remained central. Publicity of medical neglect cases prompted rapid enquiries, usually a dismissal somewhere in the organisation and an interesting culture of improvement inscribed into rules for medical men and (from the later nineteenth century) women, patients, nursing staff, cooks, cleaners and administrators. Mutual healthcare organisations were even more susceptible to complaints from patients.[35] As the relative balance of private, public and philanthropic provision changed, then, we can begin to see an emerging set of patient rights and doctoring duties. These came relatively easily for the middling orders. They were contested and created by the sick poor.

In turn, a second important staging post in the journey to legally inscribed patient rights was the resolution of the liminal position of voluntary or forced immigrants. For American communities the issue was of course particularly acute throughout the period covered by this chapter, and notably after the civil war. Yet European states also had equivalent problems, including mass migration for work purposes, forced emigration because of war or religious persecution and so called 'push' migration caused by industrial decay, rapid population growth or the unviability of agricultural land. Migrant groups posed a singular question for states and communities: what rights to welfare and healthcare should immigrants who had not made accumulated contributions actually get? One answer to this question was, as we have seen, to enter into bilateral agreements with other states where there were balancing migration flows. The impact of such agreements was to set minimum standards of welfare and medical care for both the immigrant and native population. Another was to exclude these groups completely from the welfare and attendant healthcare systems, or to make such systems sufficiently discriminatory to prevent the construction of moral or customary right, as in the case of the Irish in Britain or the ex-slave population in large parts of America.[36] For most states and immigrant groups, however, the position was somewhere between these extremes. We have already seen that

Switzerland limited rights by granting different levels of citizenship, and every European state adopted some version of this practice. On the other hand, it is also possible to see a loosening of restrictive criteria as the nineteenth century progressed and second and third generation migrants integrated into populations. Indeed, as Laura Tabili has shown persuasively, neighbourhoods and communities were often extremely supportive of immigrant families.[37] By the 1920s, this groundswell of popular support led inexorably in areas such as care for the disabled to rights for all rather than simply rights for some.

## Conclusion

The constellation of private, public, philanthropic and mutual providers of healthcare shifted in subtle ways across Europe and America between the 1650s and the later nineteenth century. The tendency for the state (and in America the local state) to play a more significant role as an organiser and funder of health services is clear. A shared conversation about the structure, organisation and ideological foundations of health and welfare initiatives in the later nineteenth century fed directly into a fracturing of this common experience, laying the foundations for the three major welfare models that still underpin conceptions of the duties of the state to its citizens in the developed world. Underneath these developments, the middling orders and respectable labouring classes had and garnered choice. For the sick poor of Europe and America the issue was much more about generating a right for their claims to be considered. In this they were remarkably successful, and the power of pauper letters, complaints about treatment and the appropriation of the voices of epistolary advocates in creating rights where none existed is striking. Some groups – for example, ex-slaves and tramps – continued to be marginalised and others were obliged to turn firmly to self-help and self-organisation to balance the neglect of states and communities and the partiality of legislation on welfare and health from the early twentieth century. Nonetheless, the ability of the very poorest to navigate the different constellations of the mixed economy of healthcare across the period 1650 to the 1960s is striking. The same cannot be said of modern European and American health systems, notwithstanding the advent of 'Obamacare'. Rule-based systems across Europe in particular have become diluted by political expediency, spiralling costs, mass migration and the creation of an economic underclass to match or exceed that which has always existed in volume in America. For these groups, the rhetoric of choice in healthcare allied with the increasingly complex, form-based, administrative systems needed to make choice has arguably stifled the voice of the sick poor and reduced their ability to navigate the mixed economy of healthcare that was supposed to benefit them. Indeed, we might argue that in Europe and America in the twenty-first century the sick poor have medicine 'done to them' (or not done at all) even more than was the case in the past.

**Further reading**

A survey spanning three centuries and two continents draws on a very wide variety of source material. Three core themes of the chapter – the healthcare experiences of highly marginal groups; the constellation and navigation of healthcare systems; and issues of rights and duties – can, however, be explored with selected further reading. On marginal groups you will find useful: H. John, 'Translating Leprosy: The Expert and the Public in Stanley Stein's Anti-stigmatization Campaigns, 1931–60', *Journal of the History of Medicine and Allied Sciences* 68 (2013): 659–87 and Jim Downs, *Sick from Freedom: African-American Illness and Suffering during the Civil War and Reconstruction* (Oxford: Oxford University Press, 2012). Three pieces focusing respectively on female health, slave institutions and patients with venereal disease also connect to themes raised in the chapter: Cheryl Krasnik Warsh, *Prescribed Norms: Women and Health in Canada and the United States since 1800* (Toronto: Toronto University Press, 2010); Stephen Kenny, '"A Dictate of both Interest and Mercy"? Slave Hospitals in the Antebellum South', *Journal of the History of Medicine and Allied Sciences*, 65 (2010): 2–47; and John Parascandola, *Sex, Sin and Science: A History of Syphilis in America* (Westport: Kreager, 2008).

On rights and duties you will find useful Beatrix Hoffman, *Health Care for Some: Rights and Rationing in the United States since 1930* (Chicago: Chicago University Press, 2012) and Ernest P. Hennock, *British Social Reform and German Precedents: The Case of Social Insurance 1880–1914* (Oxford: Clarendon Press, 1987). Three books discussing the particularities of the American experience in greater depth than can be brought out in the chapter are: Jonathan Engel, *Poor People's Medicine: Medicaid and American Charity Care since 1965* (Durham, NC: Duke University Press, 2006); Todd Savitt, *Race and Medicine in Nineteenth- and Early-Twentieth-Century America* (Kent, OH: Kent State University Press, 2007); and Paul Dutton, *Differential Diagnoses: A Comparative History of Health Care Problems and Solutions in the United States and France* (Ithaca, NY: Cornell University Press, 2007). An article by Sally Wilde deals with the complex processes through which doctoring duties intersected with matters of public trust: S. Wilde, 'Truth, Trust, and Confidence in Surgery, 1890–1910: Patient Autonomy, Communication and Consent', *Bulletin of the History of Medicine*, 83 (2009): 302–30.

On constellation and navigation, particularly in terms of the contrast between middling and poor patients, you will find useful: M. Kaartinen, 'Women Patients in the English Urban Medical Marketplace in the Long Eighteenth Century', in Deborah Simonton and Anne Montenach (eds), *Female Agency in the Urban Economy: Gender in European Towns 1680–1830* (London: Routledge, 2013), 48–67; Larry Geary, 'The Medical Profession, Health Care and the Poor Law in Nineteenth Century Ireland', in Virginia Crossman and Peter Gray (eds), *Poverty and Welfare in Ireland, 1838–1948* (Dublin: Irish Academic Press, 2011), 189–206; H. Curtis, *Faith in the Great*

*Physician: Suffering and Divine Healing in American Culture, 1860–1900* (Baltimore: The Johns Hopkins University Press, 2007); and J. Israel, 'Dutch Influence on Urban Planning, Health Care and Poor Relief: The North Sea and Baltic Regions of Europe, 1567–1720', in Ole Grell and Andrew Cunningham (eds), *Health Care and Poor Relief in Protestant Europe 1500–1700* (London: Routledge, 1997), 66–83. Two classic texts in this field are: Peter Baldwin, *The Politics of Social Solidarity and the Bourgeois Basis of the European Welfare State, 1875–1975* (Cambridge: Cambridge University Press, 1990), and Gøsta Esping-Andersen, *The Three Worlds of Welfare Capitalism* (Cambridge: Cambridge University Press, 1990).

## Notes

1 John Haller Jr, *The History of American Homeopathy: From Rational Medicine to Holistic Health Care* (New Brunswick, NJ: Rutgers University Press, 2009).
2 For reasons of brevity we take this term to be unproblematic, though of course it is not, and define the poor as the bottom 30–40 per cent of the income distribution.
3 Chris Nottingham and Piet De Rooy, 'The Peculiarities of the Dutch: Social Security in the Netherlands', in Steven King and John Stewart (eds), *Welfare Peripheries* (Oxford: Peter Lang, 2007), 39–66; Anne-Lise Head-König, 'Citizens But Not Belonging: Migrants' Difficulties in Obtaining Entitlement to Relief in Switzerland from the 1550s to the Early Twentieth Century', in Steven King and Anne Winter (eds), *Migration, Settlement and Belonging in Europe 1500–1930s* (Oxford: Berghahn, 2013), 153–72.
4 For an important survey see Robert Jütte, *Poverty and Deviance in Early Modern Europe* (Cambridge: Cambridge University Press, 1994).
5 Peter Lindert, *Growing Public: Social Spending and Economic Growth since the Eighteenth Century, Volume 1* (Cambridge: Cambridge University Press, 2004).
6 On this issue see Virginia Crossman, *Poverty and the Poor Law in Ireland 1850–1914* (Liverpool: Liverpool University Press, 2013), *passim*.
7 See Javier Moscoso, *Pain: A Cultural History* (Basingstoke: Palgrave Macmillan, 2012).
8 Susan Dinan, *Women and Poor Relief in Seventeenth-Century France: The Early History of the Daughters of Charity* (Farnham: Ashgate, 2006).
9 Tim McHugh, *Hospital Politics in Seventeenth-Century France: The Crown, Urban Elites, and the Poor* (Farnham: Ashgate, 2007).
10 Marco van Leeuwen, 'Logic of Charity: Poor Relief in Pre-industrial Europe', *Journal of Interdisciplinary History*, 24 (1994): 589–613.
11 Patricia Ferguson Clement, *Welfare and the Poor in the Nineteenth Century City: Philadelphia 1800–1854* (Cranbury, NJ: Associated University Presses, 1985).
12 Kevin Siena, *Venereal Disease, Hospitals and the Urban Poor: London's Foul Wards 1600–1800* (Rochester: University of Rochester Press, 2004).
13 Timothy Smith, *Creating the Welfare State in France, 1880–1940* (Montreal: McGill-Queen's University Press, 2003).
14 See for instance Andreas Gestrich, 'Trajectories of German Settlement Regulations: The Prussian Rhine Province, 1815–1914', in King and Winter, *Migration, Settlement and Belonging*, 254–58.
15 Graham Mooney, 'Diagnostic Spaces: Workhouse, Hospital and Home in Mid-Victorian London', *Social Science History*, 33 (2009): 357–90.
16 For Swedish treatment of VD see Anna Lundberg, *Care and Coercion: Medical Knowledge, Social Policy and Patients with Venereal Disease in Sweden, 1785–1903* (Umea: Umea Demographic Database Report 14, 1999).

17 Rosemary Stevens, *In Sickness and in Wealth: American Hospitals in the Twentieth Century* (Baltimore: The Johns Hopkins University Press, 1999).

18 A focus on failed legislation reveals a considerable European appetite for change to welfare and health care systems that was not ultimately realised until the early twentieth century. See contributions to King and Stewart, *Welfare Peripheries*.

19 Carl Axel Gemzell, 'The Welfare State: Britain and Denmark', in Jorgen Sevaldsen, Claus Bjørn and Bo Bjørke (eds), *Britain and Denmark: Political, Economic and Cultural Relations in the Nineteenth and Twentieth Centuries* (Copenhagen: Odsell, 2002), 123–44; Ernest P. Hennock, *The Origins of the Welfare State in England and Germany, 1850–1914: Social Policies Compared* (Cambridge: Cambridge University Press, 2007); Wolfgang Mommsen (ed.), *The Emergence of the Welfare State in Britain and Germany 1880–1950* (London: Croom Helm, 1981).

20 On these initial bi-lateral agreements, see Paul-André Rosental, 'Migrations, souveraineté, droits sociaux. Protéger et expulser les étrangers en Europe du 19e siècle à nos jours', *Annales HSS*, 66 (2011): 335–73.

21 Anne Digby, 'The Economic and Medical Significance of the British National Health Insurance Act, 1911', in Martin Gorsky and Sally Sheard (eds), *Financing Medicine: The British Experience since 1750* (London: Routledge, 2006), 182–98.

22 See for instance Matthieu Leimgruber, *Solidarity without the State? Business and the Shaping of the Swiss Welfare State, 1890–2000* (Cambridge: Cambridge University Press, 2009); Larry Frohman, 'Breakup of the Poor Laws – German Style: Progressivism and the Origins of the Welfare State 1900–1918', *Comparative Studies in Society and History*, 50 (2008): 981–1009.

23 John Murray, *Origins of American Health Insurance: A History of Industrial Sickness Funds* (New Haven, CT: Yale University Press, 2007).

24 Healthcare systems were of course differentially navigated by individuals according to other variables such as gender or class, but we do not have the space to explore the historiography of these issues.

25 For a broad survey of the potential of pauper narratives see Andreas Gestrich, Elizabeth Hurren and Steven King, 'Narratives of Poverty and Sickness in Europe 1780–1938', in Andreas Gestrich, Elizabeth Hurren and Steven King (eds), *Poverty and Sickness in Modern Europe: Narratives of the Sick Poor, 1780–1938* (London: Continuum, 2012), 1–34, in addition to other contributions to the volume.

26 Beate Althammer, 'Functions and Developments of the *Arbeitshaus* in Germany: Brauweiler Workhouse in the Nineteenth and Early Twentieth Centuries', in Andreas Gestrich and Lutz Raphael (eds), *Being Poor in Modern Europe: Historical Perspectives 1800–1940* (Oxford: Peter Lang, 2006), 273–98.

27 Stevens, *In Sickness and in Wealth*.

28 Smith, *Creating the Welfare State*; Jean-Pierre Gutton, *La Société et les pauvres: L'Exemple de la généralité de Lyon 1534–1789* (Paris: Les Belles Lettres, 1971).

29 Mooney, 'Diagnostic Spaces'; Emily Abel, '"In the Last Stages of Irremediable Disease": American Hospitals and Dying Patients before World War II', *Bulletin of the History of Medicine*, 85 (2011): 29–56.

30 Lynsey Cullen, 'The First Lady Almoner: The Appointment, Position, and Findings of Miss Mary Stewart at the Royal Free Hospital, 1895–99', *Journal of the History of Medicine and Allied Sciences*, 68, 4 (2013): 551–82.

31 Steven King, 'Regional Patterns in the Experiences and Treatment of the Sick Poor, 1800–40: Rights, Obligations and Duties in the Rhetoric of Paupers', *Family and Community History*, 10 (2007): 61–75.

32 See various contributions to Anne-Lise Head König and Bernd Schnegg (eds), *Armut in der Schweiz, 17.-20. Jahrhundert* (Zurich: ZPD, 1989).

33 Other key turning points included the creation of national doctoring organisations where these did not exist already, performance rules under doctoring contracts and entitlement rules based on accumulated financial and social contributions by

workers. Disability legislation also falls into this category from the early twentieth century.

34 Kim Price, '"Where is the Fault?" The Starvation of Edward Cooper at the Isle of Wight Workhouse in 1877', *Social History of Medicine*, 26 (2013): 21–37.
35 Alannah Tomkins, '"The Excellent Examples of the Working Class": Medical Welfare, Contributory Funding and the North Staffordshire Infirmary from 1815', *Social History of Medicine*, 21 (2008): 13–30.
36 See for instance Lynn Marie Pohl, 'African American Southerners and White Physicians: Medical Care at the Turn of the Twentieth Century', *Bulletin of the History of Medicine*, 86 (2012): 178–205.
37 Laura Tabili, *Global Migrants, Local Culture: Narratives and Newcomers in Provincial England 1840–1939* (Basingstoke: Palgrave Macmillan, 2011).

# 3  Children's health in public and private, 1700 to 1950

*Alysa Levene*

## Introduction

Child health was a matter of growing importance over the period 1700 to 1950. Attention was focused on children's bodies by a progressive sense of the intrinsic value of *childhood*. This shift is traditionally placed in the eighteenth century when Enlightenment humanitarianism under the influence of writers such as Jean-Jacques Rousseau started to identify childhood as a time of freedom, joy and innocence that deserved to be protected from harm, over-work and the immorality of the city. For Rousseau, childhood should not be subject to adult rules and the dissipation of town life, but instead lived in the freedom of nature, according to a moral order found by the child him or herself. Rousseau and his followers set much store by good health and hardiness, which also chimed with growing state concerns for national strength and the health of future citizens. Needless to say, this vision of childhood was not one to which the vast majority of Western society could aspire; it required considerable resources, space, and indulgence on the part of parents. Nonetheless, Rousseau's ideas (most famously set out in his 1762 novel on education, *Émile*) were widely disseminated, and formed part of a seachange in ideas about childhood. Significantly for our purposes, they informed the ideas of policy makers and charity officials and thus touched on the lives of poorer children as well as the better off. However, as many authors have noted, this ideal was one very much based on middle-class notions of privacy, moral standards and resource management. This was to have enduring implications for policy makers' views of the private sphere of poor families, and the necessity to supervise and manage it.

Social class therefore had a big impact on the degree of privacy maintained by the private sphere. The design of middle-class homes started to demarcate the public and private parts of the house more clearly, with children living mainly in the more secluded parts. By contrast, the homes of the poorer classes were highly unlikely to have this degree of separation between public and private; there was simply not the necessary space, as is shown in Crook's chapter. Other children lacked a home altogether: many of the famous nineteenth-century attempts at 'child-saving' were triggered by the sight of ragged and destitute children in the large cities of Europe and North America. These children were often regarded as the children of the state, although provision for them increasingly focused on mimicking a family setting. For the poor generally, however, any encounters with medical practitioners in the home took place in a space that was open to others, often including people outside the family such as lodgers. The crowding, poor sanitation and perceived lack of moral order in these homes was, by the nineteenth century, used as a justification for imposing order on the poor, and creating means by which they had to enter the public sphere to access health and welfare services. These were further exacerbated by surveys that revealed that infant mortality was persistently high through the nineteenth century: in 1900, around 14 per cent of all babies born in England and Wales, and also in America, died before their first birthday, while in France the equivalent rate was 16.6 per cent and in Italy 17 per cent.[1] In the large industrial cities these figures were very much higher. In New York, close to a third of babies died in their first year of life in the 1880s.[2] This was a personal tragedy, a colossal waste of human capital, and, in an age in which childhood was highly romanticized, a blow to society as a whole. Viviana Zelizer, one of the key authors on the history of childhood, summed up this attitude when she wrote, 'if child life was sacred, child death became an intolerable sacrilege, provoking not only parental sorrow but social bereavement as well'.[3] Much of this mortality was preventable, being due to poor hygiene, poor feeding practices, and infectious disease.

Before we move on to develop these themes further, we must unpick a little more what we mean by public and private in the context of child health. As has already been noted, the home is the most private of the private spheres (Habermas viewed women and children at the heart of the domestic private sphere; he called the family 'the intimate sphere'[4]). Things become more complicated as we move away from parental control in the private dwelling, however. As we saw in the introduction to this book, there are various ways that we can define the public. In this chapter, two key themes will be developed. The first concerns *space*, and in particular the distinction between the home and sites outside it. The second is the question of *compulsion* and the degree to which healthcare comes with a degree of judgement of the private family. The public/private dichotomy therefore starts with whether a medical encounter took place in the home or not; but it also hinges on the important question of whether it was deemed to be for the child's good (and who deemed it to be so), and how it treated the family. Social class will be a key motif here.

The last topic we must note before moving on to the main part of the discussion is how far we can judge the *child's* wishes and experiences in the historical record. This is notoriously one of the most difficult aspects of studying children in the past, but one to which historians are paying increasing attention. The trouble is that historical records were rarely created by children (an exception is diaries and autobiographies, but even these were frequently written retrospectively from adulthood). Our impressions of their experiences and opinions are thus mediated through the words and perceptions of the adults around them. This is true in the field of child health as much as any other, where encounters with physicians were for most of our period based on outward symptoms accompanied by a narrative from the mother or carer. Soliciting these sorts of signs from children could be difficult: as we will see, a key reason why few doctors specialized in child health until the mid-eighteenth century was the perceived inability of a small child to articulate their pain, and the likelihood of their being scared or unco-operative when faced with a doctor. Despite the efforts of historians to capture the child and the child-patient's voice, they remain largely inaudible in the historical record – re-inforcing the fact that they represent the most private of private spheres.[5]

This chapter is divided into two parts. The first considers the private sphere: domestic medicine, practitioners who attended in the home, and the way that the family was configured, and increasingly laid bare, as a unit of care. The second section moves through the concentric circles of the public sphere, taking clinics, dispensaries and specialist hospitals as examples of public sites of medical care and setting them within the themes of compulsion and judgement that were outlined above. As the examples will show, there are important differences of national (and indeed intra-national) detail, but in fact there is considerable evidence of an overarching narrative of penetration of the private sphere by medical and welfare authorities – and especially the private sphere of the poorer classes. The state may have been more active in providing healthcare in France than in America; pronatalist policies may have been at the forefront in Italy and Germany compared with Britain; the notion of citizenship was a more prominent motif in the Netherlands and Canada, while 'national efficiency' took centre stage in Britain; but across all countries we see a growing interest in making the bodies of the young public, while public bodies took on an ever-growing remit to protect their health, cure their ills and measure their growth.

## The home, the family, and the private sphere

### Domestic medicine

For most families in the past, and well into the twentieth century too, medicine and healthcare started and ended in the home. Long traditions of domestic medicine, herbology, folklore and the neighbourly sharing of advice all played a part here, alongside a shortage of medical practitioners (especially in rural or frontier areas), mistrust of the few there were, and a reluctance or inability to pay their fees. The more money a family had, the more they could 'shop around' for remedies purchased from itinerant sellers or druggists, or prescribed by physicians or other practitioners who entered the home. Others sought advice for family members (including children) without opening them up to physical scrutiny at all, by writing letters to medical practitioners or using mail order advertisements. The key characteristic here was that the medical care was actively sought: some families purchased most of their healthcare from outside 'experts', but it was based on their own priorities, and sometimes a long-standing relationship with a particular physician or healer.

Many of the homeliest of home remedies contained a strong element of superstition and had little medical value, such as the Italian tradition of fixing small bags of salt around children's necks to ward off the evil eye, or the custom in parts of pre-revolutionary America of filling bags with camphor to protect against scarlet fever. Others were more closely connected with religion, such as the cures that were based on Bible reading and prayer, or magic, utilizing substances that had special life-giving properties (such as the placenta), or reciting magical words. Nevertheless, however useless these were in medical terms, they had a strong symbolic purpose and demonstrate the ways that families tried to protect their young in a world where the risks of contagion and ill fortune were legion. Such was their power that many remained current well into the era of improved diagnostics and therapies. The idea that a mother's thoughts could be 'imprinted' on her unborn baby (to which many congenital deformities and cosmetic birthmarks were attributed) was still cited as late as 1900 in one American text.[6] And some herbal remedies were, of course, effective, although for reasons that were then not understood. Nicholas Culpeper's famous mid-seventeenth-century treatises on herbal medicine recommended frankincense for stomach problems and myrrh for thrush, both of which are still used today.

Domestic remedies remained particularly popular in America, where doctors were in short supply and medical licensing was virtually non-existent well into the nineteenth century.[7] Homeopathy (popular from the 1840s) was thought to be especially appropriate for children because of its microscopic doses and lack of adverse side effects. Whole kits could be purchased for domestic use; these carried considerably less risk than more general medical kits, which often contained no specific advice for dosing children. Hydrotherapy, acupuncture, hypnosis, and other shorter-lived fads were also popular up to the end of the nineteenth century and administered by families to all their members.[8] Midwives were much more readily available than physicians in most places, and families also used almanacks and printed guides to household medicine to diagnose and dose their children. Mona Gleason has shown that Canadian families of many different backgrounds continued to rely heavily on domestic medicine alongside more orthodox remedies right through the first half of the twentieth century.[9]

In Western Europe 'regular' or 'orthodox' practitioners were more common, and among these, as Roger Cooter has noted in the British context, women and children formed an important source of practice and income.[10] This can be explained by the high proportion of the young in the population at this time, but it also shows us that families did call in regular physicians when their children were ill, although we have until very recently known tantalizingly little about what they did or how (and if) their practice was differentiated for child patients. Hannah Newton has done some path-breaking work in this area by examining how medical texts available in England described the causes and courses of diseases in children, and what cures were recommended.[11] Importantly, she has found that physicians did make distinctions between the bodies of children and adults, especially in terms of their humoral make-up (children were 'warmer' and 'moister') and predisposition to disease (for example, worms and rickets). This was also translated into different treatments: not only taking into account a child's smaller size, but also the palatability of certain medicines, and the perceived site or cause of the bodily imbalance. This viewpoint is easily squared within the prevalent Galenic and chemical mode of thinking about disease, but Newton has been the first to examine whether and how it was adapted for children. She also takes this a step further by examining parents' and children's own experiences of disease (within the limitations of the sources, as we have already noted), noting the time and energy devoted to nursing children, and that it involved fathers as well as mothers, nurses and other family members.

One of the themes that Newton is at pains to stress is that medical treatment, whether 'orthodox' or lay, may have been painful, tiring and emotionally draining for all concerned, but it was seen to have benefits. Child patients themselves frequently thanked their carers for their attention and love. Margaret Pelling tells us that this sort of domestic work was not high status (unless the family was of high rank); in fact, the standing of physicians could be lowered by dint of their association with 'what was still a residual and deprived sphere of domestic privacy'.[12] Nonetheless, it seems from Newton's work that families valued and followed the advice of these outside experts. This was not just a matter for parents, either; wet nurses and employers did the same (although they were not necessarily the ones who were paying). The penetration of the private world by doctors and other healers was not necessarily an unwelcome intrusion, as in some of the examples we will examine below, but was seen instead as a vital means of trying to cure children and alleviate their suffering.

Despite the new light that Newton has shed on seventeenth-century family practice, it seems that it was not until the eighteenth century that orthodox practitioners started to interest themselves specifically in domestic medicine for children. As was noted above, this period saw a convergence of concerns about humanitarianism, population decline and the resources latent in every child, and it resulted in a growing interest from doctors (who, not coincidentally, realized that this could be a lucrative area of practice). A growing swell of publications aimed at mothers placed male orthodox practitioners squarely in the driving seat of children's medicine – the first of several developments tending towards the disempowerment of parents, and especially mothers, as the most qualified people to judge their children's health needs. The key English-language example was William Buchan's *Domestic Medicine*, first published in 1769 and hugely popular across Europe and North America, but there were many examples in other languages as well, most notably in French and German. The authors of these texts stressed the ignorance of

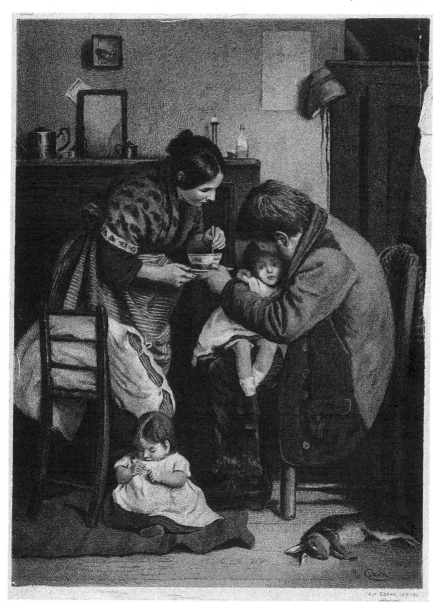

*Figure 3.1* A sick child on her father's lap. © The Wellcome Library, London.

women in matters to do with child health and the risk that they posed to their children by using traditional modes of healing instead of calling a doctor promptly. As one of the earliest widely popular texts, *An Essay upon Nursing and the Management of Children from their Birth to Three Years of Age* by William Cadogan (first published in 1748), stated:

> In my Opinion, this Business [of childrearing] has been too long fatally
> left to the Management of Women, who cannot be supposed to have a
> proper Knowledge to fit them for such a Task, notwithstanding they look
> upon it to be their own Province.[13]

In fact, it was not as simple as this. As Lisa Petermann has shown, texts like
these did shake the previous faith in the family's ability to cure and raise their
own members, but they also acknowledged the dependent relationship
between the doctor, the child and the mother (what she calls the paediatric
'triad').[14] This schema highlights the different relationship between a doctor
and a child patient compared with an adult – necessarily so, given the child's
inability to communicate their pain and symptoms as effectively. However, it
also highlights the way that child patients were protected by their adult carers,
usually their mothers. Thus the eighteenth- and nineteenth-century child
doctor becomes a figure who was invited into the private sphere but whose
judgements and actions were mediated via the mother. This is even truer of
medical texts: parents could decide what to consult and when, and how far to
follow their advice. Nonetheless, the popularity of works like these is testament to the growing incursion of outside authorities into the private sphere of
the child's sickroom.

This was not the only occasion on which the private sphere of childcare was
denigrated by orthodox practitioners. In nineteenth-century America, motherhood took on a role of paramount importance: mothers were seen as doing no
less than raising the future citizens of the republic.[15] However, as specialist
doctors gained confidence over the second half of the century (by this point
calling themselves pediatrists, and later by the more familiar term paed/pedia-
tricians), they again moved to place mothers in a position of ignorance, and in
need of outside guidance to successfully raise their precious charges. One of the
most famous child doctors and authors in nineteenth-century America was
Luther Emmet Holt, professor of paediatrics at the College of Physicians and
Surgeons, Columbia University, and founder of the specialist journals *Archives
of Pediatrics* and the *American Journal of Diseases of Children*.[16] In 1894 he
published a book called *The Care and Feeding of Children* that was aimed at
the middle classes and covered daily regime as well as healthcare. At the time
that his work was written the merits of formula milk were being stressed by
physicians, a marked contrast with the earlier emphasis on breastfeeding, which
was styled as part of the nurturing ethos of the 'Republican Mother' of the
mid-century period. In contrast, formula milk, which was composed according
to a set procedure (undermined, it must be said, by the poor quality of cows'
milk), was under the control of the doctor and at first could only be obtained
on prescription. Just like William Cadogan more than a century earlier, these
doctors cast mothers and nurses as ill equipped to provide the necessary scientific regime to successfully raise the nation's young in health.

Trends such as these, alongside the adoption of diagnostic tools such as
the stethoscope and the thermometer, and the increase in hospital beds for

children, can all be understood as undermining the confidence and self-sufficiency of the private sphere when it comes to the healthcare and nurture of the young. However, in practice, things are more complicated than this. The attempts to control the way that children were cared for in sickness and health were all informed by an idea that the private sphere was of supreme importance to the functioning of the family and the state. This was the principal justification for intervention: mothers needed to be educated to be able to perform their vital functions. There is a sense, then, that the private sphere could not fulfil its vital potential without supervision and advice from outside. However, families could mitigate this by their own actions and decisions: they could continue to call on their traditional modes of healing alongside newly professionalized paediatricians, for example, by referring to friends and neighbours, purchasing cures from druggists and itinerant sellers, and using traditional remedies. They could choose which publications to purchase or borrow, and what advice to follow. Some felt empowered by the advice they received: one New York mother wrote to the Children's Bureau (of which more later) after following the advice set out in their extremely popular pamphlet, *Infant Care* (first published in 1914 and with a distribution of over one and a half million by 1921),[17] saying that when people complimented her on the bonny health of her boy, she told them proudly, 'He's a Government baby'. This mother evidently felt more confident in her mothering skills because she was following a set of rules for childcare, even though many of the nation's grandmothers were shaking their heads at the adoption of official advice instead of inherited knowledge and instinct.[18] Other mothers felt bewildered by the array of rules on feeding, changing, sleeping, and calling the doctor, perhaps particularly those without their own mothers nearby, or who received conflicting advice from them.

### Policing the private

By the middle of the nineteenth century, it was for the first time starting to be considered acceptable for public bodies and charities to enter the home and to judge parents' ability to raise and care for their children. Roger Cooter noted this in the first significant collection of essays on the topic in English (published in 1992), referring to the recurring theme of 'the increased invasion of the state into the organization of family life in general, and child health and welfare in particular'.[19] Prior to this, family life had been seen as essentially private: it was up to parents to care for and discipline their children, and to make decisions about the balance of education and work that was best for their family. However, over the course of the late eighteenth and early nineteenth centuries, reform campaigns emerged in many Western countries in response to a perception that parents (almost always the parents of the poorer classes) were *not* always able to make the best decisions for their children's health and well-being. This was eventually played out across the Western world in legislative reforms governing children's employment, schooling and healthcare (for example, the foundation of school health clinics and health visiting services).

These incursions into the home were carried out by state and voluntary bodies alike, such as the societies for child welfare, sanitary inspectors, and housing reformers, who were all concerned with the impact of poor conditions on children. The motivation was again the convergence of concerns about population quality and humanitarianism, but now combined with a growing awareness of the ill effects of industrialization and urban conditions on child health and stature that overrode the previous sense that childrearing was a matter of personal liberty. This was often accompanied by a fear that industrial conditions were causing a decline in moral values, which were traditionally communicated from parents to children.[20] As George Behlmer has memorably written of England – but relevant in most other countries too at some stage in the nineteenth century – '[t]he Englishman's castle was to be breached for the good of the castle, and, ultimately, for the good of the Englishman as well'.[21] Furthermore, the dense courts and alleys that grew up in many industrial towns made children very visible in the public and semi-public spaces of streets and courtyards (as did their journeys to the mills, factories and workshops where they earned money to supplement the family's income, as is explained in Crook's chapter). Their ragged appearance and small stature caught the attention of a variety of bodies and was used to justify the examination and policing of the home. Countries such as the Netherlands, which industrialized later, escaped some of these problems of urban living, but arrived at a similar end-point of public scrutiny of child health and welfare.[22]

Still, many of these schemes made concessions to the fact that they were intruding into a domestic and female-dominated space, primarily by employing lady visitors and inspectors, whom, it was felt, understood the workings of this sphere, and were best placed to communicate new ideas and practices to working-class mothers. Sometimes this was misplaced: mothers often felt patronized by the middle-class 'Lady Bountifuls' who did not understand the problems of making ends meet so that children could be adequately clothed, fed and cared for.[23] In other cases a better balance was struck: the midwives and agents employed by the American Children's Bureau in the 1920s were apparently appreciated, partly because they could only give advice and small sums of money, and thus posed little threat to the integrity of the poor family (they were specifically precluded from removing children, and much of their work involved answering questions by correspondence).

This move towards female involvement in the shaping and delivery of health and welfare services is known as *maternalism*: a phenomenon seen in many countries, particularly from the 1880s to the 1920s, whereby women took their private responsibilities and areas of expertise out into the public sphere and worked to change policy for women and children; indeed, women could be the driving force behind these policy changes.[24] In countries with a tradition of *laissez faire* in matters concerning the family (such as the UK and America), such women were able to play an important role. We can see this in the American Children's Bureau (founded in 1912), which was the only federal agency headed by a woman, Julia Lathrop, herself a maternalist reformer, and which supervised the landmark Sheppard-Towner Maternity and Infancy Act of 1921 that was passed immediately after women got the vote.[25] In contrast, in countries where the state was more actively involved in welfare (such as France and Germany), such opportunities for women were fewer, although the state took on a greater role in the welfare of its citizens.[26]

The families affected by projects like these were not passive recipients, however; in fact in some cases they strongly resisted interference in their management of their children's health. One example is the opposition to the smallpox vaccination programmes that were made compulsory from the middle of the nineteenth century, in Britain in 1853 and in Germany in 1874, for example. Many parents opposed these measures because they involved what was seen as a potentially dangerous practice that they feared exposed their children to harm, and that demonstrated a lack of trust in their abilities to raise their own families. This feeling was only exacerbated by the fact that vaccination frequently took place in a public place, which not only brought risks of contagion (which would be brought back into the home) but also often had connections with charity or statutory poor relief.[27] The final insult was that because many schemes used matter from a recently vaccinated child to vaccinate others, parents could be required to take their child back to the clinic to have another procedure, effectively (in their eyes) making the child a tool of a state programme. Anti-vaccination campaigns sprang up across Europe, and in America refusal rates were particularly high in poor areas (which were unfortunately also the areas of highest exposure to the disease because of the greater population density there). Cases were even reported of parents sucking the matter back out of their children's arms to undermine the vaccination process.[28] The chaplain at the Chicago Smallpox Hospital recorded that some mothers hid their children in the house to avoid vaccination or hospitalization during an epidemic in 1893–4, while others abandoned their children because of the fear of infection.[29] In Montreal too there were anti-vaccination riots during a smallpox epidemic in the late 1880s.[30] Although these examples give us very different impressions of family relationships, the issue does offer an insight into the way that a medical measure was squared with the idea of personal freedom. As Dr C.R. Drysdale wrote to the *British Medical Journal* in 1896 on the topic of vaccination,

> As to the argument about the liberty of the subject, this is out of place in the case of children. Children are not free agents, but are always in subjection to parents or guardians. Hence it is an error to say that the compulsory vaccination of children is an attack on individual liberty. We force parents in this century to feed, clothe, and house their children, and lately to see them educated; and surely this entitles the State to demand that children should be protected against such a terrible danger as small-pox contagion is to health and life.[31]

Thus the private sphere was to be opened up to medical intervention for the benefit of the child, the family and the state. However, parents continued to resist the vaccination of their children with particular force; we see this again when diphtheria antitoxin was introduced in the 1890s, and much later, with programmes to fluoridate water supplies in the 1940s.[32]

Once the homes of the working classes had been opened up to enquiry it was a small (though extremely significant) step to deciding that some parents were not capable of raising their children at all. Crowded homes led to fears about incest and irreligion, while the breaking down of the sanctity of the domestic sphere allowed people to admit that parents could sometimes go too far in the cruel treatment of their children. In moves unthinkable just decades earlier, charity and state officials gained powers to question, examine and punish parents for causing their children harm by neglect, poor treatment, or (to use the modern term) abuse. Legislation permitting, their final sanction was the removal of a child altogether. The most famous of the voluntary bodies carrying out this sort of work were the Societies for the Prevention of Cruelty to Children, first established in New York in 1875. Legislation followed: the 1889 Prevention of Cruelty to Children Act in Britain, for example, permitted the removal of children who were thought to be the victims of abuse, and allowed for their medical examination for signs of mistreatment. In most cases this was a judgement made by forces external to the family and their peers; in some cases neighbours informed on parents, which indicates how far the barriers of private parenting were breaking down – but also, perhaps, the degree to which such investigations came to be accepted as being for the good of the child. Indeed, they were occasionally sought by parents themselves.[33]

Interestingly for our current purposes, the shelters to which such children were taken (often temporarily before they were returned to their parents, as for permanent removal was not as common as the popular image suggests) were frequently styled as 'Homes', as were institutions for poor, handicapped and orphaned children at around the same time.[34] Perhaps ironically, the need for a child to receive care in a domestic-type environment was being recognized just as the ability of their parents to provide it was called into question. For the first time, the state was acting in consistent fashion *in loco parentis* on the grounds of medical and welfare needs. Elsewhere, physical, moral and eugenic concerns were more firmly at centre stage in attitudes to the way that children were reared, and this was used as a justification for the separation of children from their parents. One of the starkest examples is, of course, the forcible removal of Australian Aboriginal children to white homes in the first half of the twentieth century, a history now painfully immortalized as the 'Stolen Generation'. Gleason has also pointed out that in Canada surveillance increased the further a family was from the white, Anglo-Protestant ideal; health differentials were markedly wider in French-speaking Catholic Quebec, for example, as well as among First Nation populations.[35] The risks of harm, neglect or degeneration were therefore present in all of these schemes, but these risks were differentiated according to class, morals and sometimes race as well. Ironically, however, attempts to *support* families via state allowances were also controversial, again because this represented an incursion into the private domain.[36]

This section has shown that the private sphere was where most of children's medical care and experiences of illness took place, although our knowledge of how this felt and how it was made sense of within wider ideas about medicine and the body is only just starting to expand. This is precisely because the home and relations within it were seen as private, and the treatment of children particularly so, while the vast majority of families (let alone children) left no records as to the type of treatment and prevention that they used, for what conditions and why. We have also seen that the private sphere was increasingly opened to scrutiny over the course of the nineteenth century across most of the Western world, and that parents – and especially the parents of the poorer classes and those outside the ethnic or racial hegemony – were subjected to advice and information in a way that often brought about unfavourable scrutiny of their childrearing. The home was not the only site subject to this sort of surveillance in this period: children were also measured and surveyed at school, in the workplace, and in child welfare clinics.

The focus on poor families can partly be explained by the fear that they were not in a position to offer their children proper guidance in moral behaviour because of material considerations and the pressures of work that took them from home. Children were on the one hand seen as the innocent victims of poverty and/or poor parenting. However, on the other, there was a fine line between innocent victim and knowing delinquent, and the child rescue charities and other welfare bodies were particularly concerned to prevent children from crossing it.[37] Given the often deprived conditions of poorer homes and the more crowded living conditions they experienced in towns, welfare measures such as these were increasingly tied up with health and childrearing more broadly. Furthermore, if children were successfully put on the path to sound morals they could promote these behaviours at home and 'rescue' the whole family. We will see that this was a common hope among those who set up children's hospitals and clinics as well. The child is thus a conduit for public concerns to be transmitted to the private sphere. Finally, as medical practitioners learnt more about child health, and the home was opened up, many more areas of welfare and child development became suffused with medical knowledge. Thus, doctors began to speak up for safe milk supplies, school medical services, nutrition, and the improvement of infant mortality rates, all ways that further focused the medical gaze on the bodies of the young. As one author has written of the American context, children's health by the end of the nineteenth century was a social science as well as a medical one.[38]

## Children's health in the public sphere

These sorts of concerns and perspectives led to the foundation of a growing number of more public sites for the prevention and cure of ill health among children, such as outpatient clinics and dispensaries, and specialized children's hospitals. We can see these as another step in removing medical care from the private sphere, and thus a further insight into the ambivalent view of the family at this time. However, it also represents the growing sense of expertise and optimism in what orthodox medicine could achieve, a concern about the persistence of high infant mortality rates, and an appreciation of the benefits of isolation and hospital therapy. As we will go on to see, the boundaries of these sites were porous, and often did not preclude a relationship with the private sphere. Nor were they altogether public, certainly not in terms of access: admission to hospital wards, for example, was regulated and restricted, and once a child was admitted, visiting rights for parents were strictly controlled. On the other hand, families often had to endure long waits and humiliating questioning regarding their finances before they could access medical expertise, a reminder that decision-making for their child was largely out of their hands.

Outpatient clinics and dispensaries were the first of these spaces to emerge. The clinics were provided by voluntary and state bodies, and offered a range of services, from parent-craft classes to advice on nutrition, dispensing of vitamins, milk, and food supplements, vaccinations, and baby weighing sessions. The dispensaries had more overtly medical functions and were often supported by home-visiting services. Both had their heyday in the late nineteenth century for the reasons already established: the growth in expertise on child development around that time (and especially the creation of 'normal' growth and weight charts that provided an important reference point), and the gradual acceptance that outside bodies could and perhaps should advise and police the family. America again lagged behind Europe somewhat here: the first children's clinic in New York was established in 1860 and momentum gained pace in the early twentieth century. In Britain such services were further underpinned by legislation such as the 1918 Maternity and Child Welfare Act, while the Netherlands passed a *Gezondheidswet*, or Health Act, that included provision for child health in 1919. The dispensary movement had a longer history: the Kinderkrankeninstitut was founded in Vienna in 1788 (Vienna was to remain an important centre for the development of paediatrics). The dispensaries seem to have been immediately popular with families, perhaps because of the paucity of other medical facilities for the young, but the clinics received more variable reactions before gradually being accepted as performing a useful function. Indeed, some of the baby clinics provided under the terms of the American Sheppard-Towner Act became hubs of community social life. Free neighbourhood health centres remained a crucial part of community care into the 1930s in American cities (especially in immigrant areas) before being eclipsed by private (paid for) services.[39]

Neither dispensaries nor clinics offered treatment that removed the child from the family (although they might refer them on elsewhere). Hospitals were quite different in this respect, although most of the general hospitals that treated children as well as the specialist children's hospitals that emerged from the early nineteenth century also had large outpatient departments – a fact less commented on in the historiography. The first specialist institution was founded in Paris in 1802: the Hôpital des Enfants Malades, and other large European cities followed suit over the next few decades.[40] England was one of the last of these, founding the Great Ormond Street Hospital for Sick Children in 1852. The late arrival of this hospital has been attributed to the greater availability of dispensaries in England compared with the Continent, and mistrust of inpatient care. Once established, however, Great Ormond Street quickly became popular with parents: it saw 140 patients in its first year, but five years later this number had tripled.[41] In America, specialist children's hospitals were built on the back of the expertise gained in the clinics: Philadelphia opened its hospital in 1855, Boston and New York followed in 1869, and by 1895 there were 26 such institutions across the country.[42] Toronto's Hospital for Sick Children was founded in 1875. By the 1920s these institutions were largely displacing the separate dispensaries.

As already suggested, the children's hospitals aimed to educate as well as cure: they often had a strong Christian ethos that they hoped would 'civilize' their patients and teach them the value of hygiene and sound morals, which they would then take home with them. As the promotional material of the Children's Hospital in Philadelphia stated, '[u]pon returning home, the children would thus become agents of reform within their families'.[43] Of course this could set up tensions where the child's family was of a different faith or denomination, and is

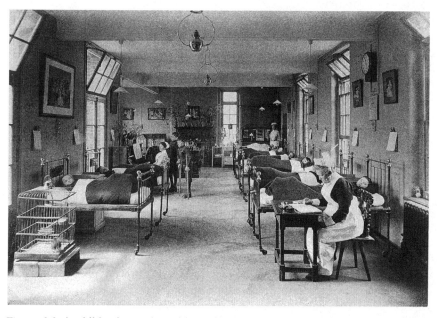

*Figure 3.2* A children's ward at Alexandra Hospital, East Clandon, Surrey, 1913.
© The Wellcome Library, London.

a further demonstration of the way that healthcare could be an insensitive instrument of cultural hegemony. Parental visiting disrupted this re-equilibrating process as well as the regimented nursing schedule (although in other hospitals not designed specifically for children, parents were required to carry out nursing duties). At the Boston Children's Hospital parents could only visit for one hour on Mondays, Wednesdays and Fridays, but financial supporters could attend at almost any time (a similar situation prevailed at Great Ormond Street).[44] In Toronto daily visiting was not permitted until 1961.[45]

Institutions such as these gave a prominent role to medical experts, and to diagnosis and care outside the home. In this respect they represent a public encounter with medicine compared with many of the examples in the previous section. However, it would be wrong to characterize them as entirely separate from the domestic sphere. The large numbers of children attending hospital outpatient departments, clinics and dispensaries were cared for at home. Parents could decide when to attend clinics and whether to continue with treatment (a bane of attending doctors). Even in hospitals, they might still manage to maintain some control over the management of their children's care. Andrea Tanner has uncovered many examples of children being removed from Great Ormond Street by their parents, often so that they could die at home. This is in itself a sad insight into the important function of family and home at the end of a child's life. Crucially, this also meant that there was no requirement for an autopsy – perhaps the greatest invasion into the private body imaginable.[46] And finally, although those running children's hospitals did frequently control the child's regimen and contact with their families during their stays, they often specifically represented themselves as acting *in loco parentis* and as custodians of a protective space for care and cure. We see a romanticized picture in the 1871 children's novel *At the Back of the North Wind* by George MacDonald, where a poor child, Nanny, receives much better 'fathering' from a benefactor while in a London children's hospital than she had from her drunkard grandmother. Moreover, the hospital has a civilizing effect on Nanny:

> If Nanny had been taken straight from the street, it is very probable she would not have been so pleasant in a decent household, or so easy to teach; but after the refining influences of her illness and the kind treatment she had had in the hospital, she moved about the house just like some rather sad pleasure haunting the mind.[47]

Children's hospitals, clinics and dispensaries did not always offer 'magic bullets'; indeed, in numerous cases the new institutions could only try to alleviate chronic suffering. However, there were many children who were able to benefit from specialist treatments or even simply an improved diet, rest, and warmth for a few weeks or months by being removed from the private domestic sphere and placed in the 'public' one. And as medical care and cure became more complicated, it could be argued that the care given in the private sphere had to open up in order for the young to benefit. X-rays, surgery, and treatments that involved intubation and intravenous lines could simply not be offered as safely or easily by domestic practitioners as they could in a hospital.

As these institutions became more overtly medical, then, the distinction between the private domestic sphere and the public one that was controlled by doctors and nurses sharpened. Medical practitioners became ever more 'expert', while parents were expected to seek and follow their advice. The Third White House Conference on Child Health and Protection in 1930 laid particular emphasis on the value of institutions at a time when many families still lacked access to healthcare.[48] America also led the way in the formulation of child guidance: a combination of medicine, psychoanalysis and psychiatric social work that aimed to 'guide' disturbed children back to acceptable and normal behaviour. This involved, among other things, examining the child's relationship with their family and correcting parenting 'problems'. Medicine and the state became involved in more and more aspects of children's lives: mass education, for example, highlighted the degree of variation in child attainment and physical health, leading to the foundation of special schools and school medical services. Attention on medicine and child welfare was also sharpened whenever concerns about population quality came to the fore, such as the times when mass conscription highlighted the poor condition of many adult males, and when evacuation programmes brought urban and rural children together (the town children were often markedly less healthy).

In all of these ways, children's healthcare was gradually brought within the remit of the public sphere – that is, delivered predominately outside the home, and organized by orthodox practitioners rather than family members. Advice literature for parents continued to flourish, but there remained a distinct line between the simple illnesses and problems that could be dealt with at home, and the more serious ones that necessitated a trip to a physician. This did not change in any lasting way until the period following the Second World War, when Benjamin Spock sparked a new zeitgeist in his *Baby and Child Care* (published 1946), a book that emphasized the value of parents' own instincts in rearing their children. At the same time psychologists and psychiatrists such as the British John Bowlby were starting to demonstrate the importance of maternal bonding on a child's emotional development. This led directly and finally to the introduction of freer visiting rights to children in hospital and a new understanding of child psychology. Children's medicine had been removed irrevocably from the home, but by the second half of the twentieth century the boundaries of public medical sites such as hospitals were starting to be broken down again.

## Conclusion

In 1992 Roger Cooter wrote that the field of child health history lacked 'intellectual richness' and was 'stuck in infancy'.[49] In particular, he noted the lack of attention to children aged 4–14, the child as a 'welfare object', and, especially, the lack of social and economic contextualization of child health and its priorities. In 2003 the editors of another collection on child health in Britain and the Netherlands that specifically referenced the Cooter volume also wrote that 'the history of the sick child has not advanced far'.[50] However, there are signs that this is now an outdated judgement. While new additions to the field are still dominated by individual institutions and charities, there has been a move toward utilizing these to make much broader points about the treatment and conceptualization of the young in sickness and in health. Alongside this, historians (and also sociologists and anthropologists) have turned their attention to questions of race, disability, and national and local differences. The child's own experience has also come to the forefront recently, a historical perspective scarcely conceived of when Cooter's edited volume appeared. We have not had the space to consider these themes in this chapter, but they have all added to our understanding of child health in the broadest sense.[51]

Instead, in this chapter we have examined child health in history from the viewpoint of 'public and private'. As the chapters in this book show, there are many ways of interpreting this dichotomy; however, in the current case we have been engaged principally in a discussion of the private sphere of the home, and the ways that medicine and healthcare interacted with it. This is an important perspective since domestic medicine is often overlooked in favour of hospitals, charities and practitioners. As Sturdy wrote in a collection of essays on medicine and the public sphere in 2002,

> Until recently, historians and sociologists have tended to adopt a rather simplistic view of the relationship between public and private spheres privileging the former as the site of the important business of politics while regarding the latter as merely a secondary and relatively deprived site concerned with little more than the work of demographic reproduction.[52]

The discussion in this chapter certainly supports his suggestion that we look again at the character of the private sphere of healthcare. In particular, it has noted how fine the gradations from the home into the public sphere are, particularly when we think about questions of who made the decisions for the child: parents or practitioners. We can now take a step back to draw out three of the most striking aspects of what has been covered.

The first is the remarkable concurrence across nations in the story of increased penetration into the private family. This happened at slightly different times in different places, as has been illustrated through the chapter, and with differing relationships to governmental policy; but the validity of the general trend is striking. This is partly because the changes in ideas about childhood and its value (both current and future) were also widely shared. Concerns about infant and child mortality were also widespread, and gained currency as they came to be used as a measure of a nation's development and humanity. A medicalized sense of welfare was thus used to justify the supervision of childrearing.

Secondly, and equally striking, is the ambivalent attitude to the domestic sphere from charities and government bodies. This is, of course, linked to the first point: the penetration of the family could only come about with an increasing acceptance that parents needed advice and safeguards in the care of their children. And this, in turn, relates to the third point, which is that the idealized image of the child that was used as a reference point in the reforms outlined in this chapter was a middle-class white one. Poor families and those outside the ethnic mainstream could not but fail to meet many of the more material criteria of good parenting when judged on these terms. However, this co-existed with a sense that the family was generally the best place for the child: charities such as the societies for preventing cruelty came to emphasize education for parents in order to rectify poor situations rather than removing their children. The same can be seen in the intentions of the child guidance movement in the interwar years, by which time there was also a sense that a balanced and happy family life was necessary for emotional as well as physical health. However, this ideal was not upheld for all families, as demonstrated by the removal of children from aboriginal families, where heredity was viewed as inferior and parents were not to be trusted with their children's care. Moreover, in other ways, medical care for children (coalescing as a clearly defined specialism of 'paediatrics' by the end of the nineteenth century) underwent its most radical changes in spaces outside the home, and in particular in specialist wards and hospitals where parents for a long time had limited access.

The third point, then, is one of class differentiation. The middle classes and above had much more scope to buy different types of medical care; however, they also escaped much of the scrutiny to which the working classes were subject. To return to George Behlmer's words, it was not actually the castles that were breached by health and welfare services in the later nineteenth century so much as the urban dwellings of the poor. It was here that the greatest levels of crowding and infectious diseases were found, where hygiene issues affected the safety of food and milk supplies leading to dysentery and marasmus (wasting), where maternal work was most likely to have an adverse impact on childcare and breastfeeding (although there is evidence of working women receiving their babies during the day to feed them), and where lack of money meant a compromised diet. However, the other side of the coin was that the poor had access to a growing range of free and subsidized health and welfare services (a notable exception was the American Sheppard-Towner provision, which was designed to be available for all classes). The Sheppard-Towner Act is also interesting because it gave permissive powers to individual states to enact their own provision. Thus, states with large black or Hispanic populations employed black and Spanish-speaking nurses, aligning provision with the requirements of local families. Still, race remained a big issue in America, Australia, New Zealand and Canada in a way that was not seen in most of Western Europe. Health provision for children (and families more generally) remained sub-standard in areas with large black, ethnic minority and aboriginal populations, resulting in a huge differential in health and mortality rates. Unfortunately, for the children of these groups of the population, the now entrenched idea of the value of childhood had yet to be translated into equal access to good healthcare. Indeed, there is evidence that the public sphere has yet to entirely embrace full support of the domestic one where these families are concerned.

**Further reading**

There is very little literature on the notion of public and private in children's healthcare, and histories tend to focus on individual nations or individual institutions. The close relationship between health and welfare is also clear in many of the more general works on the public/private provision for the young. Two of the most useful works are the edited collections: by Roger Cooter, *In The Name of the Child: Health and Welfare, 1880–1940* (London and New York: Routledge, 1992), which is particularly strong on medical-welfare issues; and Marijke Gijswijt-Hofstra and Hilary Marland, *Cultures of Child Health in Britain and the Netherlands in the Twentieth Century* (Amsterdam: Rodopi, 2003), which provides a cross-national perspective on issues such as national efficiency and citizenship in the formulation of child health. A good example of a detailed investigation of specialist hospitals for children is Elizabeth M. R. Lomax's *Small and Special: The Development of Hospitals for Children in Victorian Britain* (London: Wellcome Institute for the History of Medicine, 1996), while Charles R. King's *Children's Health in America: A History* (New York: Twayne Publishers, 1993) is an excellent introduction to children's healthcare in America. More recently, Hannah Newton's *The Sick Child in Early Modern England, 1580–1720* (Oxford: Oxford University Press, 2012) offers a new way of integrating 'children's physic' into the early modern medical canon, while at the other end of the time period, Mona Gleason's *Small Matters: Canadian Children in Sickness and Health* (Montreal and Kingston: McGill-Queen's University Press, 2013) shows how effective oral testimonies can be in putting the child at the centre of the experience of healthcare at home, at school, and in hospital. The patient perspective is provided by databases of hospital admission registers and case notes, such as the publicly available Historic Hospitals Admission Records Project (http://www.hharp.org/), which includes records from Great Ormond Street and the Royal Hospital for Sick Children in Glasgow as well as several smaller institutions.

**Notes**

1 Enrique Regidor, Cruz Pascual, David Martínez, Maria E. Calle, Paloma Ortega and Paloma Astasio, 'The Role of Political and Welfare State Characteristics in Infant Mortality: A Comparative Study in Wealthy Countries since the Late Nineteenth Century', *International Journal of Epidemiology*, 40, 5 (2001): 1187–95.
2 Charles R. King, *Children's Health in America: A History* (New York: Twayne Publishers, 1993), 106.

3 Viviana Zelizer, *Pricing the Priceless Child: The Changing Social Value of Children* (New York: Basic Books, 1981), 23.

4 Jürgen Habermas, *The Structural Transformation of the Public Sphere: An Inquiry into a Category of Bourgeois Society* (Cambridge, Mass.: MIT University Press, 1991), 55–6.

5 A recent exception is Mona Gleason's study of child health in Canada in the first half of the twentieth century, which makes use of oral testimonies. Mona Gleason, *Small Matters: Canadian Children in Sickness and Health* (Montreal and Kingston: McGill-Queen's University Press, 2013).

6 Angel Rafael Colón with Patricia Ann Colón, *Nurturing Children: A History of Pediatrics* (Westport, Conn.: Greenwood Press, 1999), 218.

7 At the time of the Declaration of Independence there were only 3,500 doctors in America; see Colón, *Nurturing Children*, 156.

8 James H. Cassedy, *Medicine in America: A Short History* (Baltimore and London: The Johns Hopkins University Press, 1991), 36–7.

9 Gleason, *Small Matters*, esp. chapters 2 and 3.

10 Roger Cooter, 'Introduction', in Roger Cooter (ed.), *In the Name of the Child: Health and Welfare, 1880–1940* (London and New York: Routledge, 1992), 10.

11 Hannah Newton, *The Sick Child in Early Modern England, 1580–1720* (Oxford: Oxford University Press, 2012).

12 Margaret Pelling, 'Public and Private Dilemmas: The College of Physicians in Early Modern London', in Steve Sturdy (ed.), *Medicine, Health and the Public Sphere in Britain, 1600–2000* (London and New York: Routledge, 2002). The quotation is taken from the editor's introduction, 5.

13 William Cadogan, *An Essay upon Nursing and the Management of Children from Their Birth to Three Years of Age* (London: J. Roberts, 1748), 1.

14 Lisa Petermann, 'From a Cough to a Coffin: The Child's Medical Encounter in England and France, 1762–1888', unpublished PhD thesis (University of Warwick, 2007).

15 See King, *Children's Health*, 25–47. The idea of 'Republican motherhood' is specifically connected to the American context, but it was an important theme in several other countries too, including France, Germany and the Netherlands.

16 Colón, *Nurturing Children*, 228.

17 King, *Children's Health*, 136.

18 King, *Children's Health*, 141; Rima D. Apple, '"Training the Baby": Mothers' Responses to Advice Literature in the First Half of the Twentieth Century', in Barbara Beatty, Emily D. Cahan and Julia Grant (eds), *When Science Encounters the Child: Education, Parenting and Child Welfare in Twentieth Century America* (New York: Teachers College Press, 2006), 195–214.

19 Cooter, 'Introduction', 7.

20 See Colin Heywood, *Childhood in Nineteenth-Century France: Work, Health and Education among the 'classes populaires'* (Cambridge: Cambridge University Press, 1988), 183–214.

21 George K. Behlmer, *Child Abuse and Moral Reform in England, 1870–1908* (Stanford, Calif.: Stanford University Press, 1982), 16.

22 For example, the Netherlands: see Gijswijt-Hofstra and Marland, *Cultures of Child Health*.

23 Jane Lewis, *Women in Britain since 1945: Women, Family, Work and the State in the Post-war Years* (Oxford: Blackwell Publishing, 1992).

24 For a classic discussion see the introduction and contributions to Seth Koven and Sonya Michel (eds), *Mothers of a New World: Maternalist Policies and the Origins of Welfare States* (New York and London: Routledge, 1993).

25 By 1923 all but 3 of the 48 state bureaux of child hygiene in America were headed by women. Molly Ladd Taylor, '"My Work Came out of Agony and Grief":

Mothers and the Making of the Sheppard-Towner Act', in Koven and Michel, *Mothers of a New World*, 323.

26 Seth Koven and Sonya Michel, 'Introduction', in Koven and Michel, *Mothers of a New World*, 1–42.

27 Logie Barrow, 'In the Beginning Was the Lymph: The Hollowing of Stational Vaccination in England and Wales, 1840–98', in Sturdy, *Medicine, Health and the Public Sphere*, 205–23; also Nadja Durbach, '"They Might as Well Brand Us": Working Class Resistance to Compulsory Vaccination in Victorian England', *Social History of Medicine*, 13 (2000): 45–62.

28 Logie Barrow, '"In the Beginning"', 212. He also notes that in English workhouses babies could be vaccinated without the parents' consent, a further reminder of the extent to which children under the care of public authorities could be viewed as citizens of the state. Vaccination was not carried out in the home in England until the 1890s, although this was common earlier in Scotland and Ireland.

29 King, *Children's Health*, 104.

30 Gleason, *Small Matters*, 56.

31 Charles R. Drysdale, 'The Royal Commission on Vaccination', *British Medical Journal*, 2, 1864 (1896): 786.

32 Amy C. Whipple, '"Into Every Home, Into Every Body": Organicism and Anti-statism in the British Anti-fluoridation Movement, 1952–1960', *Twentieth Century British History*, 21, 3 (2010): 330–49.

33 See, for example, Harry Ferguson, 'Cleveland in History: The Abused Child and Child Protection', in Cooter, *In the Name of the Child*, 146–73; Behlmer, *Child Abuse*; Harry Hendrick, *Child Welfare: England, 1872–1989* (London and New York: Routledge, 1994).

34 Ferguson, 'Cleveland in History'.

35 Gleason, *Small Matters*, passim.

36 In some cases this had a specifically pronatalist intent; as, for example, in Napo-leonic France and again after the First World War, and also in Germany and Italy in the 1930s. See John Macnicol, 'Welfare, Wages and the Family: Child Endow-ment in Comparative Perspective, 1900–50', in Cooter, *In the Name of the Child*, 244–76.

37 For a fuller discussion of children as victims and threats see Hendrick, *Child Welfare*.

38 King, *Children's Health*, 85–93, paraphrased quotation from p. 92.

39 Charles E. Rosenberg, 'Social Class and Medical Care in Nineteenth-Century America: The Rise and Fall of the Dispensary', in Judith Walzer Leavitt and Ronald L. Numbers (eds), *Sickness and Health in America: Readings in the History of Medicine and Public Health* (Madison: University of Wisconsin Press, 1978), 157–71.

40 Others included those in Berlin in 1830, St Petersburg in 1834, Vienna and Breslau in 1837, Prague in 1842, Turin in 1843, Stockholm in 1845 and Copenhagen in 1846. Colón, *Nurturing Children*, 191.

41 Andrea Tanner, 'Choice and the Children's Hospital: Great Ormond Street Hos-pital Patients and Their Families, 1855–1900', in Anne Borsay and Peter Shapely (eds), *Medicine, Charity and Mutual Aid: The Consumption of Health and Welfare in Britain, c. 1550–1950* (Aldershot, Hants: Ashgate, 2007), 144.

42 Colón, *Nurturing Children*, 192. This also accompanied the foundation of specialist professorships and learned societies, such as the Pediatric Section of the American Medical Association, which was established in 1880.

43 Tanner, 'Choice and the Children's Hospital', 143.

44 The emotional impact of separation from parents (and especially mothers) on a child was not discovered until the 1950s, at which time unrestricted hospital visiting began to be debated. See Harry Hendrick, 'Children's Emotional Well-being and

Mental Health in Early Post-Second World War Britain: The Case of Unrestricted Hospital Visiting', in Gijswijt-Hofstra and Marland, *Cultures of Child Health*, 213–42.

45 Gleason, *Small Matters*, 107.

46 Tanner, 'Choice and the Children's Hospital'.

47 George MacDonald, *At the Back of the North Wind* (Ware, Herts: Wordsworth Editions, 1994), 320.

48 King, *Children's Health*, 150–1.

49 Cooter, 'Introduction', 1 and 3.

50 Gijswijt-Hofstra and Marland, 'Introduction', 8.

51 For example, Cheryl Krasnick Warsh and Veronica Strong-Boag (eds), *Children's Health Issues in Historical Perspective* (Waterloo, Ont.: Wilfrid Laurier University Press, 2005); Anne Borsay and Pamela Dale, *Disabled Children: Contested Caring, 1850–1979* (London: Pickering & Chatto, 2012).

52 Sturdy, 'Introduction', 5.

# 4 Mental disorder, crime and the development of healthcare systems

*Katherine D. Watson*

## Introduction

It has long been the duty of organized states to promote public security by means of a system of criminal justice, to resolve disputes, protect people and property, and maintain social order.[1] Since the early modern period medicine has become increasingly essential to this objective, leading to the development of a distinctive area of practice known as forensic medicine, broadly defined as the application of medical knowledge to the investigation of crime. This definition sets it apart from other medical specialties and has proved integral to the creation of the concept of the 'expert witness'.[2] Experts differ from other witnesses because of their professional knowledge, or expertise, which enables them to testify not only to what they have observed but also to offer their own opinions as facts.[3] The central importance of expert witnesses in criminal trials has been well established since the mid-nineteenth century, particularly in the sub-specialty of forensic psychiatry. The history of this area of medico-legal practice shows that the intellectual development and day-to-day interests of forensic medicine are dependent on law and legal procedure,[4] so that the private nature of the encounter between doctor and patient is challenged by the public interest in the expert's interactions with the victims and perpetrators of criminal acts.

The way in which medical experts perform their role is determined by the justice system in which they operate. The central fact-finding responsibility of the jury and inherent distrust of the prosecution case distinguish the adversarial system, found principally in common law jurisdictions such as the United Kingdom and its former colonies, from its Continental counterpart, the inquisitorial system. The latter is characterized by pre-trial investigations directed by magistrates who weed out weak evidence, so that by the time a case reaches court there is a significant presumption of guilt. Its focus on written documents and judge-led questioning of witnesses means there is less scope for testing the prosecution case by means of examination and cross-examination of witnesses than there is in the adversarial system, which by its lawyer-centred nature tends to involve ill-natured oral confrontations between the prosecution and the defence.[5] Forensic medicine and the practices of expert witnesses have been shaped by these legal traditions. In Europe, investigating magistrates were mandated to seek out all forms of evidence that might help them establish a case, so that medical evidence became a regular part of criminal proceedings in the medieval period; doctors were understood to be more expert in medical matters than anyone else. But the modern concept of the expert witness arose in the adversarial Anglo-American context in the late eighteenth century and emerged into public prominence during the nineteenth, as lawyers came to dominate criminal trial procedure while medicine, science and technology developed into dominant social institutions.[6] Psychiatrists were quick to spot professional opportunities offered by engagement with the law, and swiftly established themselves as experts on disorders of the mind.[7] Although the professional integrity of expert witnesses has since been periodically tainted by accusations of partisanship or incompetence, the role has become firmly embedded in both adversarial and inquisitorial criminal justice systems.

What this means in practice is that forensic psychiatrists must work within a setting defined by law and legal expectations of evidence and proof, to reveal and explain hidden aspects of individuals' bodies and minds. Forensic medical expertise is thus a public, not a private act.[8] It is both a medical and a legal artefact, and as such it provides a unique means of studying the ambiguous dichotomy between the private imperative intrinsic to medical intervention on behalf of the mentally ill, and the public good championed by criminal justice institutions.

This chapter will consider the changing nature of the relationship between medicine, law and society revealed by the history of mental disorder and crime in England,[9] France, Germany and the United States since the mid-eighteenth century, examining the ways in which forensic psychiatry has consistently acted as a bridge between the private sphere of human activity and experience and the public arena. This connection has been most obviously visible in two broad areas, illicit sexuality and homicide, because of the perceived social danger they pose, and there has been a tendency to explain criminal behaviours in medical terms. This is particularly true of three groups: men who engaged in sex with other men, women who killed their own infants, and murderers whose state of mind rendered them less than fully culpable for their acts. The medicalization of crime led, especially in the case of homicide, to an expectation that the risk of offenders' future dangerousness should be assessed and managed. As such risk is most often associated with unstable mental states, the courts' growing reliance on medical opinion in turn influenced the development of the healthcare systems put in place to treat the individuals – 'criminals' redefined as 'patients' – whose conduct was thus explained or excused. Areas once considered the professional territory of general practitioners or legal officials came increasingly under the authority of the psychiatric profession during the twentieth century, creating a three-way association between the courtroom, the asylum and the prison reflected in the figure of the psychiatric expert.[10]

The four national frameworks on which the chapter concentrates highlight the types of legal cases – and the degree to which they were embedded in specific legal and forensic contexts – that have stimulated government intrusion into and regulation of the private sphere. At the same time, an underlying current of public opinion has also proven itself increasingly capable of influencing government policy. In order to show these developments, as well as the connections and contrasts between the Anglo-American, French and German contexts, the chapter is divided into three sections. The first examines the historical relationship between insanity and criminal responsibility. The second studies this connection through the example of the medicalization of the crimes of sodomy and infanticide. The final section considers mental health and dangerousness in relation to homicide, and surveys the regulation of healthcare provision for the insane criminal in each country. The state may have been more or less active in promoting specific systems of treatment both within and outside criminal custody, but across all countries we see a growing debate about the proper balance between protecting the rights of the public and those of the mentally ill offender.

## Insanity and legal culpability

By the seventeenth century an elaborate medico-legal perception of the insane individual existed. In Europe this was based on Roman law, which accepted that the insane were not accountable for their acts, modified by sixteenth-century medical insights about the effects of mental states such as depression on the ability to form the intent to commit a crime. In England, the common law also excused the 'raving' mad, who because of their derangement could not understand the nature of the acts they committed, and accepted that insanity might be temporary and yet exculpatory, but stressed the importance of knowing the difference between right and wrong.[11] These views of the insane criminal acknowledged them as both patients and legal subjects, but had little bearing on their practical situation. Once a judge or jury had decided that an accused person was insane, it was left to friends and relatives to look after them. Those not cared for at home could be confined in hospitals, workhouses or gaols without medical certification.[12]

By the end of the eighteenth century insanity was increasingly being viewed as a natural and potentially curable disease, rather than a supernatural affliction. In 1808 the German physician Johann Reil (1759–1813) coined the term *psychiatrie,* derived from the Greek words for 'soul' or 'mind' and 'doctor' (*psyche* and *iatros*). Practitioners of this new branch of medicine wanted to cure the mentally ill, leading to practical outcomes such as the separation of the mentally disordered from other prisoners or inmates and the creation of hospitals exclusively designed for psychiatric care. These developments offered new hope to the insane criminal.

Identifying the insane criminal became a key means by which early psychiatrists, known as 'alienists' following the publication of Philippe Pinel's

*Medico-Philosophical Treatise on Mental Alienation or Mania* (1801), asserted their importance in the public arena. Early modern doctors had thought of insanity as a lack of intellectual capacity caused by mental impairment ('idiocy', in the terminology of the day) or an absence of human under-standing (the 'mad beast' or 'raving lunatic'), but Pinel and his followers began to classify degrees of insanity, rather than completely different types. As chief physician at the Salpêtrière, the main Paris asylum for women, Pinel (1745–1826) was able to make clinical observations of the inmates, recogniz-ing that insanity did not always involve a disorder of the intellect but might take the form of a mental distancing – or alienation – from reality that could be present even when intellectual capabilities were fully intact. This marked the transition from total to partial insanity.

For our purposes, the most important of the classifications that Pinel iden-tified was 'mania without delirium' (*manie sans délire*), in which the patient was overcome by a kind of instinctive rage and driven by a blind impulse to commit acts of violence. This was termed 'moral derangement' by Benjamin Rush (1746–1813) in the United States in 1811, and the same condition was called 'moral insanity' by the English doctor James Cowles Prichard (1786–1848) in 1835. By the late nineteenth century American neurologists and psychiatrists had given it yet another name, 'moral imbecility', the emotional equivalent of arrested intellectual development that today would be categor-ized as a personality disorder, like psychopathy.[13] According to the historian of crime and criminology Nicole Rafter, the work of Pinel, Rush and Prichard on moral insanity can be considered part of the early history of the discipline of criminology – the study of the nature, causes, prevention and control of crime – before the subject or even the word itself became established.[14] Alienists interested in moral insanity conceived of criminality as a natural phe-nomenon that could be explained by scientific means – especially psychiatry.

With the possible manifestations of insanity now much less obvious to the untrained observer than the 'idiot' or 'raving lunatic' had been, psychiatry gained a ready-made entry point to the criminal justice system, particularly following the translation of Pinel's book into English and German in 1806. His student Jean-Étienne Esquirol (1772–1840), using 'mania without delir-ium' as a model, formulated a theory of homicidal monomania in 1819. This postulated the existence of a form of insanity that removed an offender's free will, so that they were compelled by some irresistible force to commit violent crimes. The key distinction from the sorts of insanity that had always been recognized by the law was that homicidal monomania led to premeditated killing rather than sudden impulsive homicide. It was not by chance that Esquirol's theory was applicable to a series of horrific and incomprehensible murders that had presented a new problem for French judges. The law did not need to be modified. It had inherited from Roman law a clear understanding that insanity excused an individual from punishment: the French Penal Code of 1810 stated that no crime could exist if the accused person was insane at the time of the act or was driven by an irresistible force. Rather, the judiciary had to adapt its interpretation of criminal culpability to the new psychiatric definition of insanity. The stage was set for the birth of a new discipline: forensic psychiatry.

The earliest writings on forensic psychiatry were penned by Étienne-Jean Georget (1795–1828), a student of both Pinel and Esquirol. He collected accounts of insanity defences presented in criminal trials and investigated mental diseases in civil and criminal courts, publishing his findings in four volumes before his early death.[15] His work prompted the American physician Isaac Ray (1807–1881) to write a similar book, *Treatise on the Medical Jurisprudence of Insanity* (1838), which established forensic psychiatry as a professional discipline in the United States. He too made a distinction between intellectual and moral insanity, assuming both derived from physical illness principally associated with the brain. In a clear statement of the public role of the forensic physician in revealing the hidden nature of such an illness, Ray noted that unless properly instructed by a practitioner qualified to investigate difficult cases, juries would seize on the most obvious but perhaps least important points, leading to verdicts 'deplorably at variance with the dictates of true science'.[16]

By the mid-nineteenth century psychiatry had also established itself in English and German courts. Lawyers, judges and juries were forced to grapple with the contrast between legal and medical understandings of free will, the key legal determinant of guilt. Legal tradition defined free will as the ability to form the intent to commit an act, knowing it to be wrong. Medical understanding of partial insanity allowed that defendants might not be accountable for *planned* acts if at the time of the act they were unable to distinguish right from wrong, 'incapable of understanding the blameworthiness of the act, or unable to resist the force of a preoccupying passion'.[17]

The problem of knowing right from wrong came to a head in England in 1843 when, acting under the power of a delusion directed against the government, Daniel McNaughtan (1802/3–1865) killed the prime minister's private secretary. His defence was that his delusions relieved him of responsibility even though he knew his act was wrong. The prosecution maintained that he was fully culpable because he *could* distinguish between right and wrong. Nine medical experts appeared for the defence, the prosecution offered no testimony in rebuttal, and the judge practically directed a verdict of 'not guilty on the ground of insanity'. This decision was extremely controversial and so the government sought the opinion of a panel of five common law judges, in the form of answers to five questions. Their replies constituted the so-called McNaughtan or M'Naghten Rules (the spelling varies), which directed that a successful insanity defence had to prove that 'at the time of the committing of the act, the party accused was labouring under such a defect of reason, from disease of the mind, as not to know the nature and quality of the act he was doing; or, if he did know it, that he did not know he was doing what was wrong'. These rules established the basis of the insanity defence in common law jurisdictions, including most American states, and stimulated continuing debate about the meaning of terms such as 'disease of the mind', 'wrong' and 'irresistible impulse', as well as the proper scope of an expert witness' testimony about the effects of a defendant's delusions at the time of the alleged crime.[18]

In 1909 Heinrich Oppenheimer (1870–1933), who held qualifications in both medicine and law, published an international comparative study of laws on criminal responsibility.[19] In France, Germany,[20] Hungary, Italy, Romania and Russia there was no punishable act if the accused person's mental state was disturbed at the time of the act so that they had lost their mental faculties or free will. In the Netherlands it was slightly less straightforward: judges did not have to automatically acquit the mentally afflicted, but had absolute power to excuse those whom they thought should be excused. The McNaughtan Rules were in use in American federal courts and 22 state courts; irresistible impulse was placed alongside the right-wrong test in seven states; and in six states the law revolved around the existence of a proven connection between mental

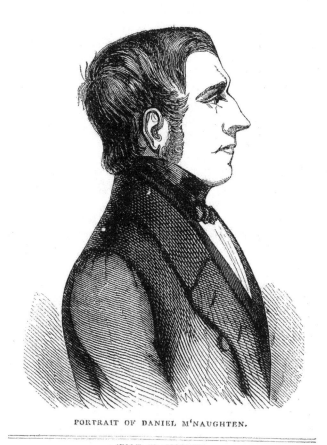

PORTRAIT OF DANIEL M'NAUGHTEN.

THE MARKETS.

*Figure 4.1* Daniel McNaughtan, 1843. © The Wellcome Library, London.

disease and crime. There seemed to be no fixed rule in the remaining states. In Canada and New Zealand partial insanity could not justify acquittal unless the delusion caused a belief in something that, if it existed, would justify the act.[21]

The McNaughtan Rules were the only test of criminal responsibility in England and Wales until the Homicide Act of 1957 replaced them with the concept of diminished responsibility, first used in Scotland in 1867. This is less controversial than a verdict of not guilty by reason of insanity because it acknowledges the defendant's guilt but accepts the existence of extenuating mental circumstances. It is available only in cases of homicide, allowing judges to reduce the punishment to one associated with a conviction for manslaughter. Depending on the circumstances, people convicted under this verdict are sent to prison or to a secure hospital.[22] The Rules dominated the insanity defence in the United States until 1954, and still remain in effect in a majority of jurisdictions today. Four states (Idaho, Kansas, Montana and Utah) do not offer defendants a special verdict of insanity, but 31 states and the federal government use the Rules in full or in part. New Hampshire has adopted a product-of-mental-illness test, while the remainder apply the American Law Institute (1962) standard: a person is not responsible for a criminal act if as a result of mental disease or defect they lack the capacity to appreciate the criminality of their conduct *or* to conform their conduct to the requirements of law.[23]

Within a century, therefore, psychiatry had established itself as an authority on the links between criminality and mental disorder, effecting changes in laws and legal practice across the western world. The next section of this chapter turns to a consideration of how medical views on mental disorder helped to shape public perceptions of culpability in relation to two different types of offender: the sodomite and the infanticidal mother. The medicalization of the latter two private crimes facilitated increasingly lenient legal consequences as the impulses that underlay them became better understood and interest shifted from criminal acts to the emotional life of the offender. Criminals became patients in a process that has at times been problematic. As medical sexual knowledge redefined sodomites as 'sexual inverts' and then as 'homosexuals', a sexual orientation now considered entirely normal was until relatively recently thought to be a form of mental illness amenable to medical cure.[24] Infanticide, on the other hand, has tended to be thought of as resulting from mental illness, so that the response of criminal justice systems has often turned on a simple dividing line between the 'mad' and the 'bad' even though the distinction is rarely this straightforward.

## Criminal culpability and the medicalization of sodomy and infanticide

The impact of law on forensic practice, and the concomitant ability of medicine to influence law, is perhaps most evident in two areas of private experience that have for centuries been subjected to public censure: the deaths of infants at the hands of their mothers and sexual acts between men. Initially considered moral offences subject to church law, infanticide and sodomy were criminalized during the early modern period, becoming capital offences in most western jurisdictions.[25] As more and more individuals found themselves on trial for their lives, prosecutors sought physical evidence to establish the fact of the crime alleged, turning to medical professionals for testimony about the physical signs left on the bodies of perpetrators and their victims. In cases of suspected sodomy, the focus of medical interest was the anus of the passive partner, who was held to be less criminally culpable than the active partner. Unusual fissures, loosening, haemorrhoids and tears were associated with illicit sexual contact between men, as was mutual venereal infection. The penis of the active partner was scrutinized for evidence that it was capable of anal penetration.[26] Women suspected of infanticide were examined for signs of recent childbirth, and infant corpses were inspected for proof of live birth and viability. The fact that medicine was not always able to make firm judgements on any of these issues did not stop the courts from seeking medical opinions, but could influence judges and juries who were frequently reluctant to convict men in the absence of evidence that a crime had occurred, or women perceived to be more sad than bad.

Following the widespread nineteenth-century removal of the death penalty from both crimes as a result of a humanitarian trend in criminal justice, the physical characteristics of sodomy and infanticide remained important factors in criminal trials but the mental state of the perpetrators grew in significance as jurists debated the proper way to deal with them – punitively or medically. In response to this legal stimulus, but also to advances in scientific knowledge about sex, psychiatric views on the moral responsibility of same-sex offenders became ever more complex. Meanwhile, popular notions about the social, environmental, cultural, and individual variables that cause infanticide led to the appropriation of medical terms to describe an offence that is rarely attributable to a demonstrable mental illness.[27]

### Infanticide

In the United States, Scotland, France and Germany the offence of 'infanticide' no longer exists: all homicides are tried as murder or manslaughter regardless of the victim's age. But some common law jurisdictions such as England and Wales, Ireland, Canada, Australia and New Zealand, and some European countries including Austria, Finland, Greece, Italy and Romania have legally defined a separate offence of infanticide as less severe than other forms of homicide.[28] Pleas of insanity had been successful in criminal courts since the eighteenth century, but judges, juries and medical witnesses often adopted a flexible definition of insanity, recognizing that it could be a mental state experienced solely at or around the time of birth by an unmarried woman subject to fear, shame, pain, confusion and isolation as a result of male seduction. This reasoning inspired the characterization of infanticide used in the 1871 Imperial German Criminal Code, which defined it as a crime committed against an illegitimate child by its mother at or immediately after birth and punished it less severely than murder or manslaughter until 1998.[29]

The supposed link between childbirth and altered mental states was also integral to the diagnosis of puerperal insanity, a nineteenth-century mental disorder that could afflict married or unmarried mothers at any time from conception to weaning. In medico-legal practice there was an acceptance that this type of insanity was transitory, usually due more to a deplorable personal situation than organic disease, yet that it still negated wilful intent; the diagnosis simply supported the existing medical and social desire to treat infanticidal women with compassion.[30] Although puerperal insanity as an independent medical concept had vanished by the early twentieth century, its effects on the law remained, most obviously in the English Infanticide Act of 1938, which remains on the statute books today.[31]

A previous law of 1922 created a new class of homicide restricted to the killing of newly born children by their mothers, and provided a foundation for an insanity plea by applying when the balance of a woman's mind was disturbed by reason of the effects of giving birth. In 1938 this law was extended to include mothers who killed infants up to the age of one year, despite a lack of 'conclusive evidence that the effects of childbirth resolved after 12 months'. The law actually applies to two different crimes: the killing of newborns by distressed women suffering from emotional and physical upheaval but who are not mentally ill; and the murder of older infants by women suffering some form of psychosis. The underlying assumptions are the same: that childbearing disturbs the balance of women's minds; and that if a woman kills an infant it is likely to be due to the mental instability associated with childbirth.[32] The 1938 Act does not presume mental illness; it allows psychiatric evidence in mitigation. It does not require proof of psychosis, merely that the balance of the mind was disturbed.[33] It thus reflects a public policy decision to deal leniently with women who kill their infants, by sentencing them to probation or hospital instead of prison or indefinite incarceration in a forensic psychiatric facility.

### Homosexuality

The homosexual, in contrast to the earlier sodomite, emerged during the late nineteenth century as a member of a specific social group that identified itself with same-sex love relationships and an associated lifestyle, but not necessarily with particular acts.[34] Forensic medical interest kept pace: nineteenth-century psychiatrists and sexologists who studied the personality and motivations of men who experienced same-sex desire testified when such men were prosecuted. Although by the early 1820s sodomy had been decriminalized in countries affected by French legal reforms (France, Belgium, the Netherlands, Bavaria, Spain), penalties against same-sex behaviours were extended elsewhere, especially Austria-Hungary (1852), Germany (1871) and Great Britain (1885). New offences against morality, such as public indecency, were widespread, and legal ages of consent were introduced. Thus, forensic doctors were increasingly confronted by sexual deviance in the courts. During the first half of the nineteenth century experts had tended to believe that such offenders experienced mental and nervous disorders as a *result* of their unnatural practices and the associated social and moral failings that such activities embodied. Around mid-century, however, prompted by the encompassing rubrics of moral insanity and degeneration,[35] psychiatrists began to suppose that (inherited) diseases of the brain and nervous system *caused* sexual deviance. Research led initially by Ambroise Tardieu (1818–1879) in France and Johann Casper (1796–1864) in Germany, who were among the first to report case studies of moral offenders, stimulated medical interest in the criminal responsibility of 'perverts', whose actions were redefined as biologically based perversions rather than perversities born of vice. What is now termed 'homosexuality' was seen as a pathological condition rather than a temporary deviation from the norm.[36]

The words 'homosexual' and 'heterosexual' were coined in 1869 by the Hungarian journalist Karl-Maria Kertbeny (1824–1882), while the psychological and neurological approach to homosexuality dates from the publication in 1870 of an article on 'contrary sexual feeling', later dubbed 'inversion', by the Berlin psychiatrist Carl Westphal (1833–1890). He explained homosexuality as a feeling, not necessarily sexual, of being entirely alienated from one's own sex, the result of pathological under-development; that is, a person born into the wrong sexed body. Gradually the biological theory began to predominate over the early learning theory, laying a foundation for the development of the science of sexology.[37] More innovative research was to flow from Germany, Austria and Britain than from elsewhere because of the criminal status of homosexuality in those countries, where its study was linked to efforts to abolish punitive laws.[38] 'Sexual forensics helped transform private sexual matters into concerns of public state officials',[39] and scientific experts such as Richard von Krafft-Ebing (1840–1902), professor of psychiatry in Vienna, and Albert Moll (1862–1939), a Berlin psychiatrist, played critical roles in this process through their ability to explain men's private desires in the public arena of a courtroom. The context was shaped by Section 175 of the German Penal Code, which criminalized same-sex acts between men (not women) but was so vaguely worded that judges found it necessary to consult forensic psychiatrists in order to interpret a defendant's motives and behaviours in relation to the 'perverse sexual acts' that the law proscribed.[40]

In his great work *Psychopathia Sexualis* (1886; 12th edition 1903), a 'medico-forensic study' based on case histories, Krafft-Ebing addressed therapeutic, societal and legal responses to sexual deviance, suggesting that the offender's mental condition, as well as his act, always had to be taken into account, because some practices were not reflections of moral defect but issues of mental illness. He took into account the insanity defence, irresistible impulses, and the question of diminished responsibility, arguing that criminalizing what was a private practice was of no benefit to society: since heredity had overridden free will homosexuals could not change their orientation. Although he opposed Section 175, Krafft-Ebing believed that homosexuality could be cured.[41]

This of course was the deleterious outcome of the medicalization of sexual behaviour. As long as psychiatry defined homosexuality as a medical condition, men might be subject to medical interventions designed to 'cure' them. This had negative consequences in England, where legal sanctions and prejudice against homosexual behaviour rose to a peak after the Second World War and 'laid the foundation on which interest in psychological interventions to alter sexuality increased sharply in the 1960s and 70s'.[42] Behavioural treatments were undertaken in NHS hospitals, including aversion therapy with electrical shock, but there was no national protocol, doubtful ethical standards, and little evidence of effectiveness. With hindsight, most of the medical professionals who carried out these 'therapies' realized that they were based on questionable social values; 'public morality and professional authority' had led to the 'medicalisation of human differences and the infringement of human rights'.[43] Participants did not benefit from treatment, and many felt an increased sense of isolation and shame.[44]

In the United States, homosexuality was initially considered a form of madness caused by degeneration, and it was only in the 1920s that some researchers began to accept it as a key variation of 'normal' sexuality.[45] During the 1930s a homosexual sub-culture began to develop in urban areas and the scope of obscenity laws was narrowed, leading to a surge of American medical interest in homosexuality as more and more men were criminalized. In 1952 the American Psychiatric Association listed homosexuality as a sociopathic personality disturbance in the first edition of its *Diagnostic and Statistical Manual of Mental Disorders* (DSM-I), and there it remained until 1973 when a revised DSM-II removed it from the list of mental disorders and relabelled it a 'sexual orientation disturbance'.[46] As in England, medical intrusion into private life had intensely negative consequences since homosexuality was seen as a potentially contagious and possibly curable illness. This led to pressure to change or psychiatric intervention, which became more common in the 1950s and 1960s, together with more extreme treatments such as aversion therapy, electroshock, castration and the then-fashionable but now discredited brain operation known as lobotomy. The research carried out by the influential biologist and sexologist Alfred Kinsey (1894–1956) undermined the association of homosexuality with disease, however, and with progressive decriminalization, the subject lost its medico-legal importance.[47] Laws prohibiting consensual male same-sex activity were successively repealed in England and Wales (1967), Austria (1971), Scotland (1980) and Germany (1994).[48] In the United States, however, despite a 2003 Supreme Court ruling against the 16 remaining state laws against 'sodomy', the decision did not encompass public conduct, did not compel compliance, and failed to label adult sexual privacy a fundamental right. The decision did, however, reaffirm the parallel evolution of law and social values.[49]

## From criminal lunatic to mentally disordered offender: Mental health and dangerousness

There was no formal legal provision made for mentally ill criminals until the case of James Hadfield (1771/2–1841) forced the English government to legislate for a new category of offender: the criminal lunatic. Following an attempt to assassinate the king in May 1800, Hadfield was found not guilty on the grounds of insanity. However, although he was clearly dangerous to himself and others it was illegal to confine him – a problem swiftly resolved by the retrospective Act for the Safe Custody of Insane Persons Charged with Offences, better known as the Criminal Lunatics Act, which received royal assent on 28 July 1800.[50] This law authorized the indefinite detention of someone who had committed a crime in a bout of insanity, and an 1816 amendment enabled the transfer to an asylum of any convict who became insane. As a result of the law, the government financed the construction of two new blocks for the criminally insane at London's Bethlem Hospital, the oldest psychiatric facility in Europe; completed in 1816, they housed 45 men and 15 women, Hadfield being among the first patients admitted.[51] Representing a meeting point between the private mental health world of a patient and the public legal world of a prisoner, English legislation on insanity, culpability and dangerousness (1800–2009) is summarized in Table 4.1. These statutes apply in England and Wales, but not in Scotland or Ireland.

By the 1830s the concept of homicidal monomania had led to the recognition that some form of custody was necessary for offenders who might remain dangerous in the future; psychiatrists agreed with lawyers that there was no question of treating such individuals as innocent or of letting a dangerous mentally ill person go free. In 1838 Esquirol noted that it was surprising that no country had a law that allowed the confinement of a mentally ill person for the good of society, and later that year precisely such a law came into effect in France. The *Loi sur les aliénés* (30 June 1838) permitted confinement in a mental asylum on three conditions: a medical certificate, notification to the judiciary, and regular visits by an administrative commission. This subsequently served as a model for legislation in other countries, including Belgium, Austria, Spain, Italy and Japan.[52] The law of 1838 survived until 1990 when it was subsumed into one (27 June 1990) designed to give the mentally ill greater protection from wrongful confinement, but criticism attached to the fact that the new law focused on the danger posed by the insane person to themselves, rather than to others. French psychiatrists remain divided about their role as potential defenders of public security, with many taking the view that their remit should be confined to the private relationship between doctor and patient.[53]

In Germany, prisoners acquitted on the grounds of mental illness under Article 51 of the Imperial Criminal Code of 1871 were committed to psychiatric care, 'distributed as widely and thinly as possible amongst the asylum population'. The Criminal Procedure Code (1877) mandated the transfer of prisoners who became mentally ill in prison to an asylum until cured and

*Table 4.1* Legislation on insanity, culpability and danger in England and Wales

| | |
|---|---|
| Criminal Lunatics Act 1800 | Direct reaction to the trial of James Hadfield: new verdict of 'not guilty on the grounds of insanity' → defendants acquitted, or found unfit for trial, to be kept in 'strict custody' indefinitely<br>Revised 1816: convicts who became insane to be removed to an asylum upon certification by two doctors, for as long as they remain insane, but to be released at the end of their sentence<br>Revised 1884: criminal lunatics to be sent to an asylum until they 'cease to be a criminal lunatic', with annual reports and case reviews every three years<br>Repealed 1981 |
| Insane Prisoners Act 1840 | Authorized the transfer of any insane prisoner (except civil prisoners) to a lunatic asylum, extending the criminal lunacy law from felony to misdemeanour cases. |
| Trial of Lunatics Act 1883 | Special verdict: guilty but insane, to be kept in custody as a criminal lunatic (until 1964) |
| Infanticide Act 1938 | Special offence: assumes balance of mother's mind disturbed by childbirth or lactation; no need to demonstrate causal link |
| Homicide Act 1957 | Special verdict: diminished responsibility due to abnormality of mind; no need to demonstrate *how* (could therefore include psychopathy) |
| Mental Health Act 1959 | Introduced the legal term 'psychopathic disorder', which was unlikely to respond to treatment after age 25 →<br>One year of treatment if defendant over 21; detention beyond age 25 only if the detainee was considered dangerous |
| Criminal Procedure (Insanity) Act 1964 | Special verdict: court-ordered hospitalization without time limit<br>Acquittal → hospital observation can be ordered because the defendant 'ought to be so detained in the interests of his own health or safety or with a view to the protection of other persons' |
| Mental Health (Amendment) Act 1975 | Removed age criteria from psychopathic disorder, opening possible detention to psychopaths of all ages |
| Mental Health Act 1983 | Five categories: mental disorder, mental illness (undefined), severe mental impairment, mental impairment, and psychopathic disorder<br>Detention of mentally ill offenders requires proof of mental condition<br>Treatability clause applied to psychopathic disorder: treatment must be 'likely to alleviate or prevent deterioration' |
| Criminal Procedure (Insanity and Unfitness to Plead) Act 1991 | Special verdict: courts can commit individual to hospital for a limited time, or order release to the community subject to restrictions<br>First specific mandate for expert medical evidence in insanity trials |
| Mental Health Act 2007 | Treatability test for detention diluted so that detention will be lawful even if treatment may not be effective (preventive detention)<br>Psychopathic disorder abolished |

*Continued*

*Table 4.1 Continued*

| Coroners and Justice Act 2009 | Revised the Homicide Act 1957 → Abnormality of mental functioning must:<br>1/ Arise from a 'recognised medical condition'<br>2/ Substantially impair the ability to (a) understand the nature of one's conduct; (b) form a rational judgment; (c) exercise self-control<br>3/ Provide an explanation for acts and omissions in doing or being a party to the killing<br>Amended provision for infanticide: it is now an alternative offence and a partial defence to murder and manslaughter |
|---|---|

Source: A. Forrester, S. Ozdural, A. Muthukumaraswamy and A. Carroll, 'The Evolution of Mental Disorder as a Legal Category in England and Wales', *Journal of Forensic Psychiatry and Psychology*, 19 (2008): 543–60; S. White, 'The Insanity Defense in England and Wales Since 1843', *Annals of the American Academy of Political and Social Science*, 477 (1985): 43–57; N. Walker, *Crime and Insanity in England, Vol. 1: The Historical Perspective* (Edinburgh: Edinburgh University Press, 1968); www.legislation.gov.uk/changes/affected/ukpga/1957/11 (accessed 24 February 2014). The full text of the earlier Acts may be found at House of Commons Parliamentary Papers, http://parlipapers.chadwyck.co.uk/marketing/index.jsp, available through university libraries.

returned to prison, or released following a legal or medical determination.[54] In 1933 detention of dangerous offenders for preventive purposes was introduced into the Penal Code, targeting two groups: the criminally irresponsible who were likely to reoffend because of their mental illness or substance abuse; and criminally responsible individuals considered likely to reoffend. These measures were intended to prevent recidivism via incapacitation and exclusion from society for a period of up to ten years, extended in 1998 to the possibility of indeterminate detention.[55]

Nineteenth-century American attitudes to the criminal responsibility of the insane were strongly influenced by Isaac Ray's 1838 treatise, in which he advocated institutionalizing mentally ill offenders where they would be 'secluded from society' until their mental and moral faculties had been restored.[56] A national programme for the building of state, county, city and private hospitals for the insane began in the 1830s, and in 1868 the Association of Medical Superintendents of American Institutions for the Insane (now the American Psychiatric Association) recommended the detention of the dangerously insane, subject to legal and medical certification, in one of these hospitals.[57] But the provisions made for doing so were not systematic, and judges (and some psychiatrists) who favoured incarceration under a more severe regimen than that found in asylums could send the criminally insane to a state prison.[58] As in England, France and Germany, insane prison inmates could be transferred to mental hospitals.

The transfer of insane convicts from prisons to asylums added to the security problems posed by a growing population of criminal lunatics, leading to calls for a separate system of mental institutions for the criminally insane. The oldest secure hospital in Europe, Dublin's Dundrum Central Criminal

Asylum, opened in 1850 with space for 80 men and 40 women,[59] followed by Rockwood Criminal Lunatic Asylum in Canada (1855), and Broadmoor Criminal Lunatic Asylum in England (1863), built to house 400 men and 100 women.[60] In Italy, the criminal asylum at Aversa, near Naples, opened in 1876. In the United States the first hospital for insane criminals opened at Auburn in New York in 1855 but provision varied between states; as in France and Germany, criminal lunatics were more usually committed to the state asylums, where separate wards were built for them, or to prison mental health wards.[61] The first secure psychiatric service in France was established in 1910, with Difficult Patient Units for those who pose a danger to others introduced in 1960. It was not until 2002 that a law provided for the creation of psychiatric units within the penitentiary system; the first opened at Lyon in 2010, and a further eight are being built to accommodate up to 440 mentally ill prisoners.[62] In Germany, forensic psychiatric hospitals were built during the twentieth century, in accordance with Section 63 of the Penal Code; in 2011 they held 6,620 patients – about 11 per cent of the total German psychiatric population.[63] The confinement of criminal lunatics was an unavoidable consequence of the nineteenth-century redefinition of the concept of dangerousness, away from the seriousness of the offence committed (the typical eighteenth-century definition) towards 'the individual criminal's biological predisposition and capacity for crime'.[64] The criminally insane were increasingly segregated from other prisoners and mental health sufferers, occupying a middle ground between patient and prisoner largely defined by their potential dangerousness to others.

Punishment now fits the criminal, rather than the crime, but this model has in recent years led to public fear of untoward lenience in relation to mentally ill offenders, 'political calls for a more rigid enforcement of criminal law and more severe punishments',[65] and a general hardening of public attitudes towards insane offenders. The number of mentally disordered prisoners has increased,[66] the number of successful insanity defences has decreased,[67] and legislative changes to make an insanity plea more difficult have followed in the wake of popular outrage over high-profile crimes committed by the mentally ill.[68] Recently, some of the most vigorous debates have concerned the status of personality disorders in relation to criminal responsibility and dangerousness.

Current legislation in England and Wales has eliminated the treatment criteria for the commitment of people suffering from psychopathy (see Table 4.1), to facilitate hospitalization for the purpose of managing the risk associated with this disorder; public protection has been placed ahead of the detainee's rights.[69] But the numbers are likely to be small: in 2006 only 655 patients out of a total of 14,681 mental health detainees in England were detained under the legal category of psychopathic disorder.[70] In Germany in 2011, over 90 per cent of people in secure detention were over 40, suggesting that previous interventions had failed; and many of this group showed characteristics of an antisocial personality disorder or of psychopathy. This is further complicated by a prison psychiatric healthcare system that has not yet

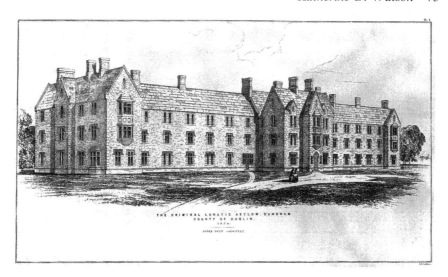

*Figure 4.2* The Criminal Lunatic Asylum, Dundrum, Dublin, Ireland, 1850. © The Wellcome Library, London.

developed effective treatments for this controversial condition, and lack of evidence that offender risk assessments are accurate. In 2004 the Federal Constitutional Court ruled that detainees are entitled to a realistic chance of release, and so must be given the opportunity to prove that they are no longer dangerous; institutions must thus make genuine efforts to rehabilitate.[71] There are clearly serious unresolved issues concerning both public safety and the individual rights of prisoner-patients.[72] In France since the Second World War there has been a trend towards assigning legal responsibility to more and more people suffering from psychiatric disorders, including behavioural problems related to psychopathy. Prison is seen as an alternative solution to mental healthcare systems – from which the dangerously mentally ill are liable to be released very early – on the grounds of security.[73] In the United States, it has long been argued that psychopaths should not be excluded from the exculpatory insanity rule but that they should be compulsorily confined until cured. This position is based on the assumption that community security might be better protected by hospitalization than by imprisonment, since convicts must be released once they have served their sentences. Under the terms of the Insanity Defense Reform Act of 1984, passed in the wake of John Hinckley Junior's insanity acquittal for attempting to kill President Reagan, the criminally insane are confined until no longer a danger to others; for some, release may be impossible.[74] Two factors make this situation even more problematic: American defendants can plead insanity for crimes other than murder, and so may end up detained for periods disproportionate to the offence or its associated prison sentence; and mentally ill prisoners can be treated such that they become competent to be executed.[75]

Despite the fact that mechanisms to divert mentally disordered offenders away from the criminal justice system towards medical care exist in the United States and in England and Wales,[76] the number of mentally ill prison inmates is continuing to rise, as it is in Europe. This is perhaps because the reduction in psychiatric hospital beds has outpaced the ability of community-based care to provide the services that noncompliant or violent patients need. Some of these difficult patients will end up within the purview of the criminal justice system where, research suggests, prisons lack the capacity to provide adequate treatment.[77] Most European countries use a mixture of prison mental health units and public healthcare systems to provide mental health services to inmates; only six countries have adopted wholly external or internal models. In England and Wales the provision for prisoners comes entirely from the public mental health system (as also in Cyprus, Ireland and Norway), while Belgium and Lithuania lie at the opposite end of the spectrum, running prison mental health services that are entirely independent of the general health system.[78] American prisons also utilize a mixed model of healthcare provision for inmates, suggesting that state funds should be transferred from general mental health services to prison health services in order to cope with the increasing demand.[79] Ultimately, the key aim in forensic psychiatric services should be to achieve the best possible balance between medical care that is tailored to the needs of the individual, as in general mental healthcare systems, but that is also evidence-based and related to the risk posed by the patient's criminal or violent inclinations.[80]

## Conclusion

This chapter has revealed a number of important facets of the relationship between public and private in matters of healthcare. First, medicine and law offer competing discourses of mental health and ill-health, predicated on each discipline's principal practical focus: the private world of a patient or the public legal world of a criminal defendant. Secondly, public opinion has a central role to play in influencing the development and implementation of legislation that, in turn, creates an area where the private and the public intersect in the figure of the patient-prisoner. Thirdly, the problem that this overlap poses to psychiatry is both goal-oriented and definitional: 'criminal responsibility' and 'insanity' are not medical but legal concepts; the punishment, care and detention of the mentally ill are conflicting goals that force medicine and law to work together.[81] However, although judges and juries may want certainty about culpability and dangerousness, psychiatrists cannot always provide it because contemporary medical practice is frequently at variance with the law's definitions. Furthermore, even if revised terms were to be introduced, they would suppose a professional agreement about diagnostic categories that does not actually exist, and would necessitate much greater conformity among psychiatrists as to the circumstances that might impair criminal responsibility.[82]

The question of mental disorder, criminal responsibility and dangerousness is one that will continue to preoccupy jurists and forensic psychiatrists in the West, and to offer a clear example of how the rights of the private individual who has committed a crime, or who may do so in the future, must be weighed against those of the public at large. The history of the legal disposition of those labelled as sexually deviant or criminally insane, and of infanticidal women, shows that the ways in which this relationship is negotiated varies according to prevailing socio-legal trends. While infanticide has been dealt with leniently due to public and legal ambivalence to the crime, and homosexual practices have been decriminalized as a result of a general liberalizing trend in society, mentally disordered offenders are subject to more restrictive and punitive practices today than at any time in the past two centuries. Since psychiatrists are often required by law to evaluate a defendant's sanity or assess the future risk of violence of mentally disordered offenders – tasks that require significant training and experience – it is obvious that forensic psychiatry must continue to operate at the boundaries between the private and the public, and the medical and the legal, as an integral element of western criminal justice systems.

## Further reading

Readers who wish to learn more about the history of madness and crime should first consult the special issue of the *International Journal of Law and Psychiatry*, 37 (2014): 1–134 edited by Harry Oosterhuis and Arlie Loughnan: twelve articles and an extended introduction offer broad overviews of developments in forensic psychiatry in ten European and North American countries. Ruth Harris, *Murders and Madness: Medicine, Law, and Society in the* fin de siècle (Oxford: Clarendon Press, 1989) provides an in-depth study of forensic psychiatry in French courts during the nineteenth century, while Joel Eigen offers a similar analysis focused on London courts in a slightly earlier period: *Witnessing Insanity: Madness and Mad-doctors in the English Court* (New Haven, CT: Yale University Press, 1995). The earliest study of the insanity defence in England, Nigel Walker, *Crime and Insanity in England, Vol. 1: The Historical Perspective* (Edinburgh: Edinburgh University Press, 1968), remains a useful overview, as does Roger Smith, *Trial by Medicine: Insanity and Responsibility in Victorian Trials* (Edinburgh: Edinburgh University Press, 1981). Richard Moran, *Knowing Right from Wrong: The Insanity Defense of Daniel McNaughtan* (New York: The Free Press, 1981) provides a thorough study of this groundbreaking case. Works in English on nineteenth-century Germany are few in number, but see Doris Kaufmann, 'Boundary Disputes: Criminal Justice and Psychiatry in Germany, 1760–1850', *Journal of Historical Sociology*, 6 (1993): 276–87. For the insanity defence in the twentieth century, see Charles Patrick Ewing, *Insanity: Murder, Madness, and the Law* (Oxford: Oxford University Press, 2008) on the United States, and Janet Colaizzi, *Homicidal Insanity, 1800–1985*

(Tuscaloosa and London: University of Alabama Press, 1989) on the problem of the dangerously insane.

There is a large body of literature on infanticide, most of which does not address the medical issues that the offence raises. However, although not a work of history, Lita Linzer Schwartz and Natalie K. Isser, *Child Homicide: Parents Who Kill* (Boca Raton, FL: CRC Press, 2007) provides a helpful overview of these matters. For an in-depth study of Victorian puerperal insanity, see Hilary Marland, *Dangerous Motherhood: Insanity and Childbirth in Victorian Britain* (Basingstoke: Palgrave Macmillan, 2004). The modern dichotomy between the mad and the sad female perpetrator is explored by Emma Cunliffe, *Murder, Medicine and Motherhood* (Oxford: Hart Publishing, 2011).

Forensic psychiatric interest in sexuality remains a relatively under-researched area within the much wider historiography of medical approaches to sexualities, but two important studies offer good starting points. Harry Oosterhuis, *Stepchildren of Nature: Krafft-Ebing, Psychiatry, and the Making of Sexual Identity* (Chicago and London: University of Chicago Press, 2000) examines the pioneering Austro-German's efforts to separate sexual deviancies from ideas of immorality. Jennifer Terry considers sex offenders in her study of the rise and fall of the notion that homosexuality is a form of insanity, *An American Obsession: Science, Medicine, and Homosexuality in Modern Society* (Chicago: University of Chicago Press, 1999).

## Notes

1 The literature on the history of western criminal justice systems is too large to cite here, but for a summary of its main areas of focus, see Louis A. Knafla, 'Structure, Conjuncture, and Event in the Historiography of Modern Criminal Justice History', in Clive Emsley and Louis A. Knafla (eds), *Crime History and Histories of Crime: Studies in the Historiography of Crime and Criminal Justice in Modern History* (Westport, CT: Greenwood Press, 1996), 33–44.
2 Stephan Landsman, 'Of Witches, Madmen, and Products Liability: A Historical Survey of the Use of Expert Testimony', *Behavioral Sciences and the Law*, 13 (1995): 131–157.
3 Mike Redmayne, *Expert Evidence and Criminal Justice* (Oxford: Oxford University Press, 2001).
4 Katherine D. Watson, *Forensic Medicine in Western Society: A History* (Abingdon: Routledge, 2011), 72–97. Medico-legal (adjective): pertaining to medicine and law or to forensic medicine.
5 David L. Weiden, 'Comparing Judicial Institutions: Using an Inquisitorial Trial Simulation to Facilitate Student Understanding of International Legal Traditions', *PS: Political Science and Politics*, 42 (2009): 759–763.
6 Tal Golan, *Laws of Men and Laws of Nature: The History of Scientific Expert Testimony in England and America* (Cambridge, MA and London: Harvard University Press, 2004).
7 Jan Goldstein, *Console and Classify: The French Psychiatric Profession in the Nineteenth Century* (Cambridge: Cambridge University Press, rev. edn, 2001); Doris Kaufmann, 'Boundary Disputes: Criminal Justice and Psychiatry in Germany, 1760–1850', *Journal of Historical Sociology*, 6 (1993): 276–287.

8 David Healy, *Bolshevik Sexual Forensics: Diagnosing Disorder in the Clinic and Courtroom, 1917–1939* (DeKalb: Northern Illinois University Press, 2009), 161–162.

9 Laws passed in England apply to both England and Wales, but this chapter is concerned primarily with events and debates that occurred in England.

10 Roger Smith, *Trial by Medicine: Insanity and Responsibility in Victorian Trials* (Edinburgh: Edinburgh University Press, 1981); James C. Mohr, *Doctors and the Law: Medical Jurisprudence in Nineteenth-Century America* (Baltimore and London: The Johns Hopkins University Press, 1993), 140–153, 164–179; Joel Peter Eigen, *Witnessing Insanity: Madness and Mad-doctors in the English Court* (New Haven, CT and London: Yale University Press, 1995); Harry Oosterhuis and Arlie Loughnan (eds), 'Historical Perspectives on Forensic Psychiatry', special issue of *International Journal of Law and Psychiatry*, 37 (2014): 1–134.

11 Watson, *Forensic Medicine*, 74–80.

12 Vincent Barras and Jacques Bernheim, 'The History of Law and Psychiatry in Europe', in Robert Bluglass and Paul Bowden (eds), *Principles and Practice of Forensic Psychiatry* (Edinburgh: Churchill Livingstone, 1990), 106.

13 Ibid., 111 and Janet Colaizzi, *Homicidal Insanity, 1800–1985* (Tuscaloosa and London: University of Alabama Press, 1989), 8.

14 Nicole Rafter, 'The Unrepentant Horse-slasher: Moral Insanity and the Origins of Criminological Thought', *Criminology*, 42 (2004): 979–1008.

15 *Examen médical des procès criminels des nommés Léger, Feldtmann, Lecouffe, Jean-Pierre et Papavoine* (1825); *Discussion médico-légale sur la folie* (1826); *Des maladies mentales, considérées dans leurs rapports avec la législation civile et criminelle* (1827); *Nouvelle discussion médico-légale sur la folie* (1828).

16 Isaac Ray, *Treatise on the Medical Jurisprudence of Insanity* (London: G. Henderson, 1839), 212. Following a lengthy list (179–248) of case studies, he concluded that those who commit seemingly motiveless murders must be suffering from mental alienation, 249. For his comments on the brain, see 122–129.

17 Eigen, *Witnessing Insanity*, 31–57; Kaufmann, 'Boundary Disputes'; Arlie Loughnan and Tony Ward, 'Emergent Authority and Expert Knowledge: Psychiatry and Criminal Responsibility in the UK', *International Journal of Law and Psychiatry*, 37 (2014): 25–36; Joel Peter Eigen, 'Delusion in the Courtroom: The Role of Partial Insanity in Early Forensic Testimony', *Medical History*, 35 (1991): 25–49 (quotation on 27).

18 Richard Moran, *Knowing Right from Wrong: The Insanity Defense of Daniel McNaughtan* (New York: The Free Press, 1981); Ciara J. Toole, 'Medical Diagnosis of Legal Culpability: The Impact of Early Psychiatric Testimony in the Nineteenth Century English Criminal Trial', *International Journal of Law and Psychiatry*, 35 (2012): 82–87; Loughnan and Ward, 'Emergent Authority', 27–28. There are at least 12 different spellings of McNaughtan's name, but Moran (xi–xiii) has confirmed this one as the correct version.

19 Heinrich Oppenheimer, *The Criminal Responsibility of Lunatics: A Study in Comparative Law* (London: Sweet & Maxwell, 1909).

20 Late nineteenth-century psychiatrists lobbied for greater flexibility in the German law, which recognized only mental health and mental illness, not mental impairment. See Eric J. Engstrom, *Clinical Psychiatry in Imperial Germany: A History of Psychiatric Practice* (Ithaca, NY and London: Cornell University Press, 2003), 197–198.

21 Oppenheimer, *Criminal Responsibility*, 37–79.

22 Watson, *Forensic Medicine*, 89.

23 Timothy Harding, 'A Comparative Survey of Medico-legal Systems', in John Gunn and Pamela J. Taylor (eds), *Forensic Psychiatry: Clinical, Legal and Ethical Issues* (Oxford: Butterworth-Heinemann, 1993), 118–166; Charles Patrick Ewing, *Insanity: Murder, Madness and the Law* (Oxford: Oxford University Press, 2008), xx;

The Insanity Defense among the States, http://criminal.findlaw.com/criminal-procedure/the-insanity-defense-among-the-states.html (accessed 29 April 2014).

24 Jennifer Terry, *An American Obsession: Science, Medicine, and Homosexuality in Modern Society* (Chicago: University of Chicago Press, 1999); Chiara Beccalossi, *Female Sexual Inversion: Same-Sex Desires in Italian and British Sexology, c. 1870–1920* (Basingstoke: Palgrave Macmillan, 2012).

25 Tom Betteridge (ed.), *Sodomy in Early Modern Europe* (Manchester: Manchester University Press, 2002); Watson, *Forensic Medicine*, 106.

26 Ivan D. Crozier, 'The Medical Construction of Homosexuality and its Relation to the Law in Nineteenth-Century England', *Medical History*, 45 (2001): 61–82.

27 Michelle Oberman, 'Mothers Who Kill: Cross-cultural Patterns in and Perspectives on Contemporary Maternal Filicide', *International Journal of Law and Psychiatry*, 26 (2003): 493–514; Roberto Catanesi, Gabriele Rocca, Chiara Candelli, Biagio Solarino and Felice Carabellese, 'Death by Starvation: Seeking a Forensic Psychiatric Understanding of a Case of Fatal Child Maltreatment by the Parent', *Forensic Science International*, 223 (2012): e13–e17; Joy Lynn E. Shelton, Yvonne Muirhead and Kathleen E. Canning, 'Ambivalence toward Mothers Who Kill: An Examination of 45 US Cases of Maternal Neonaticide', *Behavioral Sciences and the Law*, 28 (2010): 812–831.

28 This section is a revised and updated version of Watson, *Forensic Medicine*, 108–111.

29 Kerstin Michalik, 'The Development of the Discourse on Infanticide in the Late Eighteenth Century and the New Legal Standardization of the Offense in the Nineteenth Century', in Ulrike Gleixner and Marion W. Gray (eds), *Gender in Transition: Discourse and Practice in German-Speaking Europe, 1750–1830* (Ann Arbor: University of Michigan Press, 2006), 51–71.

30 Daniela Tinková, 'Protéger ou punir? Les voies de la décriminalisation de l'infanticide en France et dans le domaine des Habsbourg (XVIIIe–XIXe siècles)', *Crime, History & Societies*, 9 (2005): 43–72; Hilary Marland, *Dangerous Motherhood: Insanity and Childbirth in Victorian Britain* (Basingstoke: Palgrave Macmillan, 2004), 28–35.

31 Arlie Loughnan, 'The "Strange" Case of the Infanticide Doctrine', *Oxford Journal of Legal Studies*, 32 (2012): 685–711; Anne-Marie Kilday, *A History of Infanticide in Britain c. 1600 to the Present* (Basingstoke: Palgrave Macmillan, 2013), 166–181; James M. Donovan, 'Infanticide and the Juries in France, 1825–1913', *Journal of Family History*, 16 (1991): 157–176; Michelle Oberman, 'Understanding Infanticide in Context: Mothers Who Kill, 1870–1930 and Today', *Journal of Criminal Law and Criminology*, 92 (2002): 707–737; Jeffrey S. Richter, 'Infanticide, Child Abandonment, and Abortion in Imperial Germany', *Journal of Interdisciplinary History*, 28 (1998): 511–551; Tony Ward, 'The Sad Subject of Infanticide: Law, Medicine and Child Murder, 1860–1938', *Social & Legal Studies*, 8 (1999): 163–180.

32 Ian Lambie, 'Mothers Who Kill: The Crime of Infanticide', *International Journal of Law and Psychiatry*, 24 (2001): 71–80 (quotation on 74).

33 Robin Ogle and Daniel Maier-Katkin, 'A Rationale for Infanticide Laws', *Criminal Law Review* (Dec. 1993): 903–914.

34 Arthur N. Gilbert, 'Conceptions of Homosexuality and Sodomy in Western History', in Salvatore J. Licata and Robert P. Petersen (eds), *Historical Perspectives on Homosexuality* (New York: The Haworth Press, 1981), 57–68. This section is a revised and updated version of Watson, *Forensic Medicine*, 117–122.

35 Daniel Pick, *Faces of Degeneration: A European Disorder, c. 1848–c. 1918* (Cambridge: Cambridge University Press, 1989).

36 Beccalossi, *Female Sexual Inversion*, 51–62; Crozier, 'Medical Construction', 62; Terry, *American Obsession*, 40–73; Vern L. Bullough, 'Homosexuality and the Medical Model', *Journal of Homosexuality*, 1 (1974): 99–110; Gert Hekma, 'A

History of Sexology: Social and Historical Aspects of Sexuality', in Jan Bremmer (ed.), *From Sappho to De Sade: Moments in the History of Sexuality* (London and New York: Routledge, 1989), 173–193; Harry Oosterhuis, 'Medical Science and the Modernisation of Sexuality', in Franz X. Eder, Lesley A. Hall and Gert Hekma (eds), *Sexual Cultures in Europe: National Histories* (Manchester: Manchester University Press, 1999), 221–241.

37 Gilbert, 'Conceptions of Homosexuality', 61; Hekma, 'History of Sexology', 178–181; Oosterhuis, 'Medical Science', 226–227; Bullough, 'Homosexuality', 105–107. Westphal's article is online at Born Eunuchs Library, www.well.com/user/ aquarius/ westphal.htm.

38 Oosterhuis, 'Medical Science', 230; Crozier, 'Medical Construction', 67; Terry, *American Obsession*, 79–80.

39 Matthew Conn, 'Sexual Science and Sexual Forensics in 1920s Germany: Albert Moll as (S)expert', *Medical History*, 56 (2012): 201–216.

40 Ibid., 204.

41 Richard von Krafft-Ebing, *Psychopathia Sexualis, with Especial Reference to the Antipathetic Sexual Instinct: A Medico-forensic Study* (London: Staples Press, 12th edn, 1965); Harry Oosterhuis, *Stepchildren of Nature: Krafft-Ebing, Psychiatry, and the Making of Sexual Identity* (Chicago: University of Chicago Press, 2000).

42 Michael King, Glenn Smith and Annie Bartlett, 'Treatments of Homosexuality in Britain since the 1950s – an Oral History: The Experience of Professionals', *British Medical Journal*, 328 (2004): 429–431; Glenn Smith, Annie Bartlett and Michael King, 'Treatments of Homosexuality in Britain since the 1950s – An Oral History: The Experience of Patients', *British Medical Journal,* 328 (2004): 427–429. See also Roger Davidson and Gayle Davis, *The Sexual State: Sexuality and Scottish Governance, 1950–80* (Edinburgh: Edinburgh University Press, 2012), Chapters 3 and 4 on medical opinions towards homosexuality in Scotland.

43 King, Smith and Bartlett, 'Treatments of Homosexuality', 431.

44 Smith, Bartlett and King, 'Treatments of Homosexuality', 429.

45 Terry, *American Obsession*, 74–119.

46 Robert L. Spitzer, 'The Diagnostic Status of Homosexuality in DSM-III: A Reformulation of the Issues', *American Journal of Psychiatry*, 138 (1981): 210–215.

47 Terry, *American Obsession*, 275–296. Lobotomy is a surgical operation that involves severing connections in the brain's prefrontal lobe (associated with behaviour and personality) as a treatment for mental illness.

48 Wayne R. Dynes (ed.), *Encyclopedia of Homosexuality* (London: St James Press, 1990), www.williamapercy.com/wiki/index.php?title=Encyclopedia_of_Homosexuality.

49 Sara Rosenbaum and Taylor Burke, 'Lawrence v. Texas: Implications for Public Health Policy and Practice', *Public Health Reports*, 118 (2003): 559–561.

50 Richard Moran, 'The Origin of Insanity as a Special Verdict: The Trial for Treason of James Hadfield (1800)', *Law and Society Review*, 19 (1985): 487–519.

51 Jonathan Andrews, Asa Briggs, Roy Porter, Penny Tucker and Keir Waddington, *The History of Bethlem* (Abingdon: Routledge, 1997), 405.

52 Watson, *Forensic Medicine*, 86; Margaret Gwynne Lloyd and Michel Bénézech, 'The French Mental Health Legislation of 1838 and Its Reform', *Journal of Forensic Psychiatry*, 3 (1992): 235–250.

53 Caroline Protais, 'Psychiatric Care or Social Defense? The Origins of a Controversy Over the Responsibility of the Mentally Ill in French Forensic Psychiatry', *International Journal of Law and Psychiatry*, 37 (2014): 17–24; Valeria Savoja, Pierre François Godet and Jacques Dubuis, 'Compulsory Treatments in France', *International Journal of Mental Health*, 37 (2008–9): 17–32.

54 Eric J. Engstrom, 'Topographies of Forensic Practice in Imperial Germany', *International Journal of Law and Psychiatry*, 37 (2014): 63–70.

55  Kirstin Drenkhahn, 'Secure Preventive Detention in Germany: Incapacitation or Treatment Intervention?', *Behavioral Sciences and the Law*, 31 (2013): 312–327.
56  Ray, *Medical Jurisprudence of Insanity*, 250.
57  *Propositions and Resolutions of the Association of Medical Superintendents of American Institutions for the Insane* (Philadelphia: The Association, 1876), 20–21.
58  Henry M. Hurd (ed.), *The Institutional Care of the Insane in the United States and Canada*, Vol. 1 (Baltimore: The Johns Hopkins Press, 1916), 348–349.
59  Pauline M. Prior, *Madness and Murder: Gender, Crime and Mental Disorder in Nineteenth-Century Ireland* (Dublin: Irish Academic Press, 2008), 24–33.
60  Mark Stevens, *Broadmoor Revealed: Victorian Crime and the Lunatic Asylum* (Barnsley: Pen & Sword Social History, 2013).
61  Oosterhuis and Loughnan, 'Introduction', 7; Hurd, *Care of the Insane*, 349–351; Engstrom, 'Topographies', 65–66.
62  Protais, 'Psychiatric Care?', 19, 21.
63  Statistics for patient numbers 1970–2011 can be found in Norbert Konrad and Birgit Völlm, 'Forensic Psychiatric Expert Witnessing within the Criminal Justice System in Germany', *International Journal of Law and Psychiatry*, 37 (2014): 149–154.
64  N. Rafter, 'The Murderous Dutch Fiddler: Criminology, History and the Problem of Phrenology', *Theoretical Criminology*, 9 (2005): 65–96.
65  Oosterhuis and Loughnan, 'Introduction', 11.
66  Ibid.
67  Watson, *Forensic Medicine*, 95.
68  Protais, 'Psychiatric Care?', 23; Ewing, *Insanity*; A. Forrester, S. Ozdural, A. Muthukumaraswamy and A. Carroll, 'The Evolution of Mental Disorder as a Legal Category in England and Wales', *Journal of Forensic Psychiatry and Psychology*, 19 (2008): 543–560; James L. Knoll and Phillip J. Resnick, 'Insanity Defense Evaluations: Basic Procedure and Best Practices', *Psychiatric Times*, 1 Dec. 2008, http://www.psychiatrictimes.com/insanity-defense-evaluations-basic-procedure-and-best-practices (accessed 18 April 2014).
69  Landy F. Sparr, 'Personality Disorders and Criminal Law: An International Perspective', *Journal of the American Academy of Psychiatry and Law*, 37 (2009): 168–181; Forrester et al., 'Evolution of Mental Disorder', 553.
70  Ibid., 555.
71  Drenkhahn, 'Secure Preventive Detention', 315, 321–322.
72  Konrad and Völlm, 'Forensic Psychiatric', 151–153.
73  Protais, 'Psychiatric Care?', 17, 23–24.
74  Abraham L. Halpern, 'The Insanity Verdict, the Psychopath, and Post-acquittal Confinement', *Psychiatric Quarterly*, 63 (1992): 209–243.
75  Ibid., 233–234.
76  Henry J. Steadman, Allison D. Redlich, Patricia Griffin, John Petrila and John Monahan, 'From Referral to Disposition: Case Processing in Seven Mental Health Courts', *Behavioral Sciences and the Law*, 23 (2005): 215–226; David V. James, 'Diversion of Mentally Disordered People from the Criminal Justice System in England and Wales: An Overview', *International Journal of Law and Psychiatry*, 33 (2010): 241–248.
77  Harald Dressing and Hans-Joachim Salize, 'Pathways to Psychiatric Care in European Prison Systems', *Behavioral Sciences and the Law*, 27 (2009): 801–810; Seena Fazel and Katharina Seewald, 'Severe Mental Illness in 33, 588 Prisoners Worldwide: Systematic Review and Meta-regression Analysis', *British Journal of Psychiatry*, 200 (2012): 364–373.
78  Dressing and Salize, 'Pathways', 804.
79  Anasseril E. Daniel, 'Care of the Mentally Ill in Prisons: Challenges and Solutions', *Journal of the American Academy of Psychiatry and the Law*, 35 (2007): 406–410.

80 Kevin Howells, Andrew Day and Brian Thomas-Peter, 'Changing Violent Behaviour: Forensic Mental Health and Criminological Models Compared', *Journal of Forensic Psychiatry & Psychology*, 15 (2004): 391–406.

81 Forrester et al., 'Evolution of Mental Disorder', 544.

82 Harald Dressing, Hans Joachim Salize and Harvey Gordon, 'Legal Frameworks and Key Concepts Regulating Diversion and Treatment of Mentally Disordered Offenders in European Union Member States', *European Psychiatry*, 22 (2007): 427–432 (430).

# 5 Healthcare and the design and management of public and private space

## Britain, France and the US, *c*. 1750 to *c*. 1950

*Tom Crook*

### Introduction

It would be claiming too much to say that healthcare has been responsible for constituting the distinction between public and private space – a distinction, in any case, that scholars have used to examine the built form of societies from antiquity up to the present.[1] Here, as elsewhere, much depends on what we mean by 'public' and 'private'. As the introduction to this volume has detailed, the meanings of 'public' and 'private' are many and profoundly historical, and this extends to their spatial applications. But a good case can be made for locating the birth of our modern – and Western – architecture of public and private space in the period covered by this chapter, roughly 1750 to 1950. For it was during these two centuries that the spatial fabric of both institutional and everyday environments was transformed, so that they came to embody a number of features still present today: among others, strict adherence to regulatory standards of construction; a commitment to strong codes of bodily privacy; the incorporation of relative technological complexity; and the provision of clearly defined public spaces, dedicated either to the circulation of goods and people, or to recreational pursuits.

How might we explain this transformation? Existing histories resort to various factors, from the civilizing and disciplinary processes described by Norbert Elias and Michel Foucault to those associated with the birth of the public sphere (Habermas) and the modern self and family (Taylor, most recently).[2] Yet, if a not key causal driver, the care of health certainly has its place here and for at least two reasons: first, because it is impossible to differentiate entirely from any of the above factors; second, because healthcare has helped to render the boundary between public and private space more precise. In particular, as will be argued here, healthcare has helped to fill out the details, so to speak: to determine the micro-technologies and tactics that comprise public and private space; the minimum standards and dimensions that render them liveable; and the way they combine with natural variables such as air, light and water. We are all beneficiaries of the way considerations of health have shaped our environment. Indeed, that we now take this environment largely for granted is testament to the way it has shaped so much of our routine, daily habits: the use of taps in a private bathroom; walks to work along streamlined, sewered streets; a good night's sleep in an airy bedroom.

This chapter develops this reading by examining Britain, France and the US. This is a partial selection, of course; but besides overlapping with the geographical scope of other chapters in this volume, it also allows for a productive consideration of some of the complexities at stake. To be sure, the commonalities were many in what was already an era of transnational dialogue and borrowing; and as Andrew Lees long ago argued, all three states confronted the problem of mass urbanization at roughly the same time, during the 1830s and 1840s.[3] Yet, just as striking are the multiple variations of architectural development and spatial access. Most notably, Britain was the first to become an urban nation, doing so long before France and the US. In the 1870s, roughly 60 per cent of the British population lived in towns and cities compared to only 25 per cent in France and 20 per cent in the US. In fact, both nations would have to wait until the interwar period before they could describe themselves as urban.[4] At the same time, *within* each country, class and regional differentials generated a remarkably mixed provision of public and private spaces – to say nothing of the struggles to achieve a clear distinction between public and private space in the first place, especially in poorer districts.

Summarizing such a complex set of developments is no easy task. One option, however, is to think in terms of spatial-architectural *processes* on the one hand, and their *composite* character on the other. By 'composite' is here meant the way these processes combined various rationales, more or less pronounced in any given site, such as the disciplinary and the civilizing, as well as the sanitary. The chapter begins with a series of confined, institutional spaces and a process of cellularization. It then examines two further processes, decongesting and privatizing spaces, before finally dwelling on the emergence of more rigorous practices of hygiene.

## Cellularizations

It would be difficult to think of a time when the management of space has not been crucial, in one way or another, to the care and protection of health. Efforts to police the space between bodies have long been critical to efforts to mitigate outbreaks of infectious disease. From 1500 onwards, epidemics of plague in Britain and France – and later, in southern US ports especially, yellow fever – gave rise to a suite of tactics that included quarantine, fumigation and the isolation of the infected, whether at home or in institutions such as 'pest-houses'. In Britain between 1578 and 1665 it seems that household quarantine was imposed with unusual vigour compared to other European states. Padlocks were placed on the doors of plague-ridden houses; guards stood watch outside.[5] Equally, exceptional tactics such as this increasingly traversed a communal landscape governed by a medley of environmental regulations. One historian has even written of a 'domestication of waste' in early modern France, where a royal edict of 1539 declared that the inhabitants of Paris should henceforth build cesspools to the rear of their houses and refrain from dumping excrement and offal into the streets.[6] Meanwhile, magistrates, councillors and local officials such as beadles and hog reeves would police an assortment of so-called 'nuisances', from unruly, smelly pigpens to noisy neighbours.

It would be wrong to regard these measures as imprecise or insufficient, or even inhumane in the case of quarantine, according to later standards.[7] Early modern efforts had a coherence of their own, as governed by dominant understandings of disease causation and tolerable levels of sensory comfort. In any case, much of this would persist long into the nineteenth century, when the advent of cholera called forth crude tactics of quarantine, professionals still clung to miasmatic epidemiologies, and the category of 'nuisances' remained a capacious one. Yet, slowly but surely – and indeed long before the advent of germ theories in the mid-nineteenth century – a new regulatory precision developed with respect to the accommodation of people who were required, willingly or otherwise, to spend time in confined, closed spaces. From roughly 1750 onwards, ships, prisons, army camps and hospitals in particular attracted the attention of reformers. As the French historian Alain Corbin has argued, these spaces functioned like 'laboratories': as sites, that is, where various hygienic tactics, technologies and micro-design features were pioneered, only later to be applied to more everyday spaces.[8]

In each case this was much less about privatizing the body than providing it with a regulated unit or cell of space, where it could be posited as an object of discipline, or at least exposed to a modicum of authority and instruction. The prevention of site-specific 'fevers' such as 'hospital fever' and 'ship fever' (or what would later be distinguished, among other afflictions, as typhus and typhoid fever) was one aim; but there were many benefits besides those of health per se.[9] Fitter soldiers and sailors made for stronger armies and navies, crucial at a time when infectious diseases could be decidedly more deadly than enemy offensives. Notoriously, the British Walcheren campaign of 1809 against the French led to some 4,000 deaths by fever compared to only 100 or so in combat.[10] In prisons the concern to prevent 'moral contagion' and the transmission of criminal habits among inmates was just as strong as the desire to stop physical contagion.[11] Meanwhile, in hospitals architectural renewal was linked to the birth of clinical medicine and pathological anatomy, and the desire to obtain readier access to bodies, dead or alive.[12] Put another way, the motivations were many, and if a degree of spatial isolation made for better health it also made for pacification and observation.

The key reformers are well known, each developing and focusing existing currents of anxiety. One was the Royal Navy surgeon James Lind, now most famous for his discovery that citrus fruits can be used to cure scurvy. First published in 1757, Lind's *Essay on the Most Effectual Means of Preserving the Health of Seamen* urged the rigorous separation of the on-board sick, the daily airing of beds for those convalescing, and the cleansing and fumigation of all areas above and below deck once an outbreak of fever had passed. The burning of gunpowder and sulphur was a particular favourite of Lind's when it came to disinfecting air.[13] Another was the Scottish physician John Pringle, whose work was later promoted in the US by leading physicians such as Benjamin Rush, also one of the nation's founding fathers. In 1750 Pringle published his *Observations on the Nature and Cure of Hospital and Jayl-Fevers*, and just two years later his *Observations on the Diseases of the Army, in Camp and Garrison*, which was into its fifth edition by 1765. His recommendations were many. Tents and straw-mattresses were to be aired daily; bedsteads used where possible; penalties inflicted on those who failed to use designated 'privies' (toilets); the sick and wounded dispersed into a number of hospitals; and wards ventilated using stoves and chimneys.[14]

Naval and military hygiene gradually improved in each country after around 1780, amidst growing administrative specialization. In the US, for instance, a permanent Army Medical Department was formed in 1818.[15] Some of this impetus spilled into kindred areas. In 1803, the British Parliament passed the Passenger Vessels Act, the first of many that would seek to regulate overcrowding on ships, setting a maximum ratio of one passenger for every two registered tons of vessel. Later, the 1854 Merchant Shipping Act provided every seaman with at least 54 cubic feet of hammock space. Yet regulations of this sort were notoriously difficult to enforce on commercial ships, and even in the army and navy applying standards of hygiene could prove difficult, especially in the midst of conflict. In Britain the insufficiency of existing regulations was brought to light by the Crimean War (1853–6), which prompted a raft of government inquiries and a new phase in the development of military hygiene. Barracks at last became an object of sustained consideration. A Barrack Improvement Commission (1855) stipulated 600 cubic feet of space for each solider and an ideal of twelve men per room.[16]

Mainland military and naval hospitals were another matter, however, where alongside intensified sanitary tactics bodies were gradually accorded a more individualized, if still uniform, cell of space. In particular the Royal Naval hospitals at Haslar, near Portsmouth (opened in 1761), and Stonehouse, near Plymouth (completed in 1765), represented a novel departure. Both were unusually large, accommodating 2,000 and 1,200 patients respectively; and both were laid out around courtyards, and in the case of Stonehouse in the form of separate, three-storey pavilion blocks. Each hospital accorded beds at least 800 cubic feet of air, an increase on practices elsewhere but part of a trend towards extra space. Indeed, by the 1850s each patient was thought to require upwards of 1,500 cubic feet. Lind was the chief physician at Haslar but his meticulous tactics became common elsewhere, in general hospitals. In 1793 the French National Convention passed a decree that every hospital patient should have his or her own bed, and that beds should be separated by a distance of three feet. Just two years later the Council of Hygiene insisted that the number of beds per ward had to be fixed; that bed linen had to be fumigated regularly using burning sulphur, and walls and ceilings limewashed every year; and that toilets should be cleaned daily.[17]

Doubtless degrees of adherence varied and it is incredibly difficult to generalize, not least because of variable patterns of expansion. In the US, for instance, the boom in hospital construction had to wait until the end of the nineteenth century, when the number grew from roughly 120 in 1870 to more than 4,300 in 1910.[18] Even so, in all three countries the professionalization of nursing and hospital medicine ensured more rigorous standards of hygiene and patient care. In terms of broad architectural principles, there was also a degree of convergence around the 'pavilion plan', something that would last long into the twentieth century (see Figure 5.1).

The plan was developed in France by the surgeon Jacques-René Tenon, who was partly inspired by Plymouth's Stonehouse hospital noted above. First outlined in his *Mémoire sur les hôpitaux de Paris* (1788), Tenon's plan was characterized by a greater degree of segregation than was then common, featuring wards in long, rectangular pavilions that branched off from a single central corridor. The beds were placed in opposing pairs, each beneath one of the plentiful windows, which provided cross-ventilation and light.[19] Hospitals of this sort eventually followed, notably the self-styled 'model' Hôpital Lariboisière built in 1839–54 in Paris. And the plan travelled much beyond France, migrating to Britain in the 1850s, where it was promoted by the

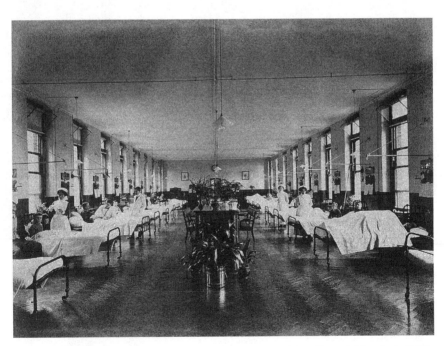

*Figure 5.1* Henry Quinn Ward in London's Great Northern Central Hospital. © The Wellcome Library, London.

nursing reformer Florence Nightingale, and then to the US in the 1880s, where the first pavilion-type establishment was the Johns Hopkins Hospital (1875–85) in Baltimore.

Hospitals were also places of inspection and classification. People of different ages and sexes were commonly set apart in different wards, as, where possible, were different afflictions. The same kinds of administrative sorting took place in prisons, where the process of cellularization found its most complete expression. The one person who did most to advance existing concerns was the county sheriff John Howard, who in 1777 published his *State of Prisons in England and Wales*. Rampant overcrowding and fever, ill-discipline and the indiscriminate mixing of offenders: Howard's conviction that such problems were partly architectural ones informed much of the reform that followed, when there was greater resort to individual cells. Designed by one of the leading prison architects of the time, William Blackburn, Gloucester County Gaol (opened in 1791) contained a number of features that would later become standard, such as grilled windows for ventilation and durable iron bedsteads rather than wooden ones. Inmates were bathed on entrance; heads were shaved; and cells were whitewashed.[20] Just as important was the goal of moral reformation. Once isolated for much of the day, so the theory went, prisoners would invariably develop a more reflective, conscientious self. The assumption was crucial: correctly deployed, space could help to forge an upstanding individual.

Reform was patchy and it did not always proceed on a strictly individual-cellular basis. New York's first state prison, Newgate, built in 1797, housed an impressive 432 inmates, but in 54 eight-man cells.[21] Regimes also softened slightly after the mid-century peak of austerity, when there was much debate in all three countries regarding the disciplinary merits of ensuring complete quiet among inmates or prolonged isolation: the so-called 'silent' and 'separate systems' pioneered in Auburn, New York, and Philadelphia respectively. There was, however, one point of commonality, namely the growing sanitary sophistication of cells. London's Pentonville Prison, opened in 1842, is a case in point, for this 'model' institution was widely revered and emulated in all three countries. Light was let in via a grilled window; but uniquely, each of the 520 cells contained a compact ablutionary unit with a tap feeding into a copper washbasin and a glazed earthenware lavatory. A combined heating and ventilation system irrigated each cell, where warmed fresh air entered via a duct above the door and foul air was let out via another at floor level. As one historian has written, 'no other prison or penitentiary had ever been so meticulously contrived'.[22] Air and light, water and waste: each natural variable was provided for in a series of cellular, self-sufficient units. Food, meanwhile, was passed through a trap in the door, which also contained a spyhole for the warders.

## Decongestions

Regardless of how they might have been paid for – another source of the public/private distinction, as the introduction has detailed – disciplinary sites pioneered what might be called a practical hygiene of collective, if also confined, spaces. It was about inculcating habits of cleanliness and ventilation, and ensuring a uniform distribution of bodies. Such sites would continue to diversify and innovate in the period through to 1950. In 1857, the French army converted hydropathic 'rain douches' into more powerful showers, of the sanitary sort we use today. These were the quickest way to obtain cleanliness and saved on water. Initially soldiers passed in a line under the same vertical jet; later, individual showers were grouped into sheds of wood and corrugated iron.[23] Still more rigorous methods of segregation were developed in hospitals, especially in isolation hospitals, where partitions were used to divide patients (often children) suffering from infectious diseases such as diphtheria, scarlet fever and smallpox. In 1911, it was reported that the hospital at the Institut Pasteur in Paris and Walthamstow's isolation hospital in London had installed 'self-contained chambers', entirely cut off from others and featuring their own toilets.[24] Tactics and technologies continued to spill over into kindred spaces. Showers, for instance, became common fixtures in prisons, boarding schools and collieries. By 1890, state-of-the-art police stations in Britain contained holding cells that contained ventilating grates and heated benches, as well as water-closets.[25]

In some respects cellularization doubled as a process of decongestion. Space was cleared around beds, and air was made to flow between walls. It was in cities, however, that a process of decongestion took place on a grand scale, becoming something like the master principle of urban reform, as Richard Sennett has argued.[26] Equally, the basic assumption first explored in disciplinary settings that space had the capacity to shape morality as much as health – the much-vaunted link between 'the moral and the physical' – was intensified in two complementary directions in the context of towns and cities. On the one hand, every aspect of the urban environment was now deemed ripe for sanitary reform, culminating in grandiose visions of perfectly healthy, civilized cities. In 1875, the British physician Benjamin Ward Richardson outlined a utopian city of health, which he called Hygeia, whose 100,000 citizens walked tree-lined, sun-filled streets and lived in houses equipped with a bathroom, water-closet and a garden to the rear.[27] There were no pubs, since no one desired alcohol; chimneys emitted colourless, odourless smoke. These holistic ambitions were later rekindled in texts such as Ebenezer Howard's *Garden Cities of To-morrow* (1898) and the birth of an internationalist town planning movement during the early 1900s.

On the other hand, social investigators and local officials highlighted just how and to what extent such ambitions were being thwarted, especially among the poor. The crucial decades were the 1820s–40s, when urbanization began to gather pace in all three countries. Britain may have been the first urban nation, but even in the then sparsely populated US, the growth of cities was pronounced from this point onwards. Boston's city-centre population grew by 61 per cent during the 1840s alone; New York's by almost 65 per cent.[28] The consequences were detailed at length. In 1845, the physician and

city inspector John H. Griscom published a landmark US investigation entitled the *Sanitary Condition of the Labouring Population of New York*. It was
inspired by Edwin Chadwick's earlier *Sanitary Report* on Britain (1842) and
Alexandre J.B. Parent-Duchâtelet's investigatory labours on Paris during the
1830s. It made for similarly grim reading. Filth-ridden streets; families hud-
dled in cellars; rooms without ventilation; narrow alleyways and 'pent-up
courts'; a lack of sanitary conveniences and clean water: such was 'the
condition of a great part of the population of this city', Griscom concluded,
'such the physical, and such the moral evils, which continually flow in a
deepening ... stream of misery, pollution and death'.[29]

The gap between ideal and reality was never closed. A mass of social
commentaries, epidemiological inquiries and official statistics in all three
countries attests to this. But in many ways this is precisely the point: a new
inquiring, reforming zeal was at work, and if there were pockets of the urban
environment that went unreformed or were left neglected then this rarely went
unnoticed – and there were many of these pockets, as we shall see below. In
terms of broad morphological patterns the most distinctive is that of the US,
where there was a preference for grid-like structures. Nonetheless, there was a
common commitment to a process of decongestion and enabling goods,
people and natural substances such as air and water to circulate more freely
than before. Crucially, this entailed instituting a clearer demarcation between
public and private spaces. The two worked together: building clearly defined
streets and public parks and installing hydraulic infrastructures at once
reflected and enabled the building of more discrete private spaces, notably
self-contained houses. Once again, the process was a composite one. Wider,
cleaner streets may have made for better health, but they were also more
pleasing to the eye and encouraged the more efficient distribution of goods.
Replacing open cesspools with hidden pipes was more sanitary, but it was also
more civilized. Indeed, the process of decongestion was partly born of disgust
and an aversion to the smell of dung-strewn streets and other people's
domestic waste.

One of the most ambitious projects of the mid-century, Baron Haussmann's
rebuilding of Paris, combined a number of these elements. Clearing away some
of the dense alleyways and dead ends of the medieval city centre, Haussmann's
plan replaced them with boulevards, some up to 30 metres in width. Beneath
the ground a vast system of sewers was built, amounting to 348 miles in length
in 1870, four times the total in 1851. Public parks were also established, their
total acreage increasing from a meagre 47 to some 4,500. The number of trees
along streets doubled.[30] Similar schemes were enacted elsewhere. In 1876 the
British city of Birmingham began a decade-long improvement scheme. Partly
inspired by Haussmann's Paris, the council refashioned some 43 acres of city-
centre land, condemning insanitary slum housing, installing streamlined streets
and accelerating work on new sewerage and water supply systems. In major
cities the scale of these systems required considerable ingenuity. Joseph Bazalgette's main drainage scheme for London, completed between 1859 and 1875,

comprised two principal works, one north of the Thames and one south, coupled with 'high', 'middle' and 'low level' main sewers within each, which drained into a set of intercepting sewers. Four pumping stations lifted sewage from lower level sewers to a point from which they could flow by gravity to the outfalls. In the end the scheme included 1,300 miles of main sewers and 82 miles of intercepting sewers. Roughly 318 million bricks were used together with over 880,000 cubic yards of concrete.[31]

It seems the process of decongestion was a fraught one wherever it took place. Local taxpayers complained about the costs, and the technological choices were many. There was debate in all three countries about the relative merits of 'combined systems', where the sewers collected both rainwater and wastewater (as in London), or 'separate systems', where the two were kept apart (as in Paris, initially). Equally, the engineering demands were intense, and not only with respect to sewerage systems: water supply systems might require the construction of reservoirs. The difficulties faced make the expansion that took place all the more remarkable. In the US the number of waterworks increased from 244 in 1870 to over 9,800 by 1924, enabling a surge in daily per capita water consumption, which more than doubled in major cities such as Chicago and Philadelphia. Likewise, the number and extent of sewerage systems underwent a considerable expansion. Between 1880 and 1905 the miles of sewer mains in Chicago increased from 337 to 1,633; in San Francisco from 128 to 332; and in Pittsburgh from 23 to 365.[32]

Something of an underground revolution took place in British, French and US cities and it was based on a new culture of engineering precision. Pipes, bricks, joints and glazes: no material detail was left unexamined in terms of securing optimum flow and maximum durability. A similar kind of regulatory intensity operated above ground. Streets were now governed by meticulous standards regarding features such as the number and placement of drains and the height of kerbstones. Municipal street cleansing squads picked horse dung and hosed down dust. In 1881 New York established its first specialist Street Cleaning Department, employing more than 200 men to 'scavenge' the city's streets.[33] In the mid-1880s, Scotland's largest city, Glasgow, was employing 175 men and 16 machines to keep its streets dirt-free; and these machines were increasingly sophisticated.[34] British models such as the Hercules Street-Cleansing Machine, first used in 1890, applied water to the road in advance of a revolving, screw-shaped brush. Operated by a single driver, the horse-drawn Hercules could clean upwards of 7,000 square yards per hour.[35]

Meanwhile, public parks – or what some termed the 'lungs of the city' – were established more extensively than ever before and were now made available to all classes. The major parks are well known: Victoria Park in London (opened in 1845); Bois de Boulogne (1858) and Bois de Vincennes in Paris (1866); and Central Park in New York (1873). Yet these were but the largest manifestations of a multifaceted project that involved installing open spaces, of varying size, throughout cities. The British industrial centre of Manchester is a case in point, for it was home to one of the first clean air movements of the nineteenth century, the Manchester Association for the Prevention of Smoke, established in 1842. By the early 1900s the city was home to some 39 open spaces, ranging from large parks of more than 60 acres, where there were promenades, gardens and pitches for football and cricket, to small gravel spaces of less than one acre in working-class areas. Between them they provided health-conscious Mancunians with more than 400 acres of recreational space.[36]

## Privatizations

Cities and towns led the way, as they put on more and more demographic weight, becoming places of more or less delineated *nodes* – sites such as markets, parks and factories – and connecting, circulating *networks*, above ground and below. In rural areas the story was very different. It was not necessarily about playing 'catch-up', for in the absence of significant over-crowding there was no corresponding need for significant environmental reform. It is notable that during the mid-nineteenth century people routinely pointed to the superior health of rural areas – hence in fact projects such as building public parks that attempted to reclaim a bit of 'nature' for urban dwellers. But by the turn of the twentieth century the sanitary state of farms, villages and small market towns was increasingly considered backward. In France, for instance, the number of towns and cities with water supply systems stood at more than 350 in 1900; and of these, some 310 had been installed in the previous 50 years. Yet, as Jean-Pierre Goubert has noted, only a handful of rural areas in France possessed modern systems of water supply around 1900. It was only in the interwar period that this began to change, and even then only slowly. On the eve of the Second World War rural dwellers might still be relying on communal fountains and artesian wells.[37]

Variations of this sort were most pronounced when it came to a third and final process that might be considered: a process of privatizing – but also sanitizing – small units of space. Here especially geographic and socio-economic differences informed considerations of quality and access. This should be distinguished from the process of cellularization, even if it partook of some of the latter's qualities, for privatizing was more about imparting civility and decency than enabling discipline. It was a question, that is, of making individuals into subjects of self-respect and bodily care, rather than into objects of institutional upkeep and authority. Equally, as noted above, privatizing space was bound up with the composite demands of decongesting space, not least the provision of pipe-based infrastructures, for these pipes ultimately emerged above ground in the form of household taps and water-closets.

Two kinds of privatization were crucial: the privatization of families and the privatization of individual bodies. The British middle classes took the lead on both fronts during the 1820s–50s.[38] For the first time, and quite deliberately, suburban middle-class zones were created to provide a measure of spatial luxury and social exclusivity. In contrast to the residential mixing and density typical of pre-industrial towns, areas such as Edgbaston in

Birmingham and Chorlton in Manchester afforded wealthy families distance from urban centres and from adjacent houses. Inside there were multiple bedrooms for parents, children and guests, and bathrooms and toilets. 'Home, sweet home'; 'an Englishman's home is his castle': the popularity of these phrases captures the new premium placed on domestic privacy, and the way the home was imagined as a space of moral and physical recuperation, set apart from the bustling crowds and dirty air of city centres. Still, there were variations even here. The ideal middle-class home was the detached 'villa', but market forces and subsequent suburban expansion made for considerable diversity, culminating in the modest, three-bedroomed semi-detached houses of the interwar period, when over four million new dwellings were built. Further variations emerge when we look abroad, such as the bigger plots of land enjoyed in US suburbs and the attachment to apartments in France. But the key point holds for all three countries: class mattered enormously in terms of the degree and quality of private domestic space.

Indeed, the moral and physical antithesis of the middle-class suburb was the inner-city 'slum', a term that became popular in Britain and the US from the 1830s onwards. The problem in all three countries was overcrowding and a culture of generalized promiscuity that thwarted all kinds of boundaries: tens of families relying on the same rickety privy-midden and standpipe; brothers sharing beds with sisters (and often parents too); animals living amidst humans; neighbours meeting and mixing in dead-end courts that were neither wholly public nor wholly private. There were many solutions besides slum clearance, including inspection. Growing numbers of municipal inspectors were employed in all three countries, guided by a growing mass of regulations. In the wake of a national statute passed in 1850, Paris established a 'Commission on Insalubrious Dwellings' ['*Commission des logements insalubres*']. Between 1851 and 1888 the commission made almost 77,000 house visits based on reports from police officers, building surveyors and doctors. It resulted in 42,000 cases in which improvements were extracted from landlords: windows were installed; partitions in rooms were removed; dung heaps were cleared.[39] Another was the development of municipal refuse teams. In Paris, for instance, the number of men engaged in collecting domestic rubbish – ash and cinders; animal and vegetable matter; paper and textiles – numbered more than 1,100 in 1909.[40]

The other principal solution was to regulate the building of new houses. In all three countries regulations generated a shift towards an architectural form that comprised the following: one family and one toilet per dwelling; a greater number of bedrooms (at least two), of minimum cubic dimensions per sleeper; piped water to the kitchen; and technologies that encouraged ventilation such as fireplaces, air bricks and windows for every inhabitable room. Reformers were quite explicit that privatized families required the right kind of technological-spatial stimulus. Sanitary houses doubled as moral houses. Yet progress on this front was incredibly slow. In Britain local authorities had been empowered since 1875 to clear houses judged 'unfit for human habitation', but it was not until the 1930s that action of this sort really gathered pace. Between 1932 and 1939, some 80 per cent of remaining slum housing was demolished in a burst of activity; it was all but gone by the 1960s.[41] Up until this point urban investigators continued to detail a social class similar to that found in Griscom's 1845 report on New York quoted above: an 'outcast' or 'submerged' section of society that led a life of desperate poverty, overcrowding and ill-health.

What was otherwise described as a social 'residuum' did indeed become more residual in the wake of these efforts; but as working-class housing expanded in urban areas so too did it diversify. In Britain and the US especially there was immense variation between cities. Multi-storey tenements dominated Scottish cities such as Glasgow and Edinburgh and US cities such as New York and Cincinnati; and here working-class families were deprived of backyards and were forced to share communal stairwells and main entrances. By contrast, the terraced houses that proliferated in English cities such as Leicester and Liverpool and in US cities such as Philadelphia and Baltimore were more private and spacious, complete with an alleyway to the rear. Yet, amidst the mix, there were also intermediate forms, including the 'triple-deckers' of Boston and the 'Tyneside flats' of Newcastle. Meanwhile, in rural areas houses might have been largely unchanged since the late eighteenth century. In the American South, for instance, log cabins and ramshackle shanties remained in use among black farmworkers long after the civil war.

Differences between social classes remained crucial, however, determining both the placement and the quality of sanitary technologies. In Britain toilets may have become common in working-class houses by the end of the century, but they were normally situated in a backyard, in an unheated, if still venti-lated, brick-built hut; whereas in middle-class houses multiple toilets were located inside, with separate closets for servants. Similarly, though the number of water-closets may have expanded from the 1850s onwards, they did so among the middle classes first and foremost. In major cities such as Birming-ham and Manchester working-class districts were served by so-called 'pail-closet systems', where inhabitants used removable buckets, topped with ash and collected once a week by the local authority – a kind of half-way technology between the cesspool and the water-closet. 'I do not see why there should in any town be two sewage systems, one for the rich and the other for the poor', argued one British borough engineer in 1881. 'This, however, appears to be the principle: the rich man should have the water-closet, the poor man the pail'.[42] It was not until the interwar period that water-closets, connected to a sewerage system, became the standard technology for all urban classes.

The same applies to beds and baths. Despite the greater provision and size of bedrooms in working-class houses, sharing a bed with a sibling remained a standard practice in poorer families through to the 1960s, even if it now tended to exclude the mixing of brothers and sisters. Similarly, though bath-rooms had become common in middle-class dwellings in all three countries by 1900, they remained the exception in working-class houses. Alternatives thus had to suffice: a washstand topped with a bowl of water and a flannel; the kitchen sink; a portable metallic tub that otherwise hung outside when not in use; or even a dip in a river. In these circumstances privacy had to be improvised: the use of curtains was often recommended. As late as 1951 roughly a third of all British houses lacked plumbed bathrooms. The situation was even more dismal in France, where it seems that approximately 80 per cent of homes lacked a bathroom.[43]

A further alternative was to use a public baths establishment, which at this point contained individual baths as well as swimming pools. These had earlier been established in Britain in the 1840s and in the 1850s in the US and France following Britain's lead. The number of baths increased rapidly during the late nineteenth and early twentieth centuries. There were some 200 in Britain by 1900 and more than 300 in 1914; by the early 1920s all US cities possessed at least one establishment, some as many as 20 (Chicago) and 25 (New York).[44] Here too class remained crucial. In Britain, first- and second-class facilities were offered in all establishments, where the more costly first-class ones were distinguished by a modest degree of luxury, including hand-held mirrors, flesh-brushes, extra towels and shoe-horns. In the US, relatively expensive public baths were supplemented with 'People's Baths', which had been pioneered in Germany in the 1880s. Some were free, but in all cases they made for a decidedly more functional experience than could be had in the more expensive public baths or in a domestic bathroom. Showers were the preferred technology; bathers were timed and ticketed; and cubicles were anonymous and uniform. It made for an efficient kind of privacy, redolent in fact of the culture of hygiene pioneered in disciplinary institutions.[45]

## Hygienic practices

These private spaces were designed to encourage greater care of the self and of one's family, but wealth made the crucial difference in terms of degrees of elaboration. The lower one's class the less ability there was to indulge in hygienic upkeep and explore the intimate environs of the body. When it came to the poor it was about securing minimum rather than ideal standards. For the rich, by contrast, there was a whole world of sanitaryware products and domestic fixtures and fittings to purchase and combine at one's leisure. Even so, in terms of everyday practices, the hundred years after 1850 constitute a crucial transitional period, at least for the growing number of urban dwellers. Slowly but surely people of all classes came to inhabit an environment that was not only more sanitary, but also more clearly defined in terms of public and private spaces. Bodies became more personal – arguably, even more embodied – in the process, something best exemplified perhaps in the shift to all-over washing, in contrast to the early modern focus on the parts that could be seen, such as hands and faces, cuffs and collars.

More exacting standards of personal hygiene, however, were complemented by more exacting practices of spatial hygiene, and it was here that germ theories had their greatest impact. Of course, meticulous, timetabled tactics of cleanliness had long been practised in disciplinary institutions, as described above; but germ theories lent these procedures a new chemical-biological precision, amplifying what had gone before and encouraging still more rigour. They did so most of all in the institutional space of the hospital, where during the latter half of the century surgery in particular was transformed through a combination of antiseptic and aseptic techniques. In 1902, one British–US manual stipulated practices such as washing surgeons' hands with antiseptic solutions; sterilizing instruments in carbolic lotion; purifying dressings, sponges and sutures; and two rounds of skin cleansing on the patient's body where the operation was to take place.[46]

Similarly, local authorities intensified their practices. By the 1890s major cities in all three countries responded to outbreaks of infectious disease using a three-fold repertoire of tactics: early notification of disease; isolation of the sick; and then the disinfection of property. Special measures previously reserved for epidemics of cholera and yellow fever were rendered part and parcel of municipal governance and subjected to ongoing experimentation. In the US, for instance, formaldehyde seems to have displaced sulphur dioxide as the most popular disinfectant at the turn of the century. Rendered into formalin (a solution of formaldehyde gas in water), it was then sprayed or evaporated into infected rooms sealed up with gummed paper. Meanwhile, high-temperature steam machines might be used to disinfect household articles such as curtains, bedding and furniture.[47]

Such tactics were part of a broader, professionalized promotion of disinfection as a discrete sanitary science. Yet, when it came to the homes of millions it was not public health officials but housewives (or their domestic servants) who applied the new standards and substances. Indeed, if class was important in terms of the overall design and distribution of domestic space, then gender was crucial in terms of its day-to-day sanitary management; or more precisely, a particular combination of germ theories, patriarchal norms and the so-called 'science' of domestic economy. Carbolic acid (phenol) and carbolic-infused products became especially popular at the end of the century, and were now subject to mass-marketing, as in Calvert's carbolic washing powder and the Lever brothers' Lifebuoy disinfectant soap (see Figure 5.2).

At the same time, with or without these products, housewives and servants were urged to engage in regimented forms of hygiene. Laundering clothes; airing rooms; beating mattresses; scrubbing floors; cleaning windows; dusting surfaces: all of these elements and more were subject to timetabled integration. Quite how meticulously these standards were practised is difficult to gauge; but it is significant that in all three countries degrees of adherence became a source of pride – and prejudice – among communities, not least within poorer communities. 'Them as wash [clothes] on Monday have all the week to dry, them as wash on Tuesday do little that's awry', went one working-class rhyme in interwar Salford, which ended: 'But them as wash on Saturday – they are sluts indeed!'[48] In this case hygienic practices were about

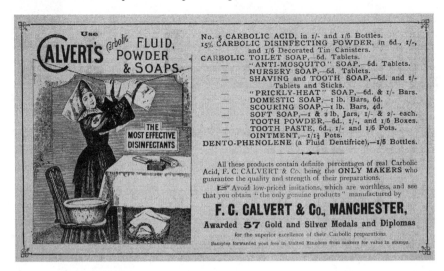

*Figure 5.2* A magazine insert advertising F.C. Calvert's carbolic cleaning products. © The Wellcome Library, London.

more than just health: they concerned a woman's status and how she was regarded by her peers.

## Conclusion

The social significance assumed by everyday practices of cleanliness is a useful reminder of one of the key themes of this chapter: simply that the improvement of health was but one of many factors that played a role in the transformation of public and private space in the period *c*. 1750 to *c*. 1950. Discipline, civility and amenity, even sensory and aesthetic refinement: all of these values combined in hugely complex ways with the desire for better health. Historians and sociologists have spoken of a 'medicalization of space' that commenced with the advent of urban societies, or what they sometimes call 'modernity'. This is a useful idea in some respects. As this chapter has argued, a concern to protect and enhance health was crucial in terms of determining some of the technologies, dimensions and tactics that have come to define public and private space. Yet, beyond the details, in terms of the general forms and interrelations of public and private space, we need to consider other factors as well. Equally, but just as crucially, we also need to bear in mind multiple variations of architectural realization and spatial access. These include variations between regions and nations; and then within these spaces the crucial variations determined by socio-economic differences.

There is no better instance of the importance of the latter than the way these variations became central to new conceptions of social hierarchy. In all three countries personal cleanliness in particular became a crucial means of distinguishing between classes. As Corbin has written of France, 'the poor' became a multifaceted, if always offensive, olfactory phenomenon during the nineteenth century, just as bourgeois standards of hygiene were raised and refined. In Britain and the US the term 'the great unwashed', initially coined in the 1830s, was used as a byword for the working classes. Ultimately, perhaps, what did or did not take place in private was a profoundly public matter. 'For the cults of religion and pedigree we have substituted the cult of soap and water', wrote the British social commentator Stephen Reynolds in 1909. 'Cleanliness is our greatest class-symbol', he went on, 'for nothing else rouses so instantaneously and violently the latent snobbery that one would fain be rid of ... . The bathroom is the inmost, the strongest fortress, of our English snobbery'.[49]

## Further reading

The development of public and private space has generated an immense amount of literature, from various historiographical genres, among them architectural, medical, cultural and social. The following books are simply those with the broadest scope or most focused on questions of space, sanitation and healthcare.

John D. Thompson and Grace Goldin's *The Hospital: A Social and Architectural History* (New Haven, CT: Yale University Press, 1975) remains a useful introductory text, featuring a chapter on the pavilion plan and including reference to Britain, France and the US. Norman Johnston's *Forms of Constraint: A History of Prison Architecture* (Urbana: University of Illinois Press, 2006) covers US and European developments, but the best account for the sanitary dimensions of prison reform remains Robin Evans, *The Fabrication of Virtue: English Prison Architecture, 1750–1840* (Cambridge: Cambridge University Press, 1982).

The literature on housing is especially extensive. Martin Daunton's *House and Home in the Victorian City: Working-Class Housing, 1850–1914* (London: Edward Arnold, 1983) is particularly attuned to the reconfiguration of public and private space and the provision of sanitary facilities. Other accounts are less focused on questions of publicity and privacy, but strong on sanitation. See especially Ann-Louise Shapiro, *Housing the Poor of Paris, 1850–1902* (Madison: University of Wisconsin Press, 1985) and Maureen Ogle, *All the Modern Conveniences: American Household Plumbing, 1840–1890* (Baltimore, MD: The Johns Hopkins University Press, 1996).

In terms of the development of hydraulic infrastructures, no book matches the comprehensive scope of Martin Melosi's survey of American developments, *The Sanitary City: Urban Infrastructure in America from Colonial Times to the Present* (Baltimore, MD: The Johns Hopkins University Press, 2000). The most useful book on France remains Jean-Pierre Goubert's *The Conquest of Water: The Advent of Health in the Industrial Age* (Oxford: Polity Press, 1986), which deals with both water and sewerage systems. In relation to Britain, Bazalgette's sewerage system for London has received the lion's share of attention (e.g. Stephen Halliday, *The Great Stink of London: Sir Joseph Bazalgette and the Cleansing of the Victorian Capital* (Stroud: Sutton, 1999)); but the development of modern water supply systems is surveyed in John Hassan's *A History of Water in Modern England and Wales* (Manchester: Manchester University Press, 1998).

The history of personal hygiene benefits from a number of accounts of broad geography and chronology, including the later chapters of Virginia Smith's *Clean: A History of Personal Hygiene and Purity* (Oxford: Oxford University Press, 2007). In terms of germ theories and how they transformed everyday practices and social perceptions, the most thorough account is Nancy Tomes's *The Gospel of Germs: Men, Women and the Microbe in American Life* (Cambridge, MA: Harvard University Press, 1998).

## Notes

1 See, for instance, Paul Veyne (ed.), *A History of Private Life: From Pagan Rome to Byzantium* (Cambridge, MA: Harvard University Press, 1992), and Richard Sennett, *Flesh and Stone: The Body and the City in Western Civilization* (London: Faber & Faber, 1994).

2 Norbert Elias, *The Civilizing Process, Volume One: The History of Manners* (Oxford: Blackwell Publishing, 1978); Michel Foucault, *Discipline and Punish: The Birth of the Prison* (London: Penguin Books, 1991); Jürgen Habermas, *The Structural Transformation of the Public Sphere: An Inquiry into a Category of Bourgeois Society* (Cambridge Mass.: MIT University Press, 1991); Charles Taylor, *A Secular Age* (Cambridge, MA: Belknap Press, 2007).

3 Andrew Lees, *Cities Perceived: Urban Society in European and American Thought, 1820–1940* (Manchester: Manchester University Press, 1985).

4 Figures cited in Lees, *Cities Perceived*, 2–3, and Jeffrey G. Williamson, *Coping with City Growth during the British Industrial Revolution* (Cambridge: Cambridge University Press, 1990), 2–5.

5 Paul Slack, *The Impact of Plague in Tudor and Stuart England* (Oxford: Clarendon Press, 1985), 210–11, 277–9.

6 Dominique Laporte, *History of Shit* (Cambridge, MA: The MIT Press, 2000), 28–30.

7 For a recent statement of the dangers of anachronism see Carole Rawcliffe, *Urban Bodies: Communal Health in Late Medieval English Towns and Cities* (Woodbridge: Boydell & Brewer, 2013).

8 Alain Corbin, *The Foul and the Fragrant: Odour and the Social Imagination* (London: Papermac, 1996), 105–110.

9 For a full discussion of the many and varied attempts to grapple with the specificities of 'fever' see L.G. Wilson, 'Fevers', in William F. Bynum and Roy Porter (eds), *Companion Encyclopaedia of the History of Medicine* (London: Routledge, 1993), 382–411.

10 Peter Mathias, 'Swords and Ploughshares: The Armed Forces, Medicine and Public Health in the Late Eighteenth Century', in Jay M. Winter (ed.), *War and Economic Development: Essays in Memory of David Joslin* (Cambridge: Cambridge University Press, 1975), 75.

11 The classic, though much disputed, account remains Foucault, *Discipline and Punish*.

12 Michel Foucault, *The Birth of the Clinic: An Archaeology of Medical Perception* (New York: Vintage, 1994); Nicholas D. Jewson 'The Disappearance of the Sick Man from Medical Cosmology, 1770–1870', *Sociology*, 10 (1976): 225–44.

13 James Lind, *Essay on the Most Effectual Means of Preserving the Health of Seamen, in the Royal Navy* (London: D. Wilson, 1762), 94–120.

14 John Pringle, *Observations on the Diseases of the Army, in Camp and Garrison* (London: A. Millar, D. Wilson and T. Durham, 2nd edn, 1753), 94–112.

15 Mary C. Gillett, *The Army Medical Department, 1818–1865* (Washington, DC: Centre of Military History, 1987), Ch. 2.

16 Edmund A. Parkes, *A Manual of Practical Hygiene, Prepared Especially for Use in the Medical Service of the Army* (London: John Churchill & Sons, 2nd edn, 1866), 284–5.

17 Graham A.J. Ayliffe and Mary P. English, *Hospital Infection: From Miasmas to MRSA* (Cambridge: Cambridge University Press, 2003), 44.

18 Morris J. Vogel, 'The Transformation of the American Hospital', in Norbert Finzsch and Robert Jütte (eds), *Institutions of Confinement: Hospitals, Asylums and Prisons in Western Europe and North America, 1500–1950* (Cambridge: Cambridge University Press, 1996), 44–5.

19 A useful overview of these developments can be found in Harriet Richardson (ed.), *English Hospitals, 1660–1948: A Study of their Architecture and Design* (Swindon: Royal Commission on the Historical Monuments of England, 1998), 5–12.

20 Robin Evans, *The Fabrication of Virtue: English Prison Architecture, 1750–1840* (Cambridge: Cambridge University Press, 1982), 147–57, 170–1.

21 David Lewis, *From Newgate to Dannemora: The Rise of the Penitentiary in New York, 1796–1848* (Ithaca, NY: Cornell University Press, 1965), 31.

22 Evans, *The Fabrication of Virtue*, 360.

23 Georges Vigarello, *Concepts of Cleanliness: Changing Attitudes in France since the Middle Ages* (Cambridge: Cambridge University Press, 1988), 220–2.

24 F. Foord Caiger, 'Cubicle Isolation: Its Value and Limitations', *Public Health*, 24 (1910–11): 336–7.

25 'A Modern Police Station', *Public Health (Supplement to the International Congress of Hygiene and Demography)* (1891): 53.

26 Sennett's *Flesh and Stone*, Part Three.

27 Benjamin W. Richardson, 'Address on Health', in Charles Wager Ryalls (ed.), *Transactions of the National Association for the Promotion of Social Science: 1875* (London: Longmans, Green, & Co., 1876), 100–20.

28 Martin Melosi, *The Sanitary City: Urban Infrastructure in America from Colonial Times to the Present* (Baltimore, MD: The Johns Hopkins University Press, 2000), 59.

29 John H. Griscom, *Sanitary Condition of the Labouring Population of New York, with Suggestions for Its Improvement* (New York: Harper & Brothers, 1845), 41.

30 For a full account see David P. Jordan, *Transforming Paris: The Life and Labors of Baron Haussmann* (New York: Simon & Schuster, 1995).

31 Joseph W. Bazalgette, *On the Main Drainage of London, and the Interception of the Sewage from the River Thames* (London: William Clowes and Sons, 1865).

32 Melosi, *The Sanitary City*, 121, 131 and 153.

33 George A. Soper, *Modern Methods of Street Cleaning* (New York: The Engineering News Publishing Company, 1909), 163.

34 John Young, 'The Scavenging of Towns', *Transactions of the Sanitary Institute*, 5 (1883–4): 248.

35 'The "Hercules" Street-Cleansing Machine', *The Builder*, 58 (1890): 179.

36 T. De Courcy Meade, 'Conference of Engineers and Surveyors to County and Other Sanitary Authorities', *Journal of the Sanitary Institute*, 21 (1900): 496–9.

37 Jean-Pierre Goubert, *The Conquest of Water: The Advent of Health in the Industrial Age* (Oxford: Polity Press, 1986), 208–11, 214–25.

38 Richard Rodger, *Housing in Urban Britain, 1780–1914* (Cambridge: Cambridge University Press, 1995), 38–43.

39 Andrew R. Aisenberg, *Contagion: Disease, Government, and the 'Social Question' in Nineteenth-Century France* (Stanford, CA: Stanford University Press, 1999), 53.

40 Soper, *Modern Methods of Street Cleaning*, 95.

41 John Stevenson and Christopher Cook, *The Slump: Britain in the Great Depression* (Abingdon: Pearson Education, 3rd edn, 2013), 29.

42 'Birmingham Sewage Works: Discussion', *Proceedings of the Association of Municipal Sanitary Engineers and Surveyors: Volume VII, 1880–81* (London: E. & F.N. Spon, 1881), 89.

43 David J. Eveleigh, *Bogs, Baths and Basins: The Story of Domestic Sanitation* (Stroud: Sutton Publishing, 2006), 166; Goubert, *The Conquest of Water*, 87.

44 Marilyn T. Williams, *Washing 'the Great Unwashed': Public Baths in Urban America, 1840–1920* (Columbus: Ohio State University Press, 1991), 8, 39.

45 W. Paul Gerhard, *Modern Baths and Bath Houses* (New York: John Wiley & Sons, 1908), Ch. 7.

46 William Rose and Albert Carless, *A Manual of Surgery for Students and Practitioners* (New York: William Wood & Company, 5th edn, 1902), 16–20.

47 Charles V. Chapin, *Municipal Sanitation in the United States* (Providence, RI: Snow & Farnham, 1901), 528–59.

48 Robert Roberts, *A Ragged Schooling: Growing up in the Classic Slum* (Manchester: Mandolin, 1976), 91.

49 Stephen Reynolds, *A Poor Man's House* (London: John Lane, 1909), 88–9.

# 6 Private and public traditions of healthcare in Central and south-eastern Europe, from the nineteenth to the (mid-)twentieth centuries

*Marius Turda*

## Introduction

Traditions of healthcare in Central and south-eastern Europe during the nineteenth and the first half of the twentieth centuries were shaped by a number of specific factors such as widespread illiteracy; predominantly rural populations; underdeveloped or non-existent infrastructure; malnutrition; frequent epidemics; numerous social problems (such as alcoholism) and sexually transmitted diseases (syphilis, in particular); high levels of infant mortality; late adoption of modern ideas of medicine; and a persistence of traditional methods of private healthcare. Beginning with the late nineteenth century – and increasingly after the First World War – a range of modern health programmes were gradually introduced throughout Central and south-eastern Europe by the newly constituted national governments attempting to re-inforce the importance of a healthy population to their nation-building ambitions. The state provided financial support for the establishment of health institutions and infrastructure, while at the same time promoting the professionalization of medicine and its corollary, the transformation of physicians into devoted supporters of the national community.

Endorsing these national efforts, international organizations such as the Rockefeller Foundation and the Health Organization of the League of Nations, for example, also proved crucial to the emergence of a new tradition of public healthcare after 1918, one based on programmes of hygiene, social assistance and preventive medicine. The establishment of institutes of hygiene and public health in Central and south-eastern Europe during the 1920s and 1930s was part of such collaborative programmes, in addition to offering training in North American methods of public health service for physicians and nurses from these regions. During the interwar period, the Rockefeller Foundation offered numerous grants and fellowships, as well as direct financial contributions towards the costs of the new institutions with the general aim of creating a group of professional experts who were to become responsible for public healthcare in their native countries.

Yet, in Central and south-eastern Europe, traditional medical practices, particularly with respect to healing and childbearing, survived into the twentieth century, especially in the rural areas (see Figure 6.7).

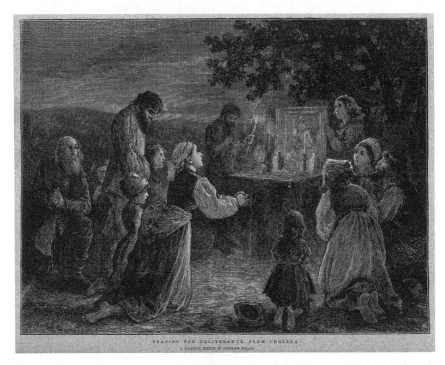

*Figure 6.1* Men, women and children praying at a shrine by the roadside during the 1873 cholera epidemic in Poland. © The Wellcome Library, London.

Any discussion of private and public traditions of healthcare in these regions, therefore, must not neglect the resilience of traditional medicine and the intense private relationship that existed between disease and the individual as well as the difference between rural and urban areas. Religion (Christianity, Islam and Judaism) played an equally important role in this context, reconfiguring the transition from private to more public forms of healthcare.

In light of such circumstances, traditions of private and public healthcare in Central and south-eastern Europe must be addressed nationally, regionally and comparatively. These are regions rich in cultural, ethnic, linguistic and religious legacies. Moreover, countries that benefited territorially from the peace treaties of 1920–1921, such as Romania, Poland, Czechoslovakia and Yugoslavia, had to address regional disparities and the different institutional traditions in the newly annexed territories. These disparities existed, for instance, between the Romanian Old Kingdom and Serbia, which had developed their health systems as independent nation states during the nineteenth century, and the regions Transylvania, Bukovina, Croatia, Bosnia and Slovenia, which had been part of the Austro-Hungarian Empire prior to November 1918. In the case of Poland, moreover, its territories were divided between three empires – Russian, German and Austro-Hungarian – all with different traditions of healthcare and institutionalized medicine.[1] It is only when these national traditions are viewed in a comparative regional (and post-imperial) framework that historical idiosyncrasies become noticeable and important.

After 1900, medicine gradually became a dominant scientific discipline in which health experts, reform-oriented politicians and intellectuals expressed their duties and responsibilities towards the nation and state.[2] One of the most important corollaries to this process in the history of these regions is the extensive social involvement of the physician, a transformation that is particularly important for the understanding of the history of public and private healthcare in Central and south-eastern Europe. It was largely due to the efforts of a number of key physicians that schemes of public healthcare were implemented in these countries during the 1920s and 1930s. These individuals also personified the emergence of a new trend in the professionalization of medicine, namely the recasting of moral and ethical questions pertaining to the nation in a medical and biological discourse. Their conceptual approaches to nationalized healthcare systems became paramount in the interwar years, when these doctors held important positions in the ministries of public health of Austria, Poland, Yugoslavia, Hungary, Romania, Bulgaria and Greece.

Although this chapter chronicles the intrinsic relationship between public and private traditions of healthcare in Central and south-eastern Europe only until 1945, it is important to note that most of these public healthcare programmes, as well as the widespread campaigns advocating personal hygiene, preventive medicine and vaccination, continued during the 1950s and 1960s. Heavily influenced by models of socialist medicine developed in the Soviet Union, the new communist regimes in Central and south-eastern Europe (apart from Greece and Austria) conceived of healthcare as part of the general transformation of society according to the principles of socialism and communism. In a classless society, healthcare was to be made available to all individuals. Similarly, the state invested a substantial amount of resources in improving the living and health conditions of the rural communities, in parallel to industrialization and the transformation of the public space. Private traditions of healthcare were gradually subsumed beneath the all-encompassing public domain until they had virtually disappeared by the late 1980s.

## On the margins of Europe

Prior to the early twentieth century, south-eastern Europe (including the Balkans) was an area where sanitary interventions were necessary to protect the general health of Europe.[3] Various quarantines were implemented to protect Europe against epidemics such as plague and cholera, such as those established in the Ottoman Empire in 1838 by Sultan Mahmud II (1785–1839). It was assumed that south-eastern Europe, especially the Danubian Principalities and Serbia, where quarantines had been effective since 1832, and the Habsburg Empire, where quarantines had been in effect since the mid-eighteenth century, would protect the rest of Europe from the spread of the Oriental plague.[4]

As noted by scholars working on the history of medicine in the Habsburg Monarchy and the Ottoman Empire, during the eighteenth and nineteenth centuries, south-eastern Europe functioned as an intermediary region, often explicitly as a *cordon sanitaire.* The constant military confrontation between the Ottoman, Habsburg and Russian empires in the eighteenth and nineteenth century provoked frequent and intense outbreaks of plague, such as during the Russo-Turkish War of 1828–1829, the Russo-Turkish War of 1877–1878 and the two Balkan Wars of 1912–1913.[5] Indeed, right from the start of these conflicts, Western medical organizations attended areas of military operations, in Macedonia, Thrace, Albania and Bulgaria.[6] All these conflicts challenged military medicine and, at the same time, provided physicians with new opportunities for medical research: field doctors studied the healing of wounds caused by new weaponry and the containment of war epidemics, of which cholera consistently ranked among the most significant.[7]

Furthermore, south-eastern Europe differed, in terms of demographic (ethnically mixed), socio-economic (predominantly rural) and religious (Greek Orthodoxy and Islam) characteristics, from Central Europe, which was mostly Catholic and Protestant. During the nineteenth century, these differences, in turn, shaped the relationship between private and public traditions of healthcare. For instance, the sanitary conditions typical of predominantly rural societies were often deemed threatening to the general health of the population by modern hygienists and health reformers.[8] As the American physician Paul Dudley White (1886–1973) once remarked: 'On the old battle-scarred valleys and mountains of Eastern Macedonia lurk some of the most dangerous of the world's diseases'.[9]

Across south-eastern Europe, local and foreign physicians alike complained about the precarious hygienic conditions among the population, malnutrition (see Figure 6.2), the spread of diseases – social (such as alcoholism), venereal (syphilis in particular) and infectious (such as malaria and typhus) – prostitution,[10] high levels of infant mortality, the rejection of modern medicine, and the persistence of religious and private traditions of hygiene and health.

Furthermore, traditions of rural hygiene and healing were perceived to be 'unhygienic habits', becoming the main target for a novel category of professionals educated in the new European scientific medicine. In some cases, folk medicine also harked back to outdated sanitary provisions, which the new states wanted to replace. These medical realities reflect, of course, a variety of different historical and cultural phenomena that defined the development of healthcare in the region. As modern nation states emerged in south-eastern Europe, beginning with Serbia and Greece during the 1810s and 1820s, attempts were made to overcome these problems.

Of particular interest are the ways in which these national states in Central and south-eastern Europe and their emerging medical elites addressed (Ottoman, Habsburg and Russian) imperial legacies while at the same time contributing to the creation of new national health systems based on the principle of national uniformity and centralized control. To give a few examples, the

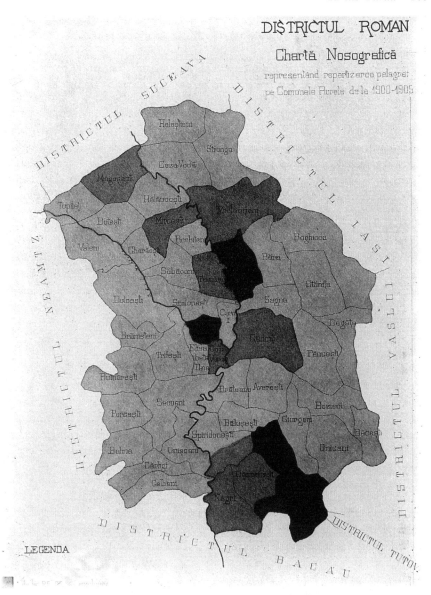

*Figure 6.2* Incidence of pellagra in Eastern Romania, 1900–1905. © The Wellcome Library, London.

Ionian Academy was founded in 1824 in Corfu and included a faculty of medicine; the Imperial School of Medicine was established in Istanbul in 1827, and it soon became a centre for medical training for generations of physicians across south-eastern Europe. In the newly established Greek state, the Royal Medical Council was established in 1834, followed by the Medical School of the National University of Athens in 1837.[11] As with other academic disciplines such as history, for example, medicine became an important instrument in the long-fought battle over the Greek state's claim to distinctive nationhood.

Until these and other institutions were established, there was a consistent lack of trained medical personnel in these countries; physicians needed to be trained abroad, and many could only afford this elite education through scholarships, initially private, from various benefactors. Well into the twentieth century, generations of medical students from Central and south-eastern Europe benefited from this transfer of knowledge by studying under leading specialists of distinct medical disciplines in various European universities. Polish and Bulgarian physicians, for instance, preferred Vienna and Berlin. Romanian doctors from Transylvania and Bukovina studied in Budapest and Vienna, while those from the Kingdom of Romania, by contrast, frequently attended French medical faculties with the support of scholarships provided by the Romanian and French governments. On their return, these physicians combined private traditions of schooling and education with public, state-sponsored initiatives. They engaged with private initiatives in combating diseases and epidemics, as well as contributing to the building of national health systems in their own countries. To some extent, the values of Western science became the standard against which medical traditions in these countries were ultimately assessed.[12]

During the late nineteenth and early twentieth centuries, the countries of Central and south-eastern Europe undoubtedly recurrently absorbed external medical knowledge, but regions and cultures are both interrelated and interdependent. The process of adopting medical values and practices was a complex movement, with the West as one source of knowledge and power. The emergence of modern traditions of public healthcare in Central and south-eastern Europe should therefore be seen as part of a larger global transformation of modern ideas of medicine, hygiene and health occurring since the Enlightenment.[13]

Preventing epidemics was one important feature of the strategies of health and hygiene introduced during this period in Central and south-eastern Europe; social assistance, and the emergence of modern ideas of child welfare and motherhood, were others.[14] Take, for example, the establishment of infant welfare institutions established in the early twentieth century in Hungary and the Polish parts of the Habsburg Empire. In the latter, these institutions were inspired by French initiatives witnessed and adopted by influential individual Polish physicians, such as Tadeusz Boy-Żeleński (1874–1941). In Hungary, on the other hand, the Stefánia Association for the Protection of Mothers and Infants, established in 1915, reacted against the proposed public unification of preventive health. In 1917, the Hungarian Parliament acknowledged a public responsibility for the protection of mothers and children, and entrusted the private organization Stefánia with carrying out the actual implementation of this new policy.[15]

Often these transfers and exchanges of knowledge and medical personnel were forced rather than voluntary, as during the Austro-Hungarian occupation of Bosnia-Herzegovina prior to the First World War. The Austrian medical journal *Wiener Medizinische Wochenschrift* (Viennese Weekly Medical Journal) published articles on Austro-Hungarian military hygienic provisions in south-eastern Europe, raising the spectre of public health threats posed by typhus, syphilis and leprosy that might infiltrate from countries with considerably inferior public and private hygiene regimes.

Medical associations and journals in Central and south-eastern Europe provided the necessary forum where local physicians could share their ideas as well as translate and invite contributions from abroad. In 1835 the Medical Society of Athens was founded, and the following year *Aesculapius*, the first Greek medical journal appeared. In Bulgaria, this crucial role in disseminating ideas of modern medicine was played by *Zdravie: Spisanie na Sofijskoto meditsinsko druzhestvo* (Strength: Journal of the Sofia Medical Society) and *Meditsinsko spisanie* (Medical Journal), while in Warsaw and Bucharest this role was fulfilled by *Zdrowie* (Health) and *Gazeta Medico-Chirurgicală* (Medico-Surgical Gazette) respectively. In Budapest, *Orvosi Hetilap* (Weekly Medical Journal), established in 1857, served a similar function, while in Prague the medical journal *Vierteljahrschrift für die praktische Heilkunde* (Quarterly for Practical Medicine) offered both German and Czech physicians an opportunity for professional interaction. There were also medical journals such as *Archives Balkanique de médicine* and *Chirurgie et leurs spécialités* (established in 1939) that aimed at trans-national co-operation and exchange of medical knowledge among the professionals in the region.

In Central and south-eastern Europe, social status and ethnicity were equally important factors determining public perceptions of health and hygiene.[16] The poor and the Roma were blamed for early nineteenth-century outbreaks of plague in Bucharest, for example, while groups such as refugees and Armenian traders were blamed for its subsequent spread. At the beginning of the twentieth century, the Roma were held responsible for transmitting diseases and infections, fuelling the growing racism in these regions, while Muslim communities in Bulgaria and Yugoslavia were often seen as opposed to modern, Christian medicine.[17] As other chapters in this volume demonstrate, however, medical representations of certain sexual, social and ethnic groups served as metaphors and symbols for wider cultural and political re-configurations of healthcare beyond the confines of the Central and south-eastern European regions.

Like much of the rest of Europe, the countries of Central and south-eastern Europe experienced profound changes after 1918. The regional crisis that had started in 1912 with the Balkan Wars, and continued after 1914, did not end with the armistice of November 1918, but extended well into the 1920s. Greece and Turkey, for instance, were not to settle their differences until 1922. The major results of this crisis were the formation of a South Slav state in the form of Yugoslavia, the establishment of Greater Romania, the expulsion of Greeks from Asia Minor and the creation of a post-imperial secular Turkish state. In the final agreements of the peace treaties, the future Yugoslavia and Romania emerged as winners; Bulgaria and Turkey were losers, as was, ultimately, Greece.

Although medical assistance and control by the Great Powers ended with the First World War, scientific knowledge including bacteriology and various methods of disinfection were still employed in the region in order to combat infectious diseases. Furthermore, the regional medical network established during the war survived in hygiene and public health projects later applied to civilians in south-eastern Europe – especially those carried out by international organizations such as the Health Organization of the League of Nations and the Rockefeller Foundation.[18] The Malaria Commission of the League of Nations similarly played an important role in Asia Minor during the early 1920s, following the Greek–Turkish war.[19] Yet this tumultuous political period also marked the beginning of a series of reforms in public health and social welfare. These reforms came to fruition in the 1930s, thus creating favourable conditions for the modern health system in this region to emerge. In fact, the difficult political situation in these countries during the interwar period offered new opportunities for social experts and welfare professionals to plan and direct the future of their nation through social policies built into their emerging health and welfare systems. During the 1920s health reformers in Greece, Bulgaria, Romania and Yugoslavia actively advocated the re-organization of the state based on modern sanitary principles, seen as the necessary requirement for the improvement of the health of the population. As these countries were predominantly rural (for example, only 20.2 per cent of Romania's population in 1930 was urban), the peasantry dominated the medical agenda.

The doctor's moral responsibilities towards the peasants – seen as symbols of untainted ethnicity – were an essential foundation of medicine's claim to authority and prestige. Yet the relationship between peasants and doctors was never straightforward. The founder of the Romanian School of Paediatrics, Mihail Manicatide (1867–1954), for instance, did not hesitate to condemn the opinion, widespread among rural doctors, that the peasant was 'a savage, a lazy person, a drunkard, a thief, someone sick and dirty, a miserable creature, but one that we need write and talk about, purposefully or otherwise; in any case, an inferior creature, on to which we bestow a great deal of favour when lowering to its level'.[20] Whereas in countries such as Britain the peasantry had all but disappeared by the end of the nineteenth century, in Central and south-eastern Europe the peasantry survived as a significant segment of the population. During the interwar period, health reformers incessantly discussed the supposed social and economic proclivities that made the peasantry susceptible to disease and thus to biological degeneration.[21] They were painfully aware of their country's health problems and medical journals poured out statistics confirming the country's hygienic deficiency. During the 1930s, therefore, public healthcare gradually became a central component of a larger biomedical agenda, and the state invested in the creation of a healthy nation and society.[22]

## The institutionalization of healthcare

The process of embracing modern traditions of healthcare did not occur simultaneously across Central and south-eastern Europe, nor was the spread of medical education – let alone the extent of medical institutionalization – similar in the individual countries. Under the Ottoman Empire, a medical school and a teaching hospital had been opened in the state shipyard in 1805, the result of a private initiative aimed solely at the military. A school for surgeons followed in 1828. These two schools were fused in 1839 as the newly established Imperial Medical School. The first non-military medical faculty in south-eastern Europe, however, was founded in 1837 in Athens, and another was established in Bucharest twenty years later. Yet the rest of the countries in the region had to wait until the twentieth century: in Bulgaria the first medical faculty was founded in 1918, in Serbia in 1920 and in Albania only in 1952. A much better situation existed in the Austro-Hungarian Empire, with Vienna, Prague and Budapest enjoying recognition in the medical community by the early twentieth century. Not surprisingly, the first ministers of welfare in Central and south-eastern Europe were established during the last years of the First World War. In Hungary the Ministry of Labour and Social Welfare was created in 1918, only to be subsequently transformed into the Commissariat for Labour and Social Welfare by the National Council of Health during the short-lived Hungarian Communist Republic. Similarly, the Austrian Ministry of Health was established in August 1918, followed in November 1918 by a Ministry of Public Health in Serbia, which became the Ministry of National Health in the first Yugoslav government only a month later.[23] Romania and Greece established a Ministry of Health and Social Care in 1922.

As Europe recovered from the economic devastation caused by the war, health reformers sought to convince their governments to accord more importance to medical projects of public health and social hygiene, all with the aim of improving the general health of the population. The countries in Central and south-eastern Europe that were expanded territorially by the ensuing peace treaties, such as Romania and Yugoslavia, had to address regional disparities and different institutional traditions in these areas. This disparity existed, for instance, between the Romanian Old Kingdom, which had developed a system of healthcare and social assistance as an independent nation-state, and Transylvania, or between independent Serbia and Croatia, Bosnia and Slovenia, which latter three had been a part of the Habsburg Empire prior to November 1918. Yet this historical discrepancy within the new states was ameliorated by sustained institutionalization and centralization. As already alluded to in the introduction, no overview of private and public traditions of healthcare in Central and south-eastern Europe can avoid considering the key role of the state, especially after 1920.

Undoubtedly the state played the most significant role in the development of healthcare and hygiene projects, but the influence of outstanding individuals should not be neglected completely. 'The physician', the Romanian health reformer Iuliu Haţieganu wrote in 1925, 'is the most useful and important social agent of the state'.[24] But it was not only the physician who underwent a radical conversion; medicine itself was seen as a 'national science' serving the state to improve the population's health and hygiene. As the Hungarian gynaecologist János Bársony (1860–1926) put it in his 1922 address to the Medical Faculty at the University of Budapest: 'the medical profession can no longer confine itself to the mere implementation of scientific knowledge. It must become the midwife in the birth of a new political mentality, which will serve the true interests of the nation'.[25]

Leading physicians and health reformers such as Julius Tandler (1869–1936) in Austria; Gustav Kabrhel (1857–1939) in Czechoslovakia; Béla Johan (1889–1983) in Hungary; Witold Chodzko (1875–1954) and Ludwik Rajchman (1881–1965) in Poland; Andrija Štampar (1888–1958) and Milan Jovanović Batut (1847–1940) in Yugoslavia; Iuliu Moldovan (1882–1966) and Gheorghe Banu (1889–1957) in Romania; Toshko Petrov (1872–1942) in Bulgaria; and, finally, Constantinos Savvas (1861–1929) and Emmanuel Lampadarios (1882–1943) in Greece played decisive roles in creating centralized systems for health and hygiene in Central and south-eastern Europe before and during the inter-war period. Their concepts of nationalized hygiene and healthcare came into the ascendency in the 1930s and 1940s, when these individuals held important ministerial positions.[26] And although Štampar was forced to resign in the 1940s, for instance, he continued to play a role as a leading expert for the Health Organization of the League of Nations; Rajchman enjoyed a similar international prestige during the 1930s. Štampar's ideas of social hygiene remained influential in south-eastern Europe, most notably among Bulgarian experts on public health.

Central to theories of health and hygiene developed during the interwar period was the idea that the biological conditions of communities could also be improved with the help of external factors such as education and a controlled environment, including the prevention and eradication of contagious diseases and parasites as well as improved sanitation and housing. The programme of healthcare promoted by the Rockefeller Foundation in Central and south-eastern Europe in particular dovetailed with the institutionalization of health and hygiene in these regions. Most public health institutions and institutes of hygiene in these regions were established with funding from the Rockefeller Foundation.[27] The general aim of these new institutions was to complement the existing ones, and together meet the challenge of combating epidemics and improving health conditions of the rural population, thus ultimately creating a modern infrastructure for the national promotion of health and hygiene in each country. The most important of these were:

- Czechoslovakia, the State Health Institute (est. 1925);
- Poland, the National Institute of Epidemiology (est. 1918) and the National Institute of Hygiene (est. 1926);

- Hungary, the National Institute of Hygiene (est. 1927);
- Romania, the Institute of Hygiene and Social Hygiene in Cluj (est. 1919), the Institute of Hygiene and Public Health in Bucharest (est. 1927), and the Institute of Hygiene and Public Health in Iaşi (est. 1930);
- Yugoslavia, the Ministerial Commission for Epidemiology (est. 1919); the Central Institute for Hygiene in Belgrade (est. 1926), and the Institute of Hygiene and the School of Public Health in Zagreb (est. 1927);
- Bulgaria, the Institute for National Health in Sofia (1929);
- Greece, the Institute of Hygiene and Bacteriology (est. 1923), the School of Hygiene (est. 1930), the School of Public Health Nursing (est. 1931), and the Athens Health Centre (est. 1939).

The intention was in each case to create a modern infrastructure for the national promotion of health and hygiene.

The other phase of institutionalization was characterized by active social and national politics, such as training in modern health techniques, the introduction of hygiene and eugenic education into the school curriculum, hygiene courses for adults and programmes improving rural sanitation. To this effect, and with the Rockefeller Foundation's and the League of Nations's support, public demonstrations of healthcare were organized in villages in Yugoslavia, Greece, Romania and Hungary during the late 1920s with the aim of familiarizing the rural population with modern hygiene methods, regular health screening and preventive medicine.[28] These international organizations also required that suitable health legislation be adopted by these countries, which included the National Popular Health Education Act in Yugoslavia (1928), the Public Health Law in Bulgaria and Hungary (1929), and the Sanitary Law in Romania (1930). On the basis of these legislative acts, public healthcare became institutionally defined and centralized.

Moreover, issues of health and disease gradually became a matter of the political and national economy. Statistical records on birth, fertility, mortality and morbidity rates provided a scientific basis for population and eugenic policies, which intensified during the 1930s and 1940s. A paramount goal was the reduction of infant mortality by means of various projects on child protection and puericulture. A number of prominent physicians were active in this field at both the national and international levels. For example, the Romanian Gheorghe Banu visited the United States in 1927. On his return he published a comprehensive overview of the North American system of public health. In the 1930s, he also became actively involved in the International Association for the Protection of Infancy as seen in his numerous contributions to the *Bulletin international de la protection de l'enfance* and his leading role in organizing various conferences on child protection, like those in Liège in 1930 and Paris in 1933. Together with Emmanuel Lampadarios, the Head of the Office for the School of Hygiene in Athens, Banu counterbalanced the influence exercised by French and Belgian activists and child reformers within international organizations. The First and the Second Balkan Congress on the

Protection of Children organized in Athens in 1936 and Belgrade in 1938, respectively, illustrate south-eastern Europe's growing importance in the field of child protection and public health.[29] Bringing together specialists from Greece, Bulgaria, Romania, Yugoslavia and Turkey, these congresses are fine examples of regional co-operation between these countries in the field of child protection and child welfare. Similarly, the ninth and eleventh International Congresses of the History of Medicine were organized by Romania and Yugoslavia in 1932 and 1938, respectively. These highly publicized events served not only to introduce foreign participants to the host country's achievements in the fields of medicine and healthcare but also to provide the local medical community with expertise and encouragement.[30]

To this process, one must add the emergence of local models of health and hygiene, such as theories of rural biology, peasant universities and rural health work in Romania, Yugoslavia and Hungary.[31] Yet the effectiveness of such projects depended on specific infrastructural conditions. Infant mortality in Bulgaria, Romania and Yugoslavia declined in the interwar period, although not at a rate comparable with that of other European countries such as Austria, France, Germany or Switzerland. On the other hand, the fact that Central and south-eastern European countries had higher birth rates than Western European countries, for instance, was considered a biological advantage as well as a particular feature of the nation's healthy racial qualities (see Table 6.1). Fertility and ethnicity were understood to be linked.[32]

Sanitized versions of local rural life – the ideal national village as a repository of specific national values and traditions – were not only an essential component of the new health policies developed after 1918 but were similarly incorporated into the emerging eugenic discourses. Projects to improve public health were perceived as a matter of politics and science. This is because health represented a socialized and socializing resource for those technologies of power employed by the state to control, supervise and discipline its subjects. The social and national pressure put on women is illustrative. Women were predominantly perceived as 'mothers of the nation' in both nationalist and eugenic discourses on reproduction. One of the key areas, then, in which the relationships between health, hygiene and eugenics were expressed was the debates surrounding marriage certificates and sterilization. This biopolitical transformation of the relationship between the state and its population favoured the broad dissemination of eugenic ideas in Central and south-eastern Europe.[33] Indeed, on the one hand, health politics aimed to improve living conditions, individual lives and the nation's welfare; on the other, physicians intervened in the lives of these individuals by recommending not only ways to improve their living conditions and general well-being, but also negative eugenic policies such as sterilization. The aspiration for a 'healthy population' thus emerged as a reflection of the ambivalence inherent in the allegedly egalitarian character of modern healthcare.

This process parallels developments occurring elsewhere at the time. By the 1930s, physicians and health reformers in Central and south-eastern Europe

*Table 6.1* Vital statistics in Central and south-eastern Europe, 1921–1938

| Years | Bulgaria | Greece | Hungary | Romania | Yugoslavia |
|---|---|---|---|---|---|
| Annual births per 1,000 population | | | | | |
| 1921–1925 | 39.0 | 23.0 | 29.4 | 37.9 | 35.0 |
| 1926–1930 | 33.1 | 30.2 | 26.0 | 35.2 | 34.2 |
| 1931–1935 | 29.3 | 29.5 | 22.4 | 32.8 | 31.8 |
| 1936 | 25.9 | 28.1 | 20.4 | 31.5 | 28.9 |
| 1937 | 24.3 | 26.4 | 20.2 | 30.8 | 27.9 |
| 1938 | 22.8 | 25.9 | 20.1 | 29.6 | 26.7 |
| 1938 as % of 1921–1925 | 58 | - | 69 | 78 | 76 |
| Annual deaths per 1,000 population | | | | | |
| 1921–1925 | 20.8 | 16.5 | 19.9 | 23.0 | 20.2 |
| 1926–1930 | 17.9 | 16.6 | 17.0 | 21.2 | 20.0 |
| 1931–1935 | 15.5 | 16.5 | 15.8 | 20.6 | 17.9 |
| 1936 | 14.3 | 15.2 | 14.3 | 19.8 | 16.0 |
| 1937 | 13.6 | 15.2 | 14.2 | 19.3 | 15.9 |
| 1938 | 13.7 | 13.3 | 14.4 | 19.2 | 15.6 |
| 1938 as % of 1921–1925 | 66 | - | 72 | 83 | 77 |
| Annual natural increase per 1,000 population | | | | | |
| 1921–1925 | 18.2 | 6.5 | 9.5 | 14.9 | 14.8 |
| 1926–1930 | 15.2 | 13.6 | 9.0 | 14.0 | 14.2 |
| 1931–1935 | 13.8 | 13.0 | 6.6 | 12.2 | 13.9 |
| 1936 | 11.6 | 12.9 | 6.1 | 11.7 | 12.9 |
| 1937 | 10.7 | 11.2 | 6.0 | 11.5 | 12.0 |
| 1938 | 9.1 | 12.6 | 5.7 | 10.4 | 11.1 |
| 1938 as % of 1921–1925 | 50 | - | 60 | 70 | 75 |
| Infant deaths per 1,000 births | | | | | |
| 1921–1925 | 156 | - | 187 | 201 | - |
| 1926–1930 | 147 | - | 172 | 192 | 151* |
| 1931–1935 | 147 | 122 | 157 | 182 | 153* |
| 1936 | 144 | 114 | 139 | 175 | 137* |
| 1937 | 150 | 122 | 134 | 178 | 141* |
| 1938 | 144 | - | 131 | 183 | 144* |
| 1938 as % of 1921–1925 | 92 | - | 70 | 91 | - |

*Approximate
Source: 'Demographic Problems of Southeastern Europe', *Population Index*, 7, 2 (1941), 86.

would have been convinced of the general connections between healthcare and nationalism. As seen in the previous section, since the establishment of nation states in the region, physicians had sought to protect national health through medical education, health reform and large-scale schemes of

preventive medicine. One of the most important corollaries to this development was the physician's extensive social and national involvement: a physician was now more than just a medical doctor caring for patients. He (and
increasingly she) gradually became an instrument of state politics, while
medicine became a medium for addressing moral and ethical questions pertaining to the health of the nation and society.

A host of further questions derive from this transformation, such as those
pertaining to the links between theories of national health, political philoso-
phies and social policies or how best to care for sick individuals in the wake
of an increased demand for a healthy society and nation. During the 1940s,
these visions of national decline and fragmentation were vividly portrayed in
eugenic discourses throughout Central and south-eastern Europe.[34] As
actively politicized eugenic discourses developed in these countries, ideas of
healthcare became part of a new political language used to describe and justify
new models of national belonging, just as much as financial constraints, political instability and domestic crises. The changes that had occurred in public
healthcare by the early 1940s were significant: the preoccupation with the
health of the nation had ceased to be the concern of a few individuals, and
become instead a central component of the national revolutions proclaimed
throughout Central and south-eastern Europe.

## The nationalization of healthcare

Apart from Hungary and Austria, all Central and south-eastern European
countries began the interwar period as victors of the First World War. In
these countries, a certain optimism characterized the health policies of the
1920s.[35] However, even in countries severely affected by the loss of their
previous status as regional powers, such as Hungary, healthcare programmes introduced during this period reflected the same engagement with
modern ideas of social hygiene, preventive medicine and large-scale vaccinations as countries such as Romania and Yugoslavia. Starting from 1922,
Hungarian medical doctors and trained nurses received Rockefeller fellowships to become specialists in various aspects of public healthcare at the
most prestigious institutions in the world.[36] Eventually, in 1925, the Hungarian Parliament legislated the establishment of the National Institute of
Public Health. The Rockefeller Foundation covered most of the initial costs,
and also supported the establishment of a school for the specialization of
public health officers (medical doctors) at the institute. Initially aimed at
providing practical training facilities for these students, a model district for
demonstration of public health organization was established in Gödöllő,
east of the capital. This centralization of public health brought together the
most important institutions devoted to urban and rural healthcare, as well
as the protection of mothers and infants and nursing care in Hungary,
including the previously mentioned National Stefánia Association and the
Green Cross Health Services, established in 1927.[37]

But there was another trend aiming to strengthen Hungary's recovery after Trianon through an elaborate system of social, economic, cultural and political measures. In this case, emphasis was laid on the need to nurture a shared scientific agenda as a necessary component of successful social and biological policies. Scientific institutes and various cultural and religious associations, as well as professional bodies such as the National Association of Hungarian Physicians, made a significant contribution to the crystallization of a eugenic discourse based on family, nation and race.

As a result of the gradual dissemination of evolutionary and racial ideas during the late nineteenth century, the nation became more than just a cultural construct: it was portrayed as a living organism, functioning according to biological laws, and embodying great physical qualities, symbols of innate virtues transmitted from generation to generation. This form of nationalism co-existed with other forms of identity such as religion, language or shared historical experiences. It is this fluid relationship between race and nation that must be noted within discussions on private and public traditions of healthcare in Central and south-eastern Europe.

It is also important to understand how public traditions of healthcare intersected with private and religious discussions of reproduction and the protection of the family. The key issue, therefore, was how to harmonize the interests of the state and the nation with the interests of individuals and families. While convincing the population of the necessity of a healthy life based on modern hygienic principles may have necessitated sustained medical education and well-implemented public health infrastructure, determining individual reproduction intersected with deep-seated religious and cultural patterns of family life that traditional communities in Central and south-eastern Europe considered unalterable. To this end, eugenics legitimated the state's intervention in the private lives of its citizens, claiming rights over reproductive practices such as contraception and abortion. In the name of a healthy nation, eugenics served as a mechanism with which the state and the church were able to orchestrate demographic policies, encouraging both large families and the protection of racial qualities.

As nation states in Central and south-eastern Europe became increasingly obsessed with their historical mission to create a racially, spiritually and linguistically homogeneous nation, they also resorted to coercive mechanisms – such as stigmatization, discrimination, segregation, and ultimately racial 'cleansing' – in order to protect their national members by eliminating those who were socially, ethnically and sexually different. It was in this context that radical biomedical agenda coupled with racism and anti-Semitism emerged during the 1940s.[38]

As recent literature has compellingly demonstrated, eugenics was not marginal in Central and south-eastern Europe; nor was it the preoccupation of a mere handful of Social Darwinist biologists, anthropologists and physicians.[39] The idea of a healthy nation was a contested eugenic concept, fought over by politicians, intellectuals, religious leaders and scientists. Competing authorities laid claim to the national body: the army, the church and the government. But eugenics knew no ideological restrictions. Socialists, conservatives and nationalists alike favoured ideas of human improvement, and so did religious groups such as the Catholics and the Protestants. The health of the nation thus politicized and ritualized echoed a wider worldview that drew on a biologized definition of identity. In this context, eugenics was intended to protect and improve not only the life of the individual but also to safeguard the social fabric, the family and the body of the nation.

The population was consistently portrayed in eugenic discourses as a biological entity whose growth, mortality, longevity and morbidity needed both regulation and supervision. Evoking a sense of an enduring threat, eugenics reconfigured the traditional understanding of individual, gender, and religious roles in society. Essentially, the boundary between private and public spheres was blurred by the idea of public responsibility for the nation, which came to dominate both. As a result, it became possible to connect notions of collective welfare with individual responsibility to the nation. But eugenic ideas of human improvement not only augmented forms of nationalism and anti-Semitism; more broadly, they endorsed the modernization of state and society in Central and south-eastern Europe. More research is needed to explore how health, social and population policies overlapped in eugenic projects in nationally specific cases in these regions. Also, one needs to assess how several medical initiatives in the fields of population policy and eugenics gradually penetrated larger intellectual circles and associations, becoming in some cases a matter of national policy. In practice this meant that the eugenic importance of reproduction and heredity was often discussed when health laws were debated in parliaments or taught in schools established for nurses or social workers.

For instance, physicians in Central and south-eastern Europe did not perceive eugenic screening for hereditary and infectious diseases as solely a medical problem. Its effects on the life of the community had long been debated. As politicians struggled to define a national consensus, their programme of social efficiency and rational planning intersected with the eugenicists' efforts to improve the health of the individuals and the family. The nation's health became essential to the country's future. To ensure it, medical and social problems would have to be controlled and managed. Within this protectionist rhetoric, the spread of venereal and infectious diseases such as malaria was deemed disastrous to the general health of the population, particularly as physicians and others described the existing sanitary conditions in their own countries in strikingly negative terms.[40]

Existing scholarship on Central and south-eastern European eugenics has concentrated on a select group of the educated professional and political elites. But while eugenic solutions to the nation's alleged biological deterioration were in fact initially advanced by the elites and later discussed by much of the urban middle class in Central and south-eastern Europe, in the interwar period eugenic arguments were extended, to be drawn from low birth rates in urban centres compared with those in rural areas, from the growing numbers of workers and their precarious living conditions and, in some cases, such as in Romania and Yugoslavia, from the existence of ethnic minorities and political scapegoating, including racism.[41] Even when they did not profess it openly, by the late 1930s most health reformers and hygienists in Central and south-eastern Europe had become fluent in the language of eugenics and the 'racial sciences'.

These occurrences should, of course, be placed in the context of domestic and international instability, the cultural propaganda of the Third Reich in south-eastern Europe from 1933 and, not least, a world war. Thus, between 1938 and 1945, Austria became part of Nazi Germany, only to be reconfigured once again at the end of the Second World War as a republic, becoming – like Greece – part of the West. During the same period, however, Poland and Czechoslovakia ceased to exist. They were re-created after 1945, joining Yugoslavia, Hungary, Romania, and Bulgaria as part of the newly emerging Communist East. After 1947, the majority of health reformers, especially in Romania, were gradually imprisoned; university chairs and departments were dissolved, and 'bourgeois' medicine was deemed 'incompatible' with the new scientific ideologies imported from the Soviet Union. By the 1950s, with the proclamation of the communist republics in Eastern Europe, public healthcare had entered a new period, one in which the Soviet model of socialized medicine predominated.

## Concluding remarks: Towards a new historiographic model

The inclusion and juxtaposition of Central and south-eastern European traditions of private and public healthcare with their well-known Western European counterparts is one of the ambitious historiographic aims characterizing this volume.

Compared to its precursors – which were undermined by ideological manipulation – current medical scholarship in Central and south-eastern Europe not only brings together significant themes and developments in medicine as part of social history, but also forcefully engages with some of the most central topics pertaining to the national traditions of these countries. And although there still is a divide between this new generation of historians of medicine and traditional historians, the hegemonic status of the latter is clearly being challenged.[42]

While the social history of medicine is intrinsically trans-disciplinary, this essential feature is diminished when the relationship between medical ideas and their historical context is not explicitly addressed. Social historians of medicine in Central and south-eastern Europe must therefore pointedly integrate their research within wider historiographic discussions if they want to overcome the reservations of their detractors. Navigating current methodologies and theories in the history of medicine should be complemented by an awareness of local primary sources.

What is needed now is a comparative theoretical framework, so that a variety of histories about these different medical traditions can be revealed and critically examined. Monographs and edited volumes are gradually being published both in and about the countries in Central and south-eastern Europe, a trend not only driven by the emergence of a new generation of medical historians but also, equally importantly, one that is defining the crystallization of social history of medicine as a discipline in the region. A number of factors contribute directly to this process, including improved access to archives, the influx of Western scholarship and, most importantly, scholars from Central and south-eastern European countries studying abroad.[43]

In pursuit of its new identity, the history of medicine in Central and south-eastern Europe should not only bring together significant themes and developments in medicine as part of social history, political demography and cultural anthropology, but should also forcefully engage with some of the most central topics pertaining to the historical traditions of these countries more generally. This recourse to historical memory is essential if, on the one hand, the Central and south-eastern countries are to be reconciled with their troubled pasts and if, on the other, the history of medicine more generally is to be systematically analysed through its appropriate local, regional, national and international contexts.[44]

Current debates about the meaning of national history in Central and south-eastern Europe yield eloquent examples of the ability of scholars in the region to produce different, almost competing, readings of the past. The social history of medicine is also currently undergoing a remarkable transformation – one defined on the one hand by society's need to engage with scientific advances and the ethical dilemmas they raise, and by the inclusion of hitherto marginalized case studies on the other.

The time has finally come for the private and public traditions of healthcare in Central and south-eastern Europe to be firmly situated within their own historiographic canon. To be sure, there remains room for improvement, especially in terms of methodology and access to archival collections. Above all, it is imperative that works of comprehensive synthesis be produced – studies that move away from narrow definitions of medical history and are theoretically and analytically robust. Besides the task of mediating between the local canons and their international context, there is a pressing need to tackle these phenomena within a framework of the region's entangled history, more specifically to look at medical traditions, both private and public, from a regional and cross-national perspective.

## Further reading

Medical traditions of healthcare in Central and south-eastern Europe remain under-researched, although much has been accomplished since the collapse of communism in 1989. Testimony to the growing interest in these areas are two recent special issues: the first, edited by Teodora Daniela Sechel, deals with

'Networks of Medical Knowledge in Central and Eastern Europe' (*East-Central Europe*, 40, 1, 2013); the second, edited by Andreas Renner and Katharina Kreuder-Sonnen, focuses on 'Öffentliche Hygiene in Osteuropa/ Public Hygiene in Eastern Europe' (*Jahrbücher für Geschichte Osteuropas*, 61, 4, 2013). Also worth mentioning is the special issue on 'Science, Medicine and Nationalism in the Habsburg Empire from the 1840s to 1918', edited by Tatjana Buklijas and Emese Lafferton (*Studies in the History and Philosophy of Science*, Part C, 38, 4, 2007). In connection to the latter, one will certainly find useful Mitchell G. Ash and Jan Surman (eds), *The Nationalization of Scientific Knowledge in the Habsburg Empire, 1848–1918* (Basingstoke: Palgrave Macmillan, 2012). The contextualization of medical traditions in Central and Eastern Europe within its international context is attempted in Iris Borowy and Wolf D. Gruner (eds), *Facing Illness in Troubled Times: Health in Europe in the Interwar Years, 1918–1939* (Bern: Peter Lang, 2005). Iris Borowy, together with Anne Hardy, also edited *Of Medicine and Men: Biographies and Ideas in European Social Medicine between the World Wars* (Bern: Peter Lang, 2008), which includes chapters on Béla Johan and Andrija Štampar. For the transfer of German medical knowledge to Eastern Europe one may consult Paul J. Weindling, *Epidemics and Genocide in Eastern Europe, 1880–1945* (Oxford: Oxford University Press, 2000). A good introduction to the history of social assistance and public welfare in Eastern Europe is provided by Sabine Hering and Berteke Waaldijk (eds), *Guardians of the Poor – Custodians of the Public: Welfare History in Eastern Europe, 1900–1960* (Opladen: Barbara Budrich Publishers, 2006). Also important in this respect is Susan Gross Solomon, Lion Murard and Patrick Zylberman (eds), *Shifting Boundaries of Public Health: Europe in the Twentieth Century* (Rochester, NY: University of Rochester Press, 2008). Finally, essential for an understanding of the history of eugenics in the region are the volumes edited by Gerhard Baader, Veronika Hofer and Thomas Mayer, *Eugenik in Österreich: Biopolitische Strukturen von 1900–1945* (Vienna: Czernin Verlag, 2008) and Marius Turda, *The History of Eugenics in East Central Europe, 1900–1945: Sources and Commentaries* (forthcoming, Bloomsbury, 2015).

## Notes

1 See Justyna A. Turkowska, 'Im Namen der "großen Kolonisationsaufgaben": Das Hygiene Institut in Posen (1899–1920) und die preußische Hegemonialpolitik in der Ostmark', *Jahrbücher für Geschichte Osteuropas*, 61, 4 (2013): 552–73.
2 Katrin Steffen, 'Experts and the Modernization of the Nation: The Arena of Public Health in Poland in the First Half of the Twentieth Century', *Jahrbücher für Geschichte Osteuropas*, 61, 4 (2013): 574–90.
3 See Christian Promitzer, Sevasti Trubeta and Marius Turda (eds), *Health, Hygiene and Eugenics in Southeast Europe to 1945* (Budapest: CEU Press, 2011); Teodora Daniela Sechel (ed.), *Medicine within and between the Habsburg and Ottoman Empires, Eighteenth–Nineteenth Centuries* (Bochum: Winkler Verlag, 2011); and Constantin Bărbulescu and Alin Ciupală (eds), *Medicine, Hygiene and Society from the Eighteenth to the Twentieth Centuries* (Cluj-Napoca: Ed. Mega, 2012).

4  Mark Harrison, *Contagion: How Commerce Has Spread Disease* (Oxford: Oxford University Press, 2012).
5  Birsen Bulmuş, *Plague, Quarantines and Geopolitics in the Ottoman Empire* (Edinburgh: Edinburgh University Press, 2012).
6  Charles S. Ryan and John Sandes, *Under the Red Crescent. Adventures of an English Surgeon with the Turkish Army at Plevna and Erzeroum, 1877–1878* (New York: Charles Scribner's Sons, 1897).
7  Paul J. Weindling, *Epidemics and Genocide in Eastern Europe, 1890–1945* (Oxford: Oxford University Press, 2000).
8  Thoma Ionescu, *Starea sanitară a României* (Bucharest: Ed. Viaţa Medicală Românească, 1999 [first published in 1906]).
9  Paul Dudley White, 'Public Health in Eastern Macedonia', *American Journal of Public Health*, 19, 1 (1920): 14.
10  Zsuzsa Bokor, *Testtörténetek. A nemzet és a nemi betegségek medikalizálása a két világháború közötti Kolozsváron* (Kolozsvár: Nemzeti Kisebbségkutató Intézet, 2013).
11  See George Antonakopoulos, 'The Royal Medical Council of Greece, 1834–1922', in Marius Turda (ed), 'Private and Public Medical Traditions in the Greece and the Balkans', special issue of *Deltos: Journal of the History of Hellenic Medicine*, (2012): 33–6.
12  See, for example, Petr Svobodný and Ludmila Hlaváčková, *Dějiny lékařství v českých zemích* (Prague: Triton, 2004); Károly Kapronczay and Katalin Kapronczay (eds), *Az orvostörténelem Magyarországon* (Budapest: Semmelweis Orvostörténeti Múzeum, 2005); and Radu Iftimovici, *Istoria universală a medicinii şi farmaciei* (Bucharest: Editura Academiei Române, 2008).
13  Teodora Daniela Sechel, 'The Politics of Medical Translations and Its Impact upon Medical Knowledge in the Habsburg Monarchy, 1770–1830', *East Central Europe*, 40, 3 (2013): 296–318.
14  Susan Zimmermann, *Divide, Provide and Rule: An Integrative History of Poverty Policy, Social Policy, and Social Reform in Hungary under the Habsburg Monarchy* (Budapest: CEU Press, 2011).
15  Erik Ingebrigtsen, '"National Models" and Reforms of Public Health in Interwar Hungary', in György Péteri (ed.), *Imagining the West in Eastern Europe and the Soviet Union* (Pittsburgh, PA: Pittsburgh University Press, 2010), 36–58.
16  Marius Turda and Paul J. Weindling (eds), *Blood and Homeland Eugenics and Racial Nationalism in Central and Southeast Europe, 1900–1940* (Budapest: CEU Press, 2007).
17  Christian Promitzer, 'Typhus, Turks, and Roma: Hygiene and Ethnic Difference in Bulgaria, 1912–1944', in Promitzer, Trubeta and Turda (eds), *Health, Hygiene and Eugenics in Southeast Europe*, 87–125.
18  Paul J. Weindling (ed.), *International Health Organisations and Movements, 1918–1939* (Cambridge: Cambridge University Press, 1995).
19  Marta Alexandra Balińska, 'Assistance and Not Mere Relief: The Epidemic Commission of the League of Nations, 1920–1923', in Weindling (ed.), *International Health Organisations*, 99–100; and Patrick Zylberman, 'Mosquitos and the Komitadjis: Malaria and Borders in Macedonia (1919–1938)', in Iris Borowy and Wolf D. Gruner (eds), *Facing Illness in Troubled Times: Health in Europe in the Interwar Years, 1918–1939* (Bern: Peter Lang, 2005), 305–43.
20  Mihail Manicatide, 'Pentru ce medical rural nu-şi poate face datoria', *Viaţa românească*, 1, 2 (1906): 315.
21  See Constantin Bărbulescu, 'Tema degenerării rasei în literatura medicală din România la sfârşitul secolului al XIX-lea', in Nicolae Bocşan, Sorin Mitu and Toader Nicoară (eds), *Identitate şi alteritate. Studii de istorie politică şi culturală*, Vol. 3 (Cluj: Presa Universitară Clujeană, 2002), 273–90; and Marius Turda, *Eugenism şi antropologie rasială în România* (Bucharest: Cuvântul, 2008).

22 Béla Johan, 'Public Health Services in Hungary', *The Hungarian Quarterly*, 4, 3 (1938): 427–33.

23 Andrija Štampar, *Public Health in Jugoslavia* (London: School of Slavonic and East European Studies, 1938).

24 Iuliu Haţieganu, 'Rolul social al medicului în opera de consolidare a statului naţional', *Transilvania*, 54 (1925), 588.

25 Quoted in Mária M. Kovács, *Liberal Professions & Illiberal Politics: Hungary from the Habsburgs to the Holocaust* (Washington, DC: Woodrow Wilson Center Press, 1994), 67.

26 Patrick Zylberman, 'Fewer Parallels than Antitheses: René Sand and Andrija Štampar on Social Medicine, 1919-1955', *Social History of Medicine*, 17, 1 (2004): 77–92; Paul Weindling, 'A City Regenerated: Eugenics, Race and Welfare in Interwar Vienna', in Deborah Holmes and Lisa Silverman (eds), *Interwar Vienna: Culture between Tradition and Modernity* (Rochester, NY: Camden House, 2009), 81–113; and František Čapka, 'Gustav Kabrhel: The Founder of the Czech Public Health Science and His Contribution to the "School and Health" Issues', *School and Health*, 21 (2011): 19–23

27 Petru Râmneanţu, 'Fundaţia Rockefeller', *Buletin eugenic şi biopolitic*, 16, 1–12 (1945): 120–43.

28 Gábor Palló, 'Make a Peak on the Plain: The Rockefeller Foundation's Szeged Project', in William H. Schneider (ed.), *Rockefeller Philanthropy and Modern Medicine: International Initiatives from World War I to the Cold War* (Bloomington: Indiana University Press, 2002), 87–105; and on Greece, see Vassiliki Theodoru and Despina Karakatsani, 'Health Policy in Interwar Greece: The Intervention by the League of Nations Health Organisation', *Dynamis*, 28 (2008): 53–75.

29 Despina Karakatsani and Vassiliki Theodoru, *'Hygiene Imperatives': Medical Supervision and Child Welfare in Greece in the First Decades of the Twentieth Century* (Athens: Dionikos, 2010) and Haralambos Oikonomou and Manos Spyridakis (eds), *Anthropological and Sociological Perspectives on Health* (Athens: I. Sideris, 2012).

30 Henry E. Sigerist, 'Yugoslavia and the Eleventh International Congress of the History of Medicine', *Bulletin of the History of Medicine*, 7 (1939): 99–147.

31 Béla Johan, *Rural Health Work in Hungary* (Budapest: The State Hygienic Institute, 1939).

32 The data is for the year 1924, and provided by Gheorghe Banu, 'Biologia satelor', *Arhiva pentru ştiinţă şi reformă socială* 7, 1–2 (1927): 87–121.

33 Marius Turda, 'Crafting a Healthy Nation: European Eugenics in Historical Context', in Marius Turda (ed.), *Crafting Humans: From Genesis to Genetics and Beyond* (Göttingen: V&R Unipress, 2013), 109–26.

34 Marius Turda, 'Controlling the National Body: Ideas of Racial Purification in Romania, 1918–1944', in Promitzer, Trubeta and Turda (eds), *Health, Hygiene and Eugenics in Southeastern Europe*, 325–50.

35 Marta Aleksandra Balińska, 'The National Institute of Hygiene and Public Health in Poland, 1918–1939', *Social History of Medicine*, 9, 3 (1996): 427–45.

36 Paul Weindling, 'Public Health and Political Stabilisation: The Rockefeller Foundation in Central and Eastern Europe between the Two World Wars', *Minerva*, 31, (1993): 253–67.

37 Gheorghe Banu, 'Organizarea igienei sociale în Ungaria', *Revista de igienă socială*, 1, 9 (1931): 800–809.

38 Anton Weiss-Wendt and Rory Yeomans (eds), *Racial Science in Hitler's New Europe, 1938–1945* (Lincoln: University of Nebraska Press, 2013); and Marius Turda, 'In Pursuit of Greater Hungary: Eugenic Ideas of Social and Biological Improvement, 1940–1941', *The Journal of Modern History*, 85, 3 (2013): 558–91.

39 Alison Bashford and Philippa Levine (eds), *The Oxford Handbook of the History of Eugenics* (New York: Oxford University Press, 2010); Sevasti Trubeta, *Physical Anthropology, Race and Eugenics in Greece 1880s–1970s* (Leiden: Brill, 2013); and Marius Turda, *Eugenics and Nation in Early Twentieth Century Hungary* (Basingstoke: Palgrave Macmillan, 2014).
40 One example is the assistance against malaria in Bulgaria during the late 1930s provided by German public health doctors from the Hamburg Tropical Hygiene Institute such as Peter Mühlens. See Stefan Wulf, *Das Hamburger Tropeninstitut 1919 bis 1945. Auswärtige Kulturpolitik und Kolonialrevisionismus nach Versailles* (Berlin: Dietrich Reimer Verlag, 1994), 110–16.
41 See Tudor Georgescu, 'Ethnic Minorities and the Eugenic Promise: The Transylvanian Saxon Experiment with National Renewal in Inter-War Romania', *European Review of History*, 17, 6 (2010): 861–80; and Ben Thorne, 'Assimilation, Invisibility, and the Eugenic Turn in the "Gypsy Question" in Romanian Society, 1938–1942', *Romani Studies*, 21, 2 (2011): 177–205.
42 Marius Turda and Steven King, 'Journeying across Empires: An Agenda for Future Research in Central and Southeastern European History of Medicine', in Daniela Sechel (ed.), *Medicine Within and Between the Habsburg and Ottoman Empires*, 235–42.
43 Marius Turda, 'Focus on Social History of Medicine in Central and Eastern Europe', *Social History of Medicine*, 21, 2 (2008): 395–401; and Marius Turda, 'Focus on Austria and Germany', *Social History of Medicine* 23, 2 (2010): 408–12.
44 Marius Turda, 'History of Medicine in Eastern Europe, including Russia', in Mark Jackson (ed.), *The Oxford Handbook of the History of Medicine* (Oxford: Oxford University Press, 2011), 208–24.

# 7 Healthcare as nation-building in the twentieth century

## The case of the British National Health Service

*Glen O'Hara and George Campbell Gosling*

### Introduction

On the 'appointed day' of Monday 5 July 1948, Britain's Labour government introduced a whole raft of social reforms, including the inception of the National Health Service (NHS). In many respects the NHS is unique: 'alone among its capitalist partners, the United Kingdom offered comprehensive health care to its entire population'.[1] Labour created it by nationalising the nation's municipal and voluntary hospitals, as well as instituting government funding of general practitioners, dentists and other healthcare providers on a per capita basis and mandating that local government provide certain public health services.[2] This tripartite system was funded primarily from general taxation and made universally available free at the point of use. As such, the NHS has always entailed compromises between public and private: while GPs and dentists remain essentially private, the state funds NHS patients, who are thus seen without charge. For most of its history the NHS has been a free service, yet one with prescription charges. More recently it has also been a public service that has seen medical care increasingly provided either by private contractors to NHS patients, or by the NHS to private or 'self-funded' patients.[3]

There is a common tendency towards national exceptionalism in all writing about the NHS, yet we can better understand the NHS by locating it within a wider tendency to use those reforms as part of nation-building and post-war rebuilding. In this way social reform has often been associated with attempts to rejuvenate 'national spirit' in the period after a crisis, such as war or depression.[4] The reorganisations to which the NHS has been subject throughout its history should also be understood as attempts to reform the service in keeping with a changing nation, whether driving or following that change: most recently, this has been evident in the rise of a more consumer-orientated society. This chapter will seek to explore the ambitions, compromises, achievements and failures associated with the NHS, as well as its abiding popularity. In order to shed light on its complex history, the emphasis is placed firmly on the national and international context of the service, rather than its more detailed administration. Both were first and foremost true of its foundation amid a wider programme of post-war reconstruction.

**Reconstruction**

It was envisaged in the 1940s that the new NHS would bolster post-war rebuilding via a sense of communal citizenship, enjoyed as of right, an idea often associated with the sociologists T.H. Marshall and Richard Titmuss. Marshall, indeed, imagined creating a new 'class fusion', in which 'equality of status is more important than equality of income'.[5] Titmuss believed that the wartime Emergency Hospital Service had brought British citizens and medical practitioners psychologically closer together, just as much as it had demonstrated the benefits of central planning: 'in total war the troubles of individuals often multiplied until they became matters of national concern, while the demands of humanity pointed, just as often, in the same direction'.[6] Just such a renewed combination of direction and humanity would also allow, in Titmuss's 1957 view, a more even and consistent application of the new sciences without the pollution of hierarchy, which it was hoped would 'come in time from the contribution of the sociologist and the social worker to a greater understanding of the dynamics of human relationships ... the task of the future is to make medicine more "social" in its application without losing in the process the benefits of science and specialized knowledge'.[7]

In the 1990s Gøsta Esping-Andersen would specify this cluster of ideas as describing 'those countries in which the principles of universalism and de-commodification of social rights were extended also to the new middle classes'.[8] Titmuss's and Marshall's ideas gave rise, in Esping-Andersen's schema, to systems very different to the 'liberal' welfare states, such as Australia and the United States, which aimed benefits at the poor, and the 'corporatist-statist' examples on the European continent that linked rights to 'class' and 'status'. Britain may have been a relatively unsuccessful example of such a 'social democratic' model when compared to the Nordic countries: alongside Marshallian universalism, she clearly retained elements from the liberal model of limited benefits and a stigmatised poor. But Labour's intention in 1948 was to move as close to this ideal as possible.[9]

Both the Prime Minister Clement Attlee and Aneurin Bevan as his Minister of Health were very clear that they intended the NHS to reforge a sense of social citizenship. As the hugely influential 1942 Beveridge Report had opined, the 'organisation of social insurance' was 'one part only of a comprehensive policy of social progress', designed to tackle the 'five giants on the road of reconstruction': want, disease, ignorance, squalor and idleness. Contributions would be required from all, but then benefits would be granted 'as of right and without means test, so that individuals may build freely upon [them]'.[10] In his radio broadcast to the nation on the eve of social security's inception, Attlee spoke of the desire, not to treat sickness, but 'to make a healthy nation': the need 'to ensure that the provision of proper care and treatment shall not depend on financial resources', to offer 'complete cover for health by pooling the nation's resources, not dependent on insurance', and to build 'one great service' based on the fact that 'all hospitals will pass into the country's ownership'.[11] With this focus on ending the insurance principle – which Winston Churchill had described as 'bringing in the magic of averages to the aid of the millions'[12] – and a mix of public services funded through the rates (local property taxes) and the Poor Law, it is easy to see 1948 as a radical break from the past. In many respects it was. However, we should also bear in mind that a host of reforms over the course of the early twentieth century had sought to establish new foundations for the delivery of health and welfare services, including those the post-war Labour government was now determined to abolish as part of the old system.

For the beginnings of the insurance principle in British social policy, we need to look not to Britain in the early twentieth century, but to Germany in the late nineteenth century, home to the reforms of Otto von Bismarck, the Prussian Minister-President who became the first Chancellor of a unified and imperial Germany in 1871. This was done through the 1880s by compulsory insurance laws covering sickness (1883), accident (1884), as well as old age and disability (both 1889). Although unpopular in Britain at the time, the German example came by the early twentieth century to be influential for many, if by no means all, senior politicians and policymakers.[13] Three decades before his wartime report on social security would set the stage for 1940s social reform, William Beveridge worked at the Board of Trade, where he seized on the Bismarckian models of employment exchanges and sickness insurance.[14] Meanwhile the Chancellor of the Exchequer, David Lloyd George, went on a five-day visit to Germany in August 1908 to examine the possibility of a health insurance system on their model.[15] Since the landslide Liberal election victory of 1906, Britain had seen a host of social reforms under the 'New Liberal' leadership of Churchill and Lloyd George. These had included the introduction of the school medical service and old age pensions. Now, under Lloyd George at the Treasury and Churchill at the Board of Trade, Britain was to introduce health and unemployment insurance, along a distinctly German line.[16] What emerged in the 1911 National Insurance Act, despite some differences in funding and administration, was an unmistakably Bismarckian system of compulsory insurance providing workers with access to a doctor and cash benefits at times of sickness and unemployment.[17]

The decades leading up to the creation of the NHS were essentially the territory of local and voluntary initiative, such as the Pioneer Health Centre in Peckham, which pursued a preventive approach based on a social understanding of health and sickness.[18] This was an isolated experiment in social medicine, but it came at the same time as social work was expanding rapidly in hospitals across the country, bringing a social dimension to the view the medical team took of a patient.[19] The 1930s also saw a notable expansion in municipal provision of general hospital services, following new powers granted to 'appropriate' Poor Law infirmaries in the 1929 Local Government Act. This legislation, passed by Neville Chamberlain as Health Minister, aimed to end the outdated Victorian Poor Law system.[20] This development is especially significant, as it shows a break from the pattern that distinguished British

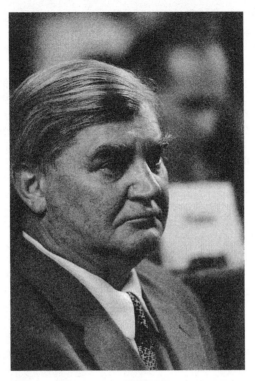

*Figure 7.1* Aneurin Bevan, Minister of Health in the post-war Labour government.
    © British Library. All Rights Reserved.

reforms to tackle poverty from German nation-building. That is to say, this Act set local authorities on a course of providing health services to the community as a whole, providing a cross-class service rather than addressing particular sections of the population with the aim of keeping the deserving out of the workhouse.

In some respects, therefore, the NHS was the culmination of early twentieth-century reforms. However, it was also a fundamental break with these. Where voluntary and municipal hospitals had been co-operating before the war, they had done so on a local level, whereas the new service was a national one, administered regionally. Where many, including most of the Labour Party, expected reforms to bring healthcare under the auspices of local government, it was nationalised. So how do we explain this change of heart? We might see the NHS as simply another of the 1945 government's nationalisations, but there were fierce fights between Bevan and Herbert Morrison, the minister responsible for local government, on the matter.[21] Many historians have seen Bevan himself as personally shaping the health service he introduced.[22] Others have looked instead to the civil servants in the Ministry of Health.[23] If one thing is clear, it is that the nationalised system that emerged was far from inevitable.

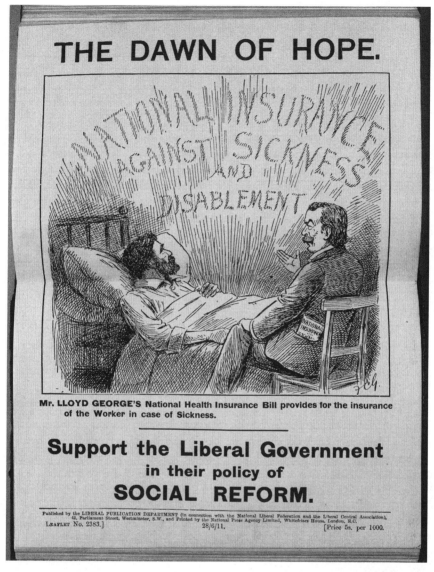

*Figure 7.2* 'The dawn of hope'. National insurance against sickness. © British Library.
All Rights Reserved.

It is also worth noting, however, that the NHS was from the start a
system that looked outwards, attempting to draw lessons from global
experiences of nation-building via state welfare schemes rather than taking
refuge in national insularity. The service's ideological father, William Beveridge had, in particular, been impressed by New Zealand's 1938 Social
Security Act, which had ended the payment of fees for hospital patients via

the introduction of hospital benefits – one of the reasons he accepted an invitation to tour the country in 1948, despite the fact that he turned 70 on the voyage out to the Southern Seas.[24] New Zealand was one of the first states in the world to end the principle of paying social insurance dues in return for healthcare rights, and to accept the idea of a universal scheme funded out of general taxation: hence Beveridge's interest and admiration, and the manner in which both doctors and politicians framed their arguments in terms of this Antipodean example.[25]

Looking inward, the creation of the Service had involved a series of compromises with the doctors, who resisted the spectre of government 'interference', and especially hated the idea of any connection with local government at all. Even the publication of Bevan's Bill was met with accusations at rather senior levels of the medical profession that this represented 'the first step ... towards National Socialism as practised in Germany', and 'the greatest seizure of property since Henry VIII confiscated the monasteries'.[26] One reason why Bevan decided very rapidly, on attaining office, to nationalise the hospitals is that this might actually reduce doctors' resistance to the new scheme, given their antipathy to local government involvement on the lines of Labour's 1944 White Paper. Sweeping away the last vestiges of the old voluntary hospital system and insurance schemes, as well as municipal hospitals built by local councils, was unpopular with a Treasury that wanted to maintain some local and charitable financial contribution to health service funding; although central government was already making a significant contribution to the running of these independent hospitals.[27]

The decisive point in this argument thus became the fact that such an income stream was unlikely to remain very buoyant. Such hospitals' charitable income and subscription schemes had been in decline for some time, since at least the First World War, leaving a gap in their finances.[28] Paul Brigden has suggested that, having failed to meet growing demand from among the middle classes, the voluntary hospitals were left without the support of this group when the debate about nationalisation came to the fore.[29] However, opinion polls from the 1940s show that the middle classes remained the strongest supporters of the voluntary hospitals.[30] An explanation for the apparent contradiction may lie in the fact that hospital treatment itself continued to be seen as undesirable into the mid-twentieth century, resulting in less demand than might have been forthcoming in terms of medical 'need' alone.[31]

## Reorganisation

How much did the introduction of the NHS in 1948 change healthcare for patients in Britain? As Helen Jones has pointed out:

> The picture of a distinctive health service which made a clean break with the past needs some modification. Most historians now point to significant continuities in healthcare provision. The creation of the NHS did

not in itself lead to the building of any new hospitals, the training of extra doctors or the evolution of new drugs and treatment.[32]

Yet it crucially created a new framework within which services could be accessed equally by all and without consideration of payment. This change was felt on the day the new service came into being. The future social work lecturer and researcher Phyllis Wilmott, at this point working as a student at St Thomas' Hospital in London, 'joyfully abandoned the little tin boxes' into which patients had always placed donations: 'it was the symbolic new beginning of a health service that was intended to be free for all'.[33]

Prime Minister Attlee was himself fully aware that a new health service would not be spared from old challenges. On the eve of the inception of the NHS he declared: 'once more we shall be faced with all kinds of anomalies, just in those areas where hospital facilities are most needed, and in those very conditions where the mass of the poor people will be unable to find the finance to supply the hospitals'.[34] A lack of co-ordination and communication between the newly unified service providers was another inherited problem. Divisions between GPs, general hospitals, teaching hospitals and those ancillary services still managed by local authorities ran deep. A lack of adequate communications was evident throughout the system, as Beveridge constantly bemoaned in the speeches he made in the House of Lords in his old age.[35] This was in large part due to the enormous inheritance of infrastructure and attitudes the NHS had to work with – vastly complex arrangements that no one Act could transform. The hospitals had indeed been nationalised, grouped together under Regional Hospital Boards; but the other two elements of the 'tripartite' structure, the self-employed general practitioners and local government working on public health, were subject to completely different arrangements. Poor co-ordination, and political jostling for position, were in these circumstances inevitable.[36]

These realities also stalled any movement towards all-purpose local health centres. These had long been imagined by health reformers as providing a truly integrated service, including dentists, chiropody, community nursing, physiotherapy, and even healthy cafés, gyms and swimming baths for all – modern, forward-thinking and progressive, on the lines of those built between the wars at the Finsbury Health Centre and the Pioneer Centre in Peckham.[37] David Stark Murray, chairman of the Socialist Medical Association, told the Labour Party Conference in 1947 that health centres could become 'the symbol to the whole of the people of this country of what a Socialist Medical Health Service really means'.[38] But they were neither tremendously popular nor immediately summoned into being by the creation of the NHS.[39] To the wider public, they appeared to threaten individual relations between general practitioner and patient, they seemed more impersonal, they might be further away, and they were thought of as more standardised and therefore bureaucratic. Sixty-nine per cent of Gallup's respondents approved of the idea of health centres in principle when they were asked about them in 1944,[40] but only a little more than a fifth of women surveyed in 1943, considered by Mass-Observation to be 'always more conservative and less progressive in outlook than men', indicated themselves to be happy to attend these, rather than the smaller and more traditional doctor's surgery. Even among men, only a third were in favour of attending these new centres.[41]

Such ambivalence was reflected in official policy, concerned as ever not to impose too many conditions on the doctors. Once he was Minister for Health, Bevan made clear to local authorities that he did not expect to see them submitting immediate plans for health centres, given the economic constraints and the needs of the rest of the NHS. Only a very few were built, mostly in new suburban settlements or in New Towns.[42] In their absence, however, conditions in general practice hardly improved: indeed, they may have deteriorated, with only 17 per cent of family doctors working from what a 1951–52 BMA survey logged as 'good well-equipped' sites, and only a further 49 per cent working at sites 'adequate' for their work.[43] It took until the 1960s to get the health centre movement going on any large scale.[44]

During this first phase of the NHS there was, in fact, as strong a degree of continuity as change – something that cannot be said of any period since the 1960s. In the 1950s the NHS had been relatively unsuccessful in the competition for government spending, losing out to areas such as education that were seen as less successful.[45] If this inhibited ambitious reform for a time, it was no longer the case once Enoch Powell became Health Minister in 1960, embracing the idea of devising plans for the coming ten to fifteen years to guide a programme of modernisation and hospital-building. While the reasons for the 1962 Hospital Plan failing to live up to its own lofty ambitions have been debated, the sheer scale of those ambitions cannot be doubted.[46] The Hospital Plan was the very embodiment of the post-war faith in central planning. Its own failure coincided with a wider loss of confidence in the state and set the stage for a rather different approach under the next Conservative government in the 1970s.

The whole system had to be reorganised in 1973–74, after which the Department of Health and Social Security remained at the apex of the decision-making pyramid. Below it, appointed regional health boards and area health authorities, now arranged according to the same borders as reorganised local government, directed the activities of district management teams; the latter were now supposed to concert the efforts of hospitals, GPs and local government alike. It was an attempt to draw together the various parts of the tripartite structure that had been left standing after Bevan's concessions. According to the new *Management Arrangements for the Reorganised National Health Service*, popularly known as the 'Grey Book', each was supposed to consult with the other, especially at area and district level.[47] But the NHS was now a multi-layered organisation indeed, and it was often thereafter criticised for being slow, unwieldy and unresponsive, its four-layered operation both bureaucratic and disjointed.[48] The number of administrative staff increased by nearly 30 per cent in three years; four-fifths of those administrators surveyed in 1977 thought that the NHS had by then too many managerial tiers; the much-heralded increases in financial autonomy never materialised, as Whitehall exerted more, not less, control over a confused and directionless system.[49]

An increasingly wealthy and assertive populace became more and more notably organised in pressure groups that demanded that greater notice be taken of patients' and families' needs: the foundation of the Patients Association in 1963, following a damaging series of revelations concerning patients being used for medical experiments without their knowledge, is the most obvious case in point.[50] By 1979 a Directory of Organisations for Patients and Disabled People listed more than 230 of these groups.[51] But it took a long time before their pressure forced administrators and doctors to agree to successive governments' attempts to build up a proper complaints and investigative machinery. The Davies Review, under the High Court Judge Sir Michael Davies, reported on hospital complaints in the mid-1970s, but his recommendations were only codified in final form in 1981; a Health Service Commissioner or 'Ombudsman', appointed to look into problems on the administrative side, only started work in 1973, after long campaigns against the idea mounted from within the NHS.[52] Formal consultative machinery, representing the rights of patients, consumers and voluntary organisations as well as the views of doctors and managers, had to wait for the appointment of community health councils in 1974. These councils gradually gathered more powers to themselves – to speak at health authority meetings, and to approve or veto hospital closures – and added at least one representative capacity to an NHS that was struggling to respond to increasingly outspoken patients and citizens.[53]

This was an unwieldy set of compromises that came under increasing attack, from any number of directions, which allowed Margaret Thatcher's Conservative government of the 1980s a large amount of ideological space in which to reshape the NHS once more. In 1982 the regional and area tiers were abolished, allowing the districts to take up most of the Service's planning and delivery; competitive tendering was introduced at the same time, while the introduction of generalist and responsible management began the following year. A sense of crisis surrounding waiting times was still evident in 1987 when a two-month-old baby, David Barber, died following heart surgery that had been postponed five times.[54] This seemed to prove the need for further reform. In 1991 more radical changes inspired by the concept of an 'internal market' allowed 'fundholding' GPs to take control of about 20 per cent of the hospital budget, chiefly involving elective surgery and outpatient appointments; more radical pilot projects were underway when Labour came to office in 1997, calling this experiment to a halt.[55]

To begin with, Tony Blair's government proceeded cautiously, replacing the Conservatives' purchaser-provider split with wider primary care groups that would be subject to strategic planning by health authorities. GP commissioning would therefore be submerged in a wider and more holistic set of contracts, while simultaneously avoiding yet another upheaval.[56] This delicate balance was later overturned by a new Blairite radicalism, itself partly caused by a search for rapid results. Blair announced in 2000 that UK health spending would rise to average EU levels, and thereafter spending rose by an unprecedented average of 7.4 per cent between 2002/3 and 2007/8.[57] In 2003/4 alone, real-terms NHS spending in the UK went up by nearly 11 per cent.[58] The quid pro quo for these historic increases was a new emphasis on quasi-market solutions: as Blair's key adviser Julian Le Grand put it:

> [F]or the choice-and-competition model to work ... there have to be competitors, actual and/or potential ... there have to be alternative providers from which to choose; there have to be easy ways for new providers to enter the market ... and there have to be ways of preventing existing providers engaging in anti-competitive behaviour. In short, the competition must be real.[59]

From around 2002, and taking their cue from the 2000 NHS Plan, Labour in office gave geographically-defined primary care trusts in England the power to commission services, and to devolve this power to GPs if they so chose – though this time, to prevent 'creaming off', costs and charges were on a fixed basis, rather than the local and competing rates of the Conservatives' internal market. This was followed by the introduction of foundation hospitals, which was the latest in a series of policies since the 1980s providing a gradual but coherent encouragement of hospitals 'opting out' from government oversight in its various forms.[60] A 'Choose and Book' computer system and the NHS Choices website were supposed to allow patients to choose which provider they wanted to be referred to.[61] Individuation and an emphasis on 'choice' did not end there. In its later years this Labour administration also began to give effect to what it termed a 'personalisation' agenda: Blair announced in 2004 that he wanted to 'change the National Health Service into a persona-lised health service for each individual'. Expert patient programmes for patients with chronic diseases, and the electronic Choose and Book system for hospital appointments, were supposed to bolster this sense of individual ownership and 'choice'.[62] The combination of vastly increased funding with structural reform appeared to lead to an improved service, both in terms of shortening waiting lists and in the eyes of the public themselves.[63] It is to this question of popularity that we now turn.

## Popularity

There was no public clamour for a national health service in the mid-1940s. Nick Hayes has examined the opinion polls of the time and found working-class opinion divided between the status quo and a reformed system, while the opposition to state-run hospitals was stronger among the middle classes.[64] Fifty-five per cent of the public were in favour of 'a publicly run health service' when asked by Gallup in July 1944, but 32 per cent were in favour of things remaining 'as they are'.[65] Asked what they thought of a state service as the Second World War came to an end, many more middle-class Britons were concerned that there would be a 'levelling down' rather than a 'levelling up'. As one young Wren told the innovative social investigators Mass-Observation:

I think it is better to have the doctor responsible for the health of the person concerned to the person and not to the State. A lazy doctor could, in the other case, make out that the person's health was up to State requirements and standard of health, and therefore clear ... himself of the obligation to the patient to cure the particular ill of the patient.[66]

There were equally divided opinions among the political class, as the Conservatives within the wartime coalition government would have much preferred a continuation of an insurance-based system, retaining much more independent freedom of choice for both doctors and patients. Had they continued in office after 1945, they would also probably have allowed hitherto self-governing voluntary hospitals to continue as independent institutions with some of their own funds.[67] Henry Willink, the Conservative Health Minister in Churchill's caretaker government, which held office between the end of the coalition and Labour's election in the summer of 1945, proposed the creation of joint area and regional planning councils. These would only extend co-operation between local authorities, voluntary hospitals and doctors. The Conservatives voted against both the second and third readings of the National Health Service Bill for just these reasons.[68]

Despite this, the NHS did gradually become a popular and established feature of British national life. By February 1948, the eve of the Service's actual operation, 61 per cent of Britons told Gallup it was a 'good thing', and only 13 per cent considered it a 'bad' idea. It was by far the most popular single action of the post-war Labour government, with 35 per cent of respondents singling the NHS out as 'the best thing' that Mr Attlee's administration had done. In 1953, 70 per cent of those polled declared themselves 'satisfied' with their treatment; that figure had risen to 80 per cent a decade later, and remained at exactly that same level when the question was asked again in 1965.[69] Healthcare provided free at the point of use was synonymous with the 'social services' for most Britons; when asked what services they associated with the phrase in 1950, the NHS was the answer given by easily the most respondents, with no other benefit receiving more than 7 per cent of the replies.[70] The NHS was so entrenched in national life by the late 1950s that one Conservative politician commented privately, 'meddle with the NHS? That's political suicide'. Even Margaret Thatcher, who distrusted the nationalised medical service in many ways, felt obliged while in government to declare that it was 'safe with us'.[71]

It is worth considering how British attitudes to the NHS compare to those towards health services in other countries. Certainly the British were not unique when it came to believing that the state should play the leading role in health-care provision. Surveys of European social attitudes, even by the end of the century, showed that Western Germans and Britons were in 'as near universal agreement as there is ever likely to be in a sample survey that health care ... should be the responsibility of the state'.[72] However, most other systems in the developed world took the form of a compulsory insurance system, involving personal or state guarantees from a multiplicity of providers: the British model, paid for mostly out of general taxation, and which essentially allowed central government to determine the level of spending, was very unusual. In Germany, for instance, most of the actual services continued to be provided by the private sector: an increased number of direct up-front payments were enacted under the Christian Democrats in 1988 and 1993.[73] Canadian and West German healthcare was for the most part administered via those countries' constituent provinces and states, mobilising insurance and sick funds with a minimum of central direction.[74] The French system was regionally decentralised, maintain-ing a distance from the machinery of the state, and administering worker and employer contributions themselves: they came under central direction only in 1967, and even then only of a limited form that required them to balance their budgets while retaining much of their independence. Patients mostly paid for care themselves, and then sought refunds from such funds.[75] This had impor-tant consequences. As Beveridge's biographer Jose Harris has pointed out, the European schemes proved more likely to attract voters' favour as systems to which they truly 'belonged', as well as allowing revenues to remain more buoyant and more resistant to public sector austerity – one key reason why British health spending stayed relatively low.[76]

UK health spending increased more slowly than almost anywhere else in the developed world, and by 1995 had fallen behind Norway and even Spain (which she had far outstripped in 1960) as a percentage of GNP.[77] UK health spending went up rather rapidly as a share of national resources: the British spent 3.2 per cent of their GDP on healthcare in the early 1960s, a figure that had risen to 5.8 per cent in 1993. But other states outstripped even this increase. The equivalent figures for France saw that country's public spending as a percentage of GDP rise from 3.1 per cent to 7.3 per cent; in the Nether-lands from 2.8 per cent to 6.7 per cent; and in Sweden from 3.6 per cent to 6.2 per cent.[78] However, even before the remarkable boost to spending at the end of the century, Britain had long been keeping up with many of the inter-national innovations and successes of both primary and invasive hospital medicine. She maintained a lead over many other countries in her general practitioner coverage, enjoying more GPs per head of population than Sweden, the Netherlands or the USA throughout the late twentieth century. British health policy might also claim notable successes against other chronic diseases, for instance heart disease, which between 1986 and 1996 fell more in the UK than it did in Ireland, the USA, Italy, Austria and Poland – though less than in the Netherlands, Sweden and Australia. By the year 2000, life expectancy at birth in England and Wales was very similar to that in France and Germany, though it had been higher in 1960; Britons were likely to live only two years less than Australians or Swedes, and a year longer than US citizens.[79] It was only a middling record, comparatively – though it was rather better than successive governments' rhetoric about the necessity of structural reform suggested.

It was British politicians' reliance on general taxation – an attempt at nation-building, as well as a measure designed to simplify the system – that marked them out amid the general trend towards universal healthcare that followed the Second World War. It is true that one reason why Britain did not adopt an insurance-based system was the limited capacity of the existing National Insurance machinery. As *The Lancet* pointed out in 1946, and as Beveridge had always assumed, the small size of the National Insurance Fund relative to general taxation meant that it could only cover a very small amount of the NHS's cost – by the early 1980s, about 10 per cent, a charge that represented some of the 'savings' gleaned by the Service for the rest of the welfare system. Anything else, as *The Lancet* put it, would be 'an extraordinarily elaborate mechanism for excluding about ten per cent of the population' – those above any arbitrarily-defined earnings limit who would still have to pay if the Edwardian insurance system was simply expanded up the income chain.[80] An alternative would have been to incorporate the mutual hospital contributory schemes into the new system, much as Lloyd George had used the friendly societies to administer his health insurance scheme. Indeed, civil servants at the Ministry of Health considered just such an option. However, significant support for a state-run service within the contributory scheme movement inhibited its national association from offering itself up. Equally, there were concerns that the schemes were too parochial to be able to effectively deliver a national system.[81] The structure adopted had the benefit of simplicity, and even more importantly the ideological attraction of rhetorical community-building; but it did not allow for the numerous sources of healthcare provision and innovation that the continental social contract systems, in particular, enjoyed.

## Conclusion

It is striking that other countries have generally not adopted the NHS as a model. In capitalist democracies third-party insurance schemes have been the standard model for funding and accessing – and for reforming – healthcare services, not the nationalised system found in Britain. This was largely the case even in Ireland, perhaps the country most likely to follow the same path as the UK. Here the institutions and traditions of medical care were largely entwined and the Beveridge Report had proved a popular stimulus for debate. However, 1948 saw not the establishment of an Irish NHS but the election defeat of Fianna Fáil, the party committed to implementing a more modest yet still radical set of reforms.[82] Various reforms, including the Mother and Child Scheme, were opposed by the Irish medical profession and Catholic Church, with the result that a mixed economy of healthcare continued. When legislation was passed to bring into existence a new Health Service Executive, 48.4 per cent of the Irish population was covered by private medical insurance in 2004.[83] Whether or not the HSE will prove to be Ireland's NHS, for better or worse, will be a question for historians of medicine in the coming decades.

The ideological space occupied by the NHS within British society continues to be a complex issue. It is both a beacon of change and a bulwark of what have become traditional values. Such potential was clear from its earliest days. As Bevan commented as he resigned from the government in 1951 amid the controversy surrounding the introduction of charges for drugs, spectacles and dentures:

> ... the National Health Service was something of which we were all very proud, and even the Opposition were beginning to be proud of it. It only had to last a few more years to become part of our traditions, and then the traditionalists would have claimed credit for all of it.[84]

As it turned out, this is exactly what happened. The NHS, with prescription charges, would be described by the Conservative Chancellor Nigel Lawson as 'the closest thing the English have to a religion'.[85] This was remarkable given that the Service remained severely constrained: rather poorly integrated, somewhat unresponsive, underfunded and (internationally) not particularly impressive even in terms of results. But that popularity did not preserve it from an ever-shifting boundary between personal, private and public care – nor the controversial attempts of historians, social theorists and policymakers themselves to dissect and understand its unique and singular nature.

## Further reading

The NHS is relatively well served in the literature. The best one-volume history remains Charles Webster, *The National Health Service: A Political History* (Oxford: Oxford University Press, 2002), perhaps augmented for the general context by the populist but useful Nicholas Timmins, *The Five Giants: A Biography of the Welfare State* (London: HarperCollins, new edn, 2001). For more detail, Charles Webster's official two-volume history is absolutely indispensable: Charles Webster, *Problems of Health Care: The National Health Service before 1957* (London: HMSO, 1988) and *The Health Services since the War, Vol. 2, Government and Health Care: The National Health Service 1958–1979* (London: TSO, 1996). The roots of the post-war Labour government's reforms are covered in Bernard Harris, *The Origins of the British Welfare State: Social Welfare in England and Wales, 1800–1945* (Basingstoke: Palgrave, 2004). A good and detailed account of the Service's creation, and contemporary and subsequent debates, is Rodney Lowe, 'The Second World War, Consensus and the Foundation of the Welfare State',

*Twentieth Century British History*, 1, 2 (1990): 152–82. Excellent guides to the theory and practice of state health and welfare services are Gøsta Esping-Andersen, *The Three Worlds of Welfare Capitalism* (Cambridge: Polity Press, 1990) and Rudolf Klein, *The New Politics of the NHS: From Creation to Reinvention* (London: Radcliffe Publishing, 6th edn, 2010). The rise of healthcare 'consumerism' can be followed in Alex Mold, 'Patient Groups and the Construction of the Patient-Consumer in Britain: An Historical Overview', *Journal of Social Policy* 39, 4 (2010): 505–21, and Christine Hogg, *Citizens, Consumers and the NHS: Capturing Voices* (Basingstoke: Palgrave, 2008). For a fuller summary of the literature on the history of the NHS see Martin Gorsky, 'The British National Health Service 1948–2008: A Review of the Historiography', *Social History of Medicine* 21, 3 (2008): 437–60.

## Notes

1 Charles Webster, *The National Health Service: A Political History* (Oxford: Oxford University Press, 2002), 1.
2 For a concise summary of the NHS's tripartite structure, see ibid., Fig. 1.1, 21.
3 Adrian O'Dowd, 'The "Self-Funding" NHS Patient: Thin End of the Wedge?', *British Medical Journal*, 345 (2012): e5128 (published on 1 August 2012).
4 Lutz Leisering, 'Nation State and Welfare State: An Intellectual and Political History', *Journal of European Social Policy*, 13, 2 (2003): 175–85.
5 Thomas H. Marshall, *Citizenship and Social Class, and Other Essays* (Cambridge: Cambridge University Press, 1950), 56. See Dorothy Porter, *Health, Civilization and the State: A History of Public Health from Ancient to Modern Times* (London: Routledge, 1999), 232–34.
6 Richard M. Titmuss, *Problems of Social Policy* (London: HMSO, 1950), 503.
7 Richard M. Titmuss, *Essays on 'The Welfare State'* (London: Unwin University Books, 2nd edn, 1963), 202.
8 Gøsta Esping-Andersen, *The Three Worlds of Welfare Capitalism* (Cambridge: Polity Press, 1990), 166–67.
9 Ibid., 65–66, 166–67.
10 Cmd. 6404, *Social Insurance and Allied Services: Report* (London: HMSO, 1942), paras 9–10, 6–7.
11 Clement Attlee, 'The New Social Services and the Citizen', BBC Home Service broadcast, 4 July 1948, available at http://www.bbc.co.uk/archive/nhs/5147.shtml, accessed 17 September 2013.
12 Speaking in Parliament on 31 October 1911, cited in Michael Freeden, *The New Liberalism: An Ideology of Social Reform* (Oxford: Clarendon Press, 1978), 237.
13 See Ernest P. Hennock, *British Social Reform and German Precedents: The Case of Social Insurance 1880–1914* (Oxford: Clarendon Press, 1987).
14 Jose Harris, *William Beveridge: A Biography* (Oxford: Clarendon Press, 1977), 153–55.
15 Bentley B. Gilbert, *The Evolution of National Insurance in Great Britain: The Origins of the Welfare State* (London: Michael Joseph, 1966), 289–353.
16 See Bernard Harris, *The Origins of the British Welfare State: Social Welfare in England and Wales, 1800–1945* (Basingstoke: Palgrave, 2004), 150–65.
17 Richard Freeman, 'A National Health Service, by Comparison', *Social History of Medicine*, 21, 3 (2008): 506.
18 Jane Lewis and Barbara Brookes, 'A Reassessment of the Work of the Peckham Health Centre, 1926–1951', *Milbank Memorial Fund Quarterly: Health and*

*Society*, 61, 2 (1983): 307–50; Lesley Hall, 'The Archives of the Pioneer Health Centre, Peckham, in the Wellcome Library', *Social History of Medicine*, 14, 3 (2001): 525–38.

19 I.F. Beck, *The Almoner: A Brief Account of Medical Social Service in Great Britain* (London: Council of the Institute of Almoners, 1948); Enid Morberly Bell, *The Story of Hospital Almoners: The Birth of a Profession* (London: Faber & Faber, 1961); Lynsey Cullen, 'The First Lady Almoner: The Appointment, Position, and Findings of Miss Mary Stewart at the Royal Free Hospital, 1895–99', *Journal of the History of Medicine and Allied Sciences*, 68, 4 (2012): 551–82.

20 Alysa Levene, Martin Powell and John Stewart, 'Patterns of Municipal Health Expenditure in Interwar England and Wales', *Bulletin of the History of Medicine*, 78, 3 (2004): 644–46; John Mohan and Martin Gorsky, *Don't Look Back? Voluntary and Charitable Finance of Hospitals in Britain, Past and Present* (London: Office of Health Economics, 2001), 38; David Owen, *English Philanthropy 1660–1960* (Cambridge: Belknap Press, 1964), 502.

21 Geoffrey Rivett, *From Cradle to Grave: Fifty Years of the NHS* (London: King's Fund, 1997), 29.

22 Not least Webster: see his *Political History*, 12–15.

23 See John Pater, *The Making of the National Health Service* (London: King's Fund, 1981).

24 Melanie Oppenheimer, 'Beveridge in the Antipodes: The 1948 Tour', in Melanie Oppenheimer and Nicholas Deakin (eds), *Beveridge and Voluntary Action in Britain and the Wider British World* (Manchester: Manchester University Press, 2011), esp. 72; Roy Porter, *The Greatest Benefit to Mankind: A Medical History of Humanity from Antiquity to the Present* (London: Fontana, 1999), 654.

25 John Stewart and Linda Bryder, '"Some Abstract Socialistic Ideal or Principle": British Reactions to New Zealand's 1938 Social Security Act', *Historical Research* (forthcoming), 2–3, 18–34. We are grateful to Professors Stewart and Bryder for allowing us an early view of this article.

26 Michael Foot, *Aneurin Bevan: A Biography, Vol. 2, 1945–1960* (London: Davis-Poynter, 1973), 142–43.

27 Frank Honigsbaum, *Health, Happiness and Security: The Creation of the National Health Service* (London: Routledge, 1989), 166–75.

28 Martin Gorsky, Martin Powell and John Mohan, 'British Voluntary Hospitals and the Public Sphere: Contribution and Participation before the National Health Service', in Steve Sturdy (ed.), *Medicine, Health and the Public Sphere in Britain, 1600–2000* (London: Routledge, 2002 pp. 123–144), Fig. 6.1, 128.

29 Paul Bridgen, 'Voluntary Failure, the Middle Classes, and the Nationalisation of the British Voluntary Hospitals, 1900–1946', in Bernard Harris and Paul Bridgen (eds), *Charity and Mutual Aid in Europe and North America since 1800* (London: Routledge, 2007), 220–26.

30 Nick Hayes, 'Did We Really Want a National Health Service? Hospitals, Patients and Public Opinions before 1948', *English Historical Review*, 127, 526 (2012): 621–61.

31 George C. Gosling, 'Charity and Change in the Mixed Economy of Healthcare in Bristol, 1918–1948', unpublished PhD thesis, Oxford Brookes University, 2011, 233–95.

32 Helen Jones, *Health and Society in Twentieth Century Britain* (London: Longmans, 1994), 124.

33 David Kynaston, *Austerity Britain, 1945–51* (London: Bloomsbury, pbk edn, 2007), 283.

34 Aneurin Bevan, 'National Health Service Bill', Second Reading Debate, 30 April 1946, *House of Commons Debates*, Vol. 422, cols. 45, 49.

35 Harris, *Beveridge*, 461.

36 Stephen Harrison and Ruth McDonald, *The Politics of Healthcare in Britain* (London: Sage, 2008), 89–90.
37 Elizabeth Darling, *Re-forming Britain: Narratives of Modernity before Reconstruction* (London: Routledge, 2007), 58–80; James Vernon, *Hunger: A Modern History* (Cambridge, Mass.: Harvard University Press, 2007), 182–87.
38 John Stewart, *The Battle for Health: A Political History of the Socialist Medical Association, 1930–51* (Aldershot: Ashgate, 1999), 197.
39 Marguerite Dupree, 'Central Policy and Local Independence: Integration, Health Centres and the National Health Service in Scotland, 1948–1990', in Mark Freeman, Eleanor Gordon and Krista Maglen (eds), *Medicine, Law and Public Policy in Scotland, c. 1850–1990* (Dundee: Dundee University Press, 2011), 180–202.
40 George H. Gallup (ed.), *The Gallup International Public Opinion Polls: Great Britain, 1937–1975*, Vol. 1 (New York: Random House, 1976), 92.
41 Mass-Observation Papers, University of Sussex, File Report 1921, 'A National Health Service', October 1943.
42 Phoebe Hall, 'The Development of Health Centres', in Phoebe Hall, Hillary Land, Roy Parker and Adrian Webb (eds), *Change, Choice and Conflict in Social Policy* (London: Heinemann, 1975), 285.
43 David Morrell, 'Introduction and Overview', in Irvine Loudon, John Horder and Charles Webster (eds), *General Practice under the National Health Service, 1948–1997* (Oxford: Clarendon Press, 1998), 3.
44 Charles Webster, *The Health Services since the War, Vol. 2, Government and Health Care: The National Health Service 1958–1979* (London: TSO, 1996), 270, 541; Glen O'Hara, *From Dreams to Disillusionment: Economic and Social Planning in 1960s Britain* (Basingstoke: Palgrave Macmillan, 2007), 190–92.
45 Tony Cutler, 'A Double Irony? The Politics of National Health Service Expenditure in the 1950s', in Sally Sheard and Martin Gorsky (eds), *Financing Medicine: The British Experience since 1750* (London: Routledge, 2007), 201–20.
46 See John Mohan, *Planning, Markets and Hospitals* (London: Routledge, 2002), 111–31; O'Hara, *Dreams to Disillusionment*, 167–204.
47 B. Watkin, *The National Health Service: The First Phase, 1948–1974 and after* (London: Allen & Unwin, 1978), 146–47.
48 See David J. Hunter, *Coping With Uncertainty: Policy and Politics in the National Health Service* (Chichester: Research Studies Press, 1980), 183–94.
49 Rudolf Klein, *The New Politics of the NHS* (London: Longman, 3rd edn, 1995), 113–15.
50 A. Mold, 'Patient Groups and the Construction of the Patient-Consumer in Britain: An Historical Overview', *Journal of Social Policy*, 39, 4 (2010), esp. 510–11.
51 Klein, *New Politics*, 105.
52 Glen O'Hara, 'The Complexities of "Consumerism": Choice, Collectivism and Participation within Britain's National Health Service, *c.* 1961–*c.* 1979', *Social History of Medicine*, 26, 2 (2013): 12–13.
53 Christine Hogg, *Citizens, Consumers and the NHS: Capturing Voices* (Basingstoke: Palgrave, 2008), 17–25.
54 Associated Press, 'Baby Whose Surgery Was Postponed Five Times Dies', 5 December 1987. Available online at www.apnewsarchive.com/1987/Baby-Whose-Surgery-Was-Postponed-Five-Times-Dies/id-a7db3de5a2d95c7291f27b874c4cc907, accessed 15 January 2014. See also Jonathan Shapiro, 'The NHS: The Story So Far', *Clinical Medicine*, 10, 3 (2010): 337.
55 John Mohan, *A National Health Service?: The Restructuring of Health Care in Britain since 1979* (New York: St. Martin's Press, 1995), 4–8; Webster, *Political History*, 193–200.
56 Calum Patron, 'New Labour's Health Policy: The New Healthcare State', in Martin Powell (ed.), *New Labour, New Welfare State?* (Bristol: Policy Press, 1999), esp. 58–63.

57  Eric Shaw, *Losing Labour's Soul?: New Labour and the Blair Government 1997–2007* (London: Routledge, 2007), 98.

58  Rachael Harker, *NHS Expenditure: Commons Library Standard Note* (London: House of Commons Library, 2012), Table 1, 9.

59  Julian Le Grand, *The Other Invisible Hand: Delivering Public Services through Choice and Competition* (Princeton: Princeton University Press, 2007), 106. For an accessible summary of health policy since the 1980s, see Christopher Ham, *Health Policy in Britain* (London: Palgrave Macmillan, 6th edn, 2009).

60  Geoffrey Finlayson, *Citizen, State and Social Welfare in Britain* (Oxford: Clarendon Press, 1994), 363.

61  Nicholas Mays, Anne Dixon and Lorelei Jones, 'Return to the Market: Objectives and Evolution of New Labour's Market Reforms', in Nicholas Mays, Anna Dixon and Lorelei Jones (eds), *Understanding New Labour's Market Reforms of the English NHS* (London: King's Fund, 2011), 6–8.

62  Catherine Needham, *Personalising Public Services: Understanding the Personalisation Narrative* (Bristol: Policy Press, 2011), 35.

63  Nicholas Timmins, 'How New Labour Succeeded with NHS Policy', *The Financial Times*, 13 March 2010.

64  Nick Hayes, 'Did We Really Want a National Health Service?', 660.

65  Gallup, *Public Opinion Polls*, Vol. 1, 92.

66  Mass-Observation Papers, University of Sussex, File Report 3140, 'A National Health Service', January 1944.

67  Finlayson, *Citizen, State and Social Welfare in Britain*, 271–72; Kevin Jeffreys, *The Churchill Coalition and Wartime Politics, 1940–1945* (Manchester: Manchester University Press, 1991), 129–30, 195–96.

68  Webster, *Political History*, 10–11, 15–16; Jefferys, *Churchill Coalition*, 212–13.

69  Gallup, *Public Opinion Polls*, Vol. 1, 170, 184, 299, 683, Vol. 2, 801.

70  Rodney Lowe, 'The Second World War, Consensus and the Foundation of the Welfare State', *Twentieth Century British History*, 1, 2 (1990): 175.

71  John Stewart, 'The Political Economy of the British National Health Service, 1945–1975: Opportunities and Constraints?', *Medical History*, 52, 4 (2008): 453. On Thatcher's private views see Norman Fowler, *A Political Suicide: The Conservatives' Voyage into the Wilderness* (London: Politico's, 2008), 22.

72  Max Kaase and Kenneth Newton, 'What People Expect From the State: *plus ça change*', in Roger Jowell, John Curtice and Alison Park (eds), *British – and European – Social Attitudes, the Fifteenth Report: How Britain Differs* (Aldershot: Ashgate, 1998), 44.

73  Roger Lawson, 'Germany: Maintaining the Middle Way', in Victor George and Peter Taylor-Gooby (eds), *European Welfare Policy: Squaring the Welfare Circle* (Basingstoke: Macmillan, 1996), 34, 38.

74  Porter, *Greatest Benefit*, 655–56.

75  Matthew Ramsey, 'Public Health in France', in Dorothy Porter (ed.), *The History of Public Health and the Modern State* (Amsterdam: Rodopi, 1994), 95–98.

76  Jose Harris, 'Enterprise and Welfare States: A Comparative Perspective', *Transactions of the Royal Historical Society*, Fifth Series, 40 (1990): 175–95.

77  Anne Hardy and E.M. (Tilli) Tansey, 'Medical Enterprise and Global Response, 1945–2000', in William F. Bynum, Anne Hardy, Stephen Jacyna, Christopher Lawrence and Tilly E.M. Tansey (eds), *The Western Medical Tradition: 1800 to 2000* (Cambridge: Cambridge University Press, 2006), Fig. 4.22, 500.

78  Rudolf Klein, 'The Crises of the Welfare States', in Roger Cooter and John Pickstone (eds), *Medicine in the Twentieth Century* (Abingdon: Harwood Academic Publishers, 2000), Table 1, 158 and Table 3, 165.

79  Hardy and Tansey, 'Medical Enterprise', Fig. 4.9, 440, Fig. 4.6, 430, and Table 4.1, 423.

80 Pater, *The Making of the National Health Service*, 184–6. See Beveridge's remarks at Cmd. 6404, *Social Insurance*, para. 437, 162.
81 Martin Gorsky and John Mohan, 'Hospital Contributory Schemes and the NHS Debates: The Rejection of Social Insurance in the British Welfare State?', *Twentieth Century British History*, 16, 2 (2005): 170–192.
82 Ruth Barrington, *Health, Medicine and Politics in Ireland 1900–1970* (Dublin: Institute of Public Administration, 2000), 193–5.
83 Statistical Yearbook of Ireland: Social Inclusion, 50. Available online at www.cso.ie/en/releasesandpublications/statisticalyearbookofireland/statisticalyearbookofireland2007edition/, accessed 12 January 2014.
84 Aneurin Bevan, resignation speech, 23 April 1951. Full transcript available online at www.sochealth.co.uk/national-health-service/the-sma-and-the-foundation-of-the-national-health-service-dr-leslie-hilliard-1980/aneurin-bevan-and-the-foundation-of-the-nhs/bevans-resignation-speech-23-april-1951/, accessed 7 December 2013.
85 Nigel Lawson, *The View From No. 11: Memoirs of a Tory Radical* (London: Bantam, 1992), 613.

# 8  South Africa's mixed economy of healthcare

*Anne Digby*

## Introduction

Western views of Africa are substantially coloured by television pictures of appalling African famine. In reality, a general African experience of periodic famine mortality had been gradually superseded as early as the late 1920s and 1930s by endemic undernutrition and malnutrition affecting certain groups (especially children and their mothers) and particular regions.[1] During the same period 'western' medicine had targeted epidemic diseases such as smallpox and sleeping sickness with some success, although action against endemic diseases such as tuberculosis, malaria, or leprosy was less effective.[2] Despite some healthcare successes, in comparative terms the disease profile of the continent of Africa remains poor. Today, infant and maternal mortality is high; over nine-tenths of the world's malaria cases and deaths occur on the continent; and there are very high rates of cholera, trachoma, yellow fever, and HIV/AIDS. Indeed, the world's highest rates of HIV/AIDS are located in ten countries in south-east and Central Africa including South Africa.[3] Sub-Saharan Africa has a massive 24 per cent of the global volume of disease but only 1 per cent of the world's financial resources for health, and 3 per cent of the world's health personnel.[4] And emigration of scarce trained health personnel, particularly of doctors and nurses, to developed countries continues to be a huge problem for already beleaguered African health systems.

Dual systems of traditional/indigenous medicine and 'western'/scientific medicine marked – and continue to mark – healthcare in Africa. In the accounts of early European settlers African indigenous medicine was usually stereotyped as witchcraft and there was a tendency to extend its perceived sinister elements into a blanket condemnation of all types of indigenous medical practices. Earlier colonial regimes on the continent legislated against certain traditional medical practices through heavily deterrent witchcraft laws,[5] with both the regions of Central and Southern Africa,[6] and the country of South Africa, fitting within this paradigm.[7] In the racially segregated society of South Africa during the early- and mid-twentieth century, knowledge about African medical beliefs and practices was difficult for white people to acquire, so that simplistic stereotyping was substituted for empirical enquiry. South Africa's medical profession was heavily dominated by a membership drawn almost exclusively from a white settler population that perceived indigenous healers as a competitive threat to their own livelihood in practising 'western' medicine. This then re-inforced the characterization of indigenous healthcare – more particularly by diviners, rather than by herbalists – as malign.[8]

South Africa is a varied and geographically large country (four times the size of the UK), having the most powerful economy in Africa, and a comparatively benign health profile with few tropical diseases. Its international image is of a 'rainbow nation' of many ethnicities, with Nelson Mandela as its first democratic president acting as an icon of reconciliation. This reconciliation was all too necessary after the country's bitterly contested, racialized past, which has shaped the challenges it faces today in providing a more equitable health system that utilizes its rich professional expertise and resources to benefit all its citizens.

South Africa is unusual in being both a developed and a developing economy, and this has influenced its mixed economy of private and public healthcare. So too has the experience and legacy of racial discrimination, at its height under apartheid policies between 1948 and 1994. Even before the advent of apartheid, however, South Africa was a racially segregated society in which race determined privilege or disadvantage for both practitioners and patients within a bureaucratic, highly complex healthcare system. The country's colonial legacy had been re-inforced during the apartheid period with measures for the continued marginalization of indigenous medicine. This was despite this form of healing being the first port of call for seven-tenths of the country's majority population of Africans. Today, there are 51.8 million people living in South Africa, of whom 79.2 per cent are African, 8.9 per cent are Coloured (mixed race), 8.9 per cent are white, and 2.5 per cent are Indian.[9] In this chapter the term 'black' is used to include Coloureds, Africans and Indians.

## Indigenous medicine

It is estimated that, globally, 60 per cent of the world's population consult a traditional or indigenous healer, whereas for the African continent the figure is 80 per cent. South Africa falls between these two benchmarks with an estimated 72 per cent. This amounts to 26.6 million consumers drawn from most sectors of the African population, who use traditional medicines an average of 4.8 times a year.[10] In 1978 the World Health Organization's (WHO) Alma Alta Conference had advocated that a high priority be given to the incorporation of traditional practitioners and traditional birth attendants into national policies and regulations. But in South Africa this had to await the post-apartheid period. Elsewhere in Africa the regulation of the traditional medicine sector came earlier than this, and is found in West Africa (Nigeria, Mali, and Ghana), East Africa (Uganda), and Central Africa

(Zambia and Zimbabwe). But even in these countries, the problem of official public recognition, professional regulation, and training of healers has been problematic, with the result that progress has been relatively slow.[11] Indeed, full recognition and integration of the traditional medicine sector into a national healthcare system was found in few countries, with Asia leading the way, because here there was successful incorporation of both sectors into a unified system in China, India, Indonesia, Thailand, and Bhutan.

In South Africa the obstacles to co-operation between those practising western medicine and those practising indigenous medicine have been formidable. There was long-established cultural suspicion between the two, with allegations of quackery and primitivism from licensed doctors against healers, together with a self-perception by doctors of their own discipline as being uniquely scientific. Some common ground was found in mutual interest in South African plant species used as medicines, which were a central element in healers' therapeutics. At the same time there were allegations concerning toxicity in plant medicines by doctors against healers and accusations of bioprospecting by healers against western pharmaceutical companies, which were held to have stolen traditional knowledge without adequate compensation of indigenous intellectual property rights. Press allegations of so-called 'muthi' (medicine) murders – when killing followed the taking of live body parts to make powerful medicaments – deepened the divide.[12] Further, South African legislation had in 1974 made it an offence for licensed western doctors to collaborate with healers and other non-registered personnel.[13] A contemporary editorial in the *South African Medical Journal* suggested the state of medical opinion at the time, as it had the revealing heading 'Colleagues or Opponents?' before stating that partnerships between healer and doctor should not be countenanced.[14]

Practitioners of indigenous medicine work within the private sector. Exact numbers of healers are unknown, although there are considered to be more than 200,000 traditional practitioners including diviners, herbalists, traditional birth attendants, and traditional surgeons. Diviners (more usually female) are often referred to as *sangomas*, and are called by the ancestors to their vocation, acting as intermediaries between the human and the spirit world in divining/diagnosing illness (broadly defined) and its unknown causes. They use divination objects, their powers as a medium, and dreams/visions to do this. Herbalists (more usually male) are trained through apprenticeships and prescribe empirically for everyday conditions from their extensive knowledge of traditional medicines. Healers typically have expertise in treating traditional or African conditions, culture-bound syndromes such as malaise caused by spirit possession, or neglect of cultural custom. The practices of each type of healer, whether for preventive, curative, protective, or purifying purposes, are increasingly overlapping.[15]

Unlike the rest of the country, the province of Natal (where there was a heavy concentration of African population) had licensed herbalists since 1891.[16] Much later, South African healers more generally were accorded legal status under the Traditional Health Practitioners Act of 2007 (Act 22 of 2007).[17] Under this Act a national council of healers was to be set up to register and regulate traditional practitioners, although the Department of Health has been very slow to implement this, despite a traditional medicine directorate having been set up within the department. Following this legislation came the South African Law Commission's initiative in 2012 to set up a review of witchcraft legislation. At the time of writing, therefore, the biomedical and traditional medical sectors are still parallel systems, having restricted co-operation between them.

The informal trade in traditional medicines and their source materials is very large in South Africa, with an estimated 20,000 tonnes involved, including some 771 plant species and 200 animal species (the latter often acquired illegally). These are sourced from locations throughout the country as well as from Swaziland, Mozambique, and Zimbabwe. The huge quantities involved mean that unless much more is done to set up indigenous plant nurseries this trade is unsustainable, and is already showing growing scarcities, increased prices, and longer distances travelled to acquire prized ingredients. These informal transactions are estimated to be worth as much as 2.9 million rands per year, or the equivalent of 5.6 per cent of the national health budget. It is thought that recourse to traditional medicines by African patients is growing, with supplies bought from 300–400 'muthi' shops, from informal street traders, and from a few large traditional medicine markets such as the two in Durban.[18]

Despite concerns over the toxicity of some traditional remedies, with hospitals treating associated cases of poisoning, there is as yet no comprehensive screening process for the safety and utility of South African plant medicines. Of an estimated 24,000 indigenous plants in South Africa, about 11,000 plant specimens have been collected for study. A Reference Centre for African Traditional Medicines was set up in 1997 to begin to address a number of issues such as the standardization and authentication of medicinal plants, and the safeguarding of the intellectual property rights of healers through the patenting of safe traditional medicines.[19] The conservation of popular herbs in sustainable cultivation is also receiving belated, but much needed, attention.[20]

As in Southern and Central Africa more widely, South African patients were, and are, pluralistic in their treatment choices, moving pragmatically between different kinds of medicine within a dual healthcare system to seek relief for their suffering from indigenous healing and/or from biomedicine. The conceptualization of the character of the disease by the African sufferer and/or his friends and relatives (the therapy group) leads to a 'hierarchy of resort' in recourse to a biomedical doctor and/or a traditional healer. A perception of a 'European', 'white man's', or 'town' disease would result in the sufferer usually seeking treatment for an acute condition at a clinic where a 'quick-fix' of symptoms is hoped for from a modern biomedical drug or injection. In contrast, 'African' diseases, chronic or puzzling conditions, as well as culturally related or psycho-social illnesses, are more likely to be taken to a healer, where the underlying or 'real' cause of the problem is sought, and holistic treatment covering both physiological and spiritual issues given. Recourse to biomedicine might be influenced by external, involuntary factors such as the need to get a sick note (available from 'western' doctors) or by the requirement to pass a biomedical examination before being cleared to work in the mines. In rural areas – where attitudes are typically more conservative and choice more constrained – patients' selection is weighted more towards indigenous medicine. The differential level of payment demanded by practitioners of different types is probably less important in patients' choices than other factors, such as the healer's reputation. The higher fees of a healer are often related to the results achieved, with payment made in stages, unlike the biomedical practitioner whose lower fees have to be paid up-front at the beginning of treatment.[21]

Traditional medicine has cultural and spiritual as well as purely medical functions. Healers adopt a wide remit in their holistic view of the patient's body and mind, with a concern to find the reasons for illness – particularly the cultural origins of a condition – as well as to treat. Healers are a diverse group drawing on different healing traditions within ethnic groups, so that there are distinctive features of, for example, the practice of a Tswana practitioner

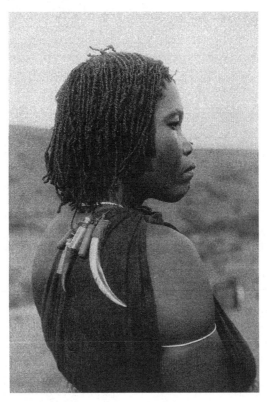

*Figure 8.1* Zululand, South Africa: A woman 'witch doctor'. © The Wellcome Library, London.

compared to a Zulu one. Mpondo healers are notable for using medicinal and charm plants both for healing humans and farm animals in south-east Africa. If customs and traditions are perceived to have been contravened, then mainly herbal remedies are employed in rituals to appease the ancestors, remove ritual impurity, or protect against evil forces.[22] For healers from all cultures there are common features, such as the custom of secrecy in regard to healing practices and medicines. This is an important difference from biomedicine where such secrecy is viewed as quackery, and another key dissimilarity is in the non-standardization of indigenous medicines. Although healers may refer their patients for allopathic treatment, there is no reciprocity in referrals from bio-medical practitioners to healers, so that asymmetry prevails.

A few examples of cross-cultural co-operation between indigenous and western medicine have been, and are still, found in South Africa. Sometimes a perception of cross-cultural practice in diagnosis came from earlier patients' perceptions of the doctor's stethoscope as the equivalent of the indigenous diviner's throwing of bones. Occasionally the doctor adopted a cross-cultural method of diagnosis in order to win the confidence of an African patient, as by giving an immediate diagnosis of disease (as would a diviner) without the preliminary taking of a case history. But others saw such methods as a betrayal of their scientific training and eschewed them. However, a pioneer initiative took place during the 1970s when missionary hospital doctors and local healers held a conference, followed by seminars at All Saints Hospital located in the Transkei (now the Eastern Cape) to discuss their respective approaches, although no practical outcomes ensued. By the late 1980s and early 1990s – with the hope of a new South Africa having a more inclusive health system – such dialogue became a little more common, but again without a successful, general bridging of gaps in perceptions and practices.[23]

In contrast to this general stand-off there was a pioneering rapprochement between western and traditional medicine at the Valley Trust in southern KwaZulu-Natal from the 1950s to the present day. Here Dr Halley Stott had set up a nutritionally focused system of social medicine within the Botha's Hill Health Centre (practising curative western primary healthcare) and the Valley Trust (where indigenous healers delivered largely preventive medi-cine). The former was publicly funded and the latter privately funded, a combination that gave sufficient independence to frustrate apartheid ideologues' opposition to indigenous medicine. Working together gave the opportunity for multiple healthcare interventions amongst the local African population to combat endemic malnutrition, whether this was through nurses, nurse aides, and health assistants attached to the health centre or through indigenous healers within the trust acting as community health workers and with their own consultancies attached to first aid posts. These were supplemented by Valley Trust dieticians and agricultural demonstra-tors working to improve local people's diet and health as well as furthering general community development. From the beginning, the health centre's staff were instructed to show respect to local healers and their practices.

Africans themselves made the choice of whom to consult over an ailment, with pluralistic consultations developing.[24]

## Biomedicine

Resources in western medicine are divided between the public and private sectors. In 1910 South Africa's Act of Union divided up the public provision and administration of healthcare between the country's four constituent provinces, municipalities, and local government, healthcare co-ordination in the latter being strengthened by the establishment of a central Department of Public Health (DPH) in 1919. This meant that curative services in the form of hospitals were provided by the four provinces of the Transvaal, Orange Free State, Natal, and the Cape, whilst preventive work was devolved to the local authorities. A further layer of complexity was added during the apartheid period in the 1970s and early 1980s when ten Bantustans, or ethnic 'Homelands', were set up, each with its own department of health and with responsibility for the newly nationalized private mission hospitals in their respective areas.[25]

The administrative outcome of this historical process was that there were fourteen different healthcare authorities at the time of the democratic transition to an elected government in 1994. Within them was a notably fragmented and geographically skewed distribution of hospitals, clinics, mobile clinics, and dispensaries. In addition to the 419 public hospitals, there were 172 private ones. Until the early 1990s public provincial hospitals had been segregated institutions; in three provinces this took the form of segregation between black and white hospitals but in the fourth (Cape Province) there was segregation within hospitals through racially separate wards. There was a conspicuous contrast between overcrowded, underfunded facilities in institutions or wards catering for black patients and more privileged facilities for white patients. Private mission hospitals catered almost exclusively for black patients and were usually located in remote, rural areas where they filled a notable gap in healthcare facilities. Missionary doctors had a humanitarian approach, as typified by one who commented, 'We were forever aware that we were treating the symptoms of an unfair, diseased society, rather than getting at the roots of all this pain'.[26]

Despite the South African constitution giving every citizen a right to access healthcare (Act 108 of 1996, section 27), there is a pronounced deficit in the rural population's access to medical care and hence prominent inequities in healthcare outcomes. Nearly half (44.7 per cent) of the South African population is defined as being rural, although this varies from provinces such as Limpopo (where 90 per cent of inhabitants are rural) or the Northern Cape (with 80 per cent) down to the Western Cape (with only 10 per cent) or Gauteng (with a mere 4 per cent).[27] Health outcomes – such as maternal or infant mortality rates, cure rates for TB or HIV prevalence – show strong differentiation between rural and urban areas. Although the rural population is more dependent on public sector healthcare, distances travelled to hospitals and clinics are much greater despite deficient patient transport and poor availability of ambulances. In rural primary healthcare facilities the basic infrastructure (safe drinking water, electricity, flush toilets, and telephone) was more likely to be missing. Shortage of health professionals has been to some extent mitigated by the presence of foreign doctors and, more recently, by qualified young healthcare professionals, who are required after graduation to do a period of community service. This has served to fill some of the gaps in the staffing of hospitals in disadvantaged areas. The inequity of this rural deficit has been inherited from the apartheid past when the rural black population was starved of resources, but democratic governments since 1994 have not acted sufficiently decisively to remedy this.[28]

South Africa has been relatively well endowed with expertise from its trained healthcare personnel. The country's efficient medical schools had an international reputation, and had been successful in quadrupling the number of trained doctors between 1950 and 1990, and improving the ratio of doctors to population from 45 to 74 per 100,000 people. During the early- and mid-twentieth century the medical profession had been almost exclusively white and male. But in order to provide a cadre of doctors to 'serve their own people', three black medical schools were set up by the apartheid state between the 1950s and 1980s. In addition the two 'open' universities of Cape Town and the Witwatersrand were permitted by the state to train black doctors during the 1940s and 1950s and again from the 1980s. Graduating black doctors generally went into townships to set up general practices with a black patient base. Given contemporary racial prejudice it was remarkably difficult for able black medical graduates either to specialize or to develop a hospital consultancy, although a small minority did so either at home or, more usually, abroad.[29] Women also entered medical training at Cape Town and Witwatersrand from the 1920s, making up 10 per cent of the profession by the 1960s.[30] Geographical inequities in the distribution of medical professionals remained, with expertise heavily concentrated in the metropolitan areas of Durban, Cape Town, and the Witwatersrand. There was, and is, a pronounced rural deficit such that in 1975 three-quarters of doctors practised in these three urban areas.[31] Overall, medical personnel were unevenly distributed. This meant that in Natal, the province with the most inequitable distribution, doctor:patient ratios varied from an average of one doctor to 834 urban patients to only one doctor to 9,565 rural patients.[32]

On the African continent more generally nursing has usually been done by men, whereas in South Africa the nursing profession has always been overwhelmingly female. During the early twentieth century nurses were white, and included a central core of skilled immigrants from Britain who served in both public and mission hospitals. Black nurses began to be trained in mission hospitals and in some large segregated urban institutions during the mid-twentieth century. Whereas the medical profession remained overwhelmingly white, a deficit in the supply of white entrants to the nursing profession meant that by 1990 over half the trained nurses were black. The professional experiences of black nurses in the public hospitals of South Africa differed. In Groote Schuur Hospital in the Cape Province transformation was a slow, contested process; Coloured (mixed race) nurses were not recruited until 1961 and African nurses not until 1985. Even then their progress up the professional ladder to the rank of sister or matron was difficult. And until the hospital took an innovating lead through instituting the country's first hospital racial integration in 1987 (four years before it was instituted nationwide in 1991), black nurses performed their duties for Coloured and African patients in segregated black wards, whilst white nurses did the same for white patients in white wards.[33] In the huge Baragwanath Hospital catering mainly for black patients from Soweto, black nurses faced overcrowded wards, periodically came into conflict with the white-dominated nursing administration, and were also drawn into the wider political disputes of the apartheid period.[34] Generally, from 1960 to 1994 the South African nursing profession expanded rapidly with professional and registered enrolled nurses increasing fourfold. Distribution of nurses between the public and private sectors was relatively equitable, whereas for other types of healthcare, personnel were disproportionately located in the private sector.[35] However, there were still some pronounced disparities. As late as 1998 the geographical distribution of nurses was remarkably uneven with, for example, 40 nurses per 10,000 people in a well-endowed province such as the Western Cape compared to 20 per 10,000 in poorer provinces such as the Northern Cape or Mpumalanga.[36]

Since 1994 a decrease in the numbers of doctors and nurses qualifying and a continued emigration of skilled healthcare personnel have worsened entrenched difficulties in getting people to work in disadvantaged rural areas. Low morale and burn-out amongst health workers, resulting from the HIV/AIDS pandemic's huge impact on an overstressed public healthcare system, have worsened the situation. Together these factors continued to weaken the development of a reformed national system with universal access to public healthcare.[37] However, creative thinking has led to an interest in training mid-level health workers in medicine, pharmacy, and other health-related disciplines, because their shorter and less expensive training could provide staffing more expeditiously than is feasible through training doctors or nurses.[38] However, apart from the longstanding enrolled nursing assistants (of whom about 51,000 existed in 2004) and the pharmacy assistants (of whom 3,063 are registered with the Pharmacy Council), numbers of mid-level personnel have remained small, with fewer than a thousand in each occupation. Plans for creating a cadre of medical assistants have gone through a predictably complicated and contested process, with doctors insisting that the assistant work under the supervision of a medic and not replace the doctor as an independent worker. This repeated the history of a much earlier project for medical aids.[39]

The democratic government began to address some of these intractable issues of racial and geographical inequity in the 'White Paper for the Transformation of the Health System in South Africa' (1997). This focused on the public provision of a national health service based in a district health system, with administrative responsibility later located in nine provincial governments.[40] This national health service plan was the first for half a century. An earlier plan based on local health centres and focused particularly on the black population had been put forward by the Gluckman Commission in 1944, but had foundered both on provincial opposition and on the apartheid government's reluctance to spend money on services for the black population.[41] In 1997 the projected reform was also intended to redress an inequitable situation whereby a disproportionate amount of expenditure went on the urban tertiary hospital sector, which had very expensive academic hospitals providing high-tech medicine largely to patients from the very small white minority. Indeed it was in one such tertiary institution, Groote Schuur Hospital, that the world's first heart transplant by Christiaan Barnard and his team took place in 1967, displaying to the world the superlative surgical standards that could be reached in apartheid South Africa.[42] Contrasting with this was a grossly underfunded system of primary healthcare serving a majority black population that largely inhabited townships and rural areas.

## Paying for healthcare

There was considerable disparity in the funding available to the public and private sectors. Public healthcare in clinics and hospitals was funded by taxation and during the early 1990s amounted to little more than two-fifths of expenditure on health despite catering for slightly more than three-quarters of the population.[43] Private health expenditure involved medical aids schemes that monopolized nearly three-quarters of private funds. The racial composition of their membership was overwhelmingly white, but from 1977 until 1991 declined (from 77 to 58 per cent) whilst black membership grew rapidly (from 7 to 21 per cent) and Coloured and Indian membership also rose.[44] Much private healthcare was concentrated in the three largest metropolitan areas of Durban, Cape Town, and the central Witwatersrand, reflecting the concentration of institutions and medical personnel there. Overall, three-fifths of all health expenditure was located in this private sector (2002/3 figures) despite the fact that medical aids membership had declined to only about one in eight of the population.[45] Until recently this private funding was exclusively directed at biomedicine and is still overwhelmingly of this type, accessing 60 per cent of specialists and 85 per cent of pharmacists in the country.[46] However, there are a few private sector social insurance companies that have recognized the needs of the users and practitioners of traditional medicine. For example, Medscheme and the Medical and Burial Savings Scheme have limited benefits for those consulting approved traditional healers, and Eskom (the nationalized electricity company), the Chamber of Mines, and the Union of Mineworkers are large employers or unions that allow periods of leave for employees/members to consult traditional healers.[47]

In private schemes membership is, and was, confined to the better-off sectors of society, whilst both private and public schemes suffer from spiralling cost inflation. These limitations, together with the fragmentation of private medical aids payment schemes, mean that there is a widely perceived need for fundamental reform of South Africa's strategies of parallel payment systems. A shift to a single national scheme is envisaged in a proposed national health insurance structure, which signifies a radical health policy shift from an inequitable two-tiered private/public system to an ambitious national single-payer system. It is envisaged that there will be universal coverage, free at the point of care, and accessible to all citizens.[48] This social insurance plan is an important, but delayed, aspect of post-1994 transformation in South Africa aiming to provide more equitable, responsive healthcare to replace the fragmented and skewed existing situation. This reflects the fact that (as we have seen) the 1996 South African Constitution enshrined the right to healthcare for every citizen and required the government to take reasonable steps to secure this. Therefore, in 2011 the first step was taken in what is envisaged as a long-term process of providing an envisioned national health insurance scheme (NHI) to fund essential healthcare for all South Africans. A 14-year project involving necessary preparatory work will lead up to the practical inception of social insurance in 2027. Already a green paper on the NHI has been published for public comment, and pilot sites have been established. Preliminary reaction from South Africans has been very positive, and is growing, with backing especially strong amongst women, a section of the population underrepresented in private medical scheme membership.[49]

## Health and disease

In comparison to the rest of the continent, South Africa is, and was, a relatively healthy country, having only a small, northern area where tropical diseases such as malaria – with heavy ensuing mortality – were a real problem. However, by the beginning of the twentieth century a number of diseases were thought to be a sufficiently serious threat to public health that even the healthiest, southern part of the country – Cape Colony – made them notifiable by doctors, including smallpox, typhus, yellow fever, cholera, syphilis, leprosy, diphtheria, typhoid (enteric), scarlet fever, puerperal fever, (tick borne) relapsing fever, and tuberculosis. But by mid-century medical interventions were becoming more effective for these illnesses – particularly with sulfone treatment for leprosy, immunization against diphtheria, and BCG for TB sufferers.

Public health and sanitation issues were perceived during the early twentieth century to be intimately related to a racial hierarchy in what has been termed 'the sanitation syndrome'.[50] As a result, the living conditions of Coloured, Indian, and African people became the target of public health officials' drastic remedial actions because they were seen as reservoirs of infection that could endanger the white population (see below). Related racially constructed interpretations of disease were found, as in a stereotyped view of syphilis, where drastic segregation was enforced against Africans under the Public Health Act of 1919.[51] The continuing prevalence of this in public debate was suggested by a statement from the influential General Smuts, who asserted in 1937 that, 'The Africans of this country are becoming rotten with disease and [are] a menace to civilisation'.[52]

Discussion of the African population's health was usually linked to the need for an efficient male black work force on which the country's economy depended. However, the occupational history of South Africa has left it with certain serious disease issues. One of these is silicosis amongst gold miners, the product of the high levels of dust including toxic silica in the mines, and another is asbestosis amongst those who have formerly worked in asbestos mines. Respiratory disease is then often associated with tuberculosis amongst miners and retired miners (and their families), which constitutes an intractable problem such that South Africa has one of the worst TB epidemics in the world.[53] And amongst agricultural workers who have been employed in the vineyards, where pay was traditionally partly in alcohol (the so-called 'dop system'), the incidence of foetal alcohol syndrome is the highest in the world.[54] More generally the traumatized society that emerged from four decades of apartheid's brutal inequalities has contributed to a remarkably high rate of violence, trauma, and injury, which is evident today in the overcrowded emergency departments of South African public hospitals, such that foreign doctors come to gain training experience there.

Past and present epidemics featured prominently in South Africa's morbidity and mortality. From the late eighteenth century vaccination reduced the mortality rate of outbreaks of smallpox, previously a deadly disease akin in its demographic impact to earlier outbreaks of plague in Europe.[55] Nor did South Africa escape plague as this dreaded disease entered the country via international shipping between 1901 and 1907, spreading inland from its ports. What Howard Phillips has termed 'racialised tunnel vision' on the part of urban public health officials then resulted in them pathologizing the African and Indian populations with authoritarian quarantine measures and residential segregation into permanent locations outside towns and cities. Less permanent in their effects (yet even more frightening in their scale) were two devastating waves of the 'Spanish' flu epidemic of 1918–19, which spread rapidly through inland areas via the newly expanded rail network, impacting with noticeably differential mortality between population groups, and with particularly high rates amongst Africans and Coloureds. This was part of a global pandemic, where the South African mortality of 6 per cent was the third highest in the world.[56]

Beginning in the early 1980s the HIV/AIDS epidemic began in a small white homosexual population but from 1987 spread rapidly to the much larger heterosexual African population. As Shula Marks aptly characterized it, this epidemic had been 'waiting to happen'[57] because a principal contributory factor was the oscillatory migrant labour system of Southern Africa, whereby male African migrants were recruited from their rural homes in South Africa and from the neighbouring countries of Botswana, Lesotho,

Mozambique, and Malawi to travel hundreds of miles to work in South Africa's gold and platinum mines.[58] Here they lived in male mining compounds, where concurrent sexual partnerships flourished and disease was transmitted, before returning to their home areas.[59] Although such circular migration patterns had been expected to dwindle after 1994, recent research has revealed its continuation, and hence the perpetuation of disease transmission from mines to miners' homes in Southern Africa's rural communities.[60] Indeed, the incidence of HIV amongst gold miners is almost double that of the general population, at 30 per cent for the former compared to 16 per cent for the latter.[61]

Given government hostility to and dilatoriness in instituting remedial measures for this pandemic, a roll-out of effective, biomedical treatment did not occur before 2003. Indeed, for a time the Minister of Health, Dr Manto Tshabalala-Msimang, preferred a policy of indigenous medicaments – such as African potato – as a treatment rather than, more appropriately, using it as an immune-boosting supplement. When anti-retrovirals were finally made freely available in what became the largest such public health programme in the world, the results were spectacular. These public measures ran parallel to private NGO (Non-Governmental Organization) activity, especially in preventive healthcare and education. And the activity of indigenous healers also impacted positively as they learned that, although their earlier hopes of indigenous cures were false, they had a valuable role to play both in referrals of patients to biomedical clinics and in giving immune-boosting supplements to enable individuals to withstand the ravages of the disease.[62] This replicated a pattern in developing countries worldwide where it is estimated that two-thirds of those suffering from HIV/AIDS have used traditional medicines to manage and gain relief from the opportunistic infections arising from HIV/AIDS.[63] Within

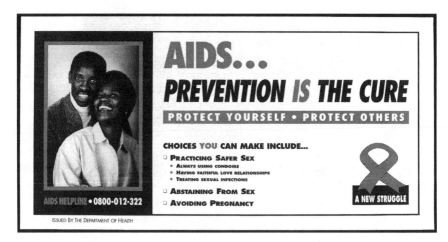

*Figure 8.2* 'AIDS: Prevention is the cure', South African Department of Health, *c*.1996. © The Wellcome Library, London.

South Africa there have been some initiatives to link the dual biomedical and indigenous spheres of healthcare to combat the pandemic. In Cape Town, for example, private medical care is supported by public grants given by the city to traditional healers who assist HIV/AIDS patients.[64]

South African life expectancy has recently increased by a remarkable 10 per cent – from 54 years in 2005 to 60 in 2011. This has partially offset an earlier ten year drop in life expectancy, which the WHO estimated as being the result of the HIV/AIDS pandemic. However, HIV prevalence remains amongst the highest in the world, and amongst pregnant women in 2012 it was still as high as 30 per cent.[65] The pandemic has claimed as many as 3.3 million lives in South Africa, with mortality especially heavy amongst young adults, and it has also created 2 million orphans.[66] Thus, its demographic impact will be long lasting.

The reaction of people in South Africa to this series of deadly epidemics served to highlight their respective attitudes to biomedicine and to indigenous medicine. The influenza epidemic was particularly illuminating in this context. In the public sphere faith in biomedicine was robust and one of the notable results of the epidemic was the creation of a central Public Health Department empowered for the first time to implement nationwide measures. But popular belief in biomedicine was weakened by its failure to provide effective remedies for influenza so that faith in alternatives also remained strong. This was shown both by recourse to folk nostrums, patent medicines and indigenous remedies and by action against 'evil' forces. Indeed, in African communities attempts at 'smelling out' the malign witches and wizards alleged to be responsible for the epidemic showed a notable increase, and the penal code for one area with a dense African population, the Transkei, was amended to lay down stiffer penalties for doing so.[67]

Morbidity and mortality cannot be separated from wider political, economic, and social issues, as we have already seen with the HIV/AIDS pandemic. By the end of the apartheid regime South Africa had very pronounced socio-economic inequality positively correlated with ethnicity, so that at the time of the democratic transition in 1994 there was a racially skewed distribution of income. Since then the growth of a stratified class society in the 'new' South Africa has to some extent increased inequality within a hierarchy where the wealth of a newly created affluent black middle-class minority contrasts with the continued impoverishment of the majority of Africans.[68] This is despite the fact that, following 1994, the democratically elected ANC government attacked the social legacy of apartheid with its privileging of the minority white population and its neglect of the black one. Government interventions to redress this situation have resulted in a rise in general living standards between 1994 and 2012: household access to electricity rose from 5.2 to 11.9 million; households with piped water increased from 7.2 to 12.7 million; and those living in formal housing increased from 5.8 to 11 million. Free clinic care is being provided for younger children and pregnant women. During the same period social welfare transfer payments (notably child

20 Myles Mander, *Marketing of Indigenous Medicinal Plants in South Africa – A Case Study in Kwazulu-Natal* (Rome: Food and Agriculture Organization of the United Nations, 1998).

21 Digby, *Division and Diversity*, 384–6, 299–300, 392–4; Mander *et al.*, 'Economics', 13.

22 Sinegugu Zukulu, Tony Dold, Tony Abbott and Domitilla Raimondo, *Medicinal and Charm Plants of Pondoland* (Pretoria: South African National Biodiversity Institute, 2012), 11.

23 Digby, *Diversity and Division*, 337–8, 352–3, 439–41.

24 Anne Digby and Helen Sweet, 'Social Medicine and Medical Pluralism: The Valley Trust and Botha's Hill Health Centre, South Africa, 1940s to 2000s', *Social History of Medicine*, 25 (2012): 425–45.

25 Anne Digby, '"The Bandwagon of Golden Opportunities"?: Healthcare in South Africa's Bantustan Periphery', *South African Historical Journal*, 64, 4 (2012): 827–51.

26 The missionary was Anthony Barker who worked in Zululand in the 1940s, and was quoted in Stanley G. Browne, 'The Contribution of Medical Missionaries to Tropical Medicine', *Transactions of the Royal Society of Tropical Medicine and Hygiene*, 73 (1979): 357–60.

27 Pieter Kok and Mark Collinson, *Migration and Urbanisation in South Africa* (Pretoria: Statistics South Africa, 2006).

28 Marije Versteeg, 'The State of the Right to Health in Rural South Africa', *South African Health Review* (Durban: Health Systems Trust, 2011), 100–6.

29 Anne Digby, 'Early Black Doctors in South Africa', *Journal of African History*, 46, 3 (2005): 427–54; Anne Digby, 'Black Doctors and Discrimination under South Africa's Apartheid Regime', *Medical History*, 57, 2 (2013): 269–90.

30 Digby, *Diversity and Division*, 200.

31 Ibid., 191.

32 Max Price, 'Health Care beyond Apartheid: Economic Issues in the Reorganisation of South Africa's Health Services', *Critical Health*, March 1987: 58.

33 Anne Digby and Howard Phillips with Harriet Deacon and Kirsten Thomson, *At the Heart of Healing: Groote Schuur Hospital, 1938–2008* (Johannesburg: Jacana, 2008), chapter 7.

34 Simonne Horwitz, *Baragwanath Hospital, Soweto: A History of Medical Care 1941–1990* (Johannesburg: University of Witwatersrand Press, 2013).

35 Sakhela Buhlungi, John Daniel, Roger Southall and Jessica Lutchman (eds), *State of the Nation: South Africa 2007* (Cape Town: HSRC Press, 2007), 292.

36 Shula Marks, *Divided Sisterhood: Race, Class and Gender in the South African Nursing Profession* (Johannesburg: University of Witwatersrand Press, 2001); 'Editorial', *South African Health Review* (Durban: Health Systems Trust, 1998), 1.

37 Buhlungi *et al.*, *State of the Nation*, 298–9.

38 Anne Digby, 'The Mid-level Health Worker in South Africa: The In-between Condition of the "Middle"', in Ryan Johnson and Amna Khalid (eds), *Public Health in the British Empire: Intermediaries, Subordinates, and Public Health Practice, 1850–1960* (London: Routledge, 2011).

39 Jannie Hugo, 'Mid-level Health Workers in South Africa: Not an Easy Option', *South African Health Review* (Durban: Health Systems Trust, 2005), 148–59; Karin Shapiro, 'Doctors or Medical Aids – The Debate over the Training of Black Medical Personnel for the Black Rural Population in South Africa in the 1920s and 1930s', *Journal of Southern African Studies*, 13 (1987): 234–55.

40 www.polity.org.za/polity/govdocs/white_papers/health.html

41 Anne Digby, 'Evidence, Encounters and Effects of South Africa's Reforming Gluckman National Health Services Commission, 1942–1944', *South African Historical Journal*, May 2012: 187–205.

42 Digby *et al.*, *At the Heart of Healing*.

43 Buhlungi *et al.*, *State of the Nation*, 291, 296.

44 Preeta Rama and Heather McLeod, *An Historical Study of Trends in Medical Schemes in South Africa: 1974–1999* (Centre for Actuarial Research: University of Cape Town, 2001), i–ii, 19.
45 'Private Health Care in South Africa' (Health Systems Trust), accessed Health Systems website at www//hst.org.za on 28 January 2013.
46 'Editorial', *South African Health Review* (Durban: Health Systems Trust, 1998), 1.
47 Pretorius, 'Traditional Healers', 254.
48 Meredith Evans and Olive Shisana, 'Gender Differences in Public Perceptions on National Health Insurance', *South African Medical Journal*, 12 (2012): 919–23.
49 Popo Maja, 'A Painstaking Journey', *Mail & Guardian*, 14–20 December 2012.
50 Maynard W. Swanson, 'The Sanitation Syndrome: Bubonic Plague and Urban Native Policy in the Cape Colony, 1900–1909', *Journal of African History*, 18 (1977): 387–410.
51 Karen Jochelson, *The Colour of Disease: Syphilis and Racism in South Africa, 1880–1950* (London: Palgrave, 2001).
52 [South African] *Sunday Times*, 2 October 1937. Smuts was prime minister from 1919 to 1924 and again from 1939 to 1948.
53 Randall M. Packard, *White Plague, Black Labor: Tuberculosis and the Political Economy of Health and Disease in South Africa* (Durban: University of Natal Press, 1989); 'Silent Killer Lurks in Miners' Lungs', *Mail & Guardian Health Supplement*, 25–31 January 2013; 'Editorial', *South African Health Review* (Durban: Health Systems Trust, 1997), 1; Jock McCulloch, *Asbestos Blues: Labour, Capital, Physicians and the State in South Africa* (Oxford: James Currey, 2002); Elaine Katz, *The White Death: Silicosis on the Witwatersrand Gold Mines* (Johannesburg: Witwatersrand University Press, 1994).
54 'South Africans in Addiction Free Fall', *Mail & Guardian Health Supplement*, 14–20 January 2012.
55 Howard Phillips, *Plague, Pox and Pandemics* (Auckland Park: Jacana, 2012), 26–7, 37.
56 Ibid., 80–81.
57 Shula Marks, 'An Epidemic Waiting to Happen?: The Spread of HIV/AIDS in South Africa in Social and Historical Perspective', *African Studies*, 61, 1 (2002): 13.
58 Charles H. Feinstein, *An Economic History of South Africa: Conquest, Discrimination and Development* (Cambridge: Cambridge University Press, 2005), 62–70.
59 Catherine Campbell, *'Letting Them Die': Why HIV/AIDS Prevention Programmes Fail* (Oxford: James Currey, 2003).
60 Lisa Steyn, 'Measuring the Waves of Migration', *Mail & Guardian Business*, 11–17 January 2013.
61 'Class Action for Silicosis Payout Tarnishes Gold Industry', *Mail & Guardian*, 26–31 January 2013.
62 Joanne Wreford, 'Loosening the Bonds of Historical Prejudice: Traditional Practitioners as Agents of Reconciliation and Change in Contemporary South Africa', in Anne Digby, Waltraud Ernst and Projit Mukharji (eds), *Crossing Colonial Historiographies: Histories of Colonial and Indigenous Medicines in Transnational Perspective* (Newcastle upon Tyne: Cambridge Scholars Publishing, 2010), 220–42.
63 *UN AIDS Report*, 2002.
64 *National Reference Centre for African Traditional Medicines: A South African Model*, 14.
65 'ARVs Raise Life Expectancy', *Mail & Guardian Health Supplement*, 7–13 December 2012.
66 Phillips, *Plague*, 112, 147, 149.
67 Ibid., 77.
68 Sampie Terreblanche, *A History of Inequality in South Africa 1652–2002* (Pietermaritzburg: University of Natal Press, 2002), 30–34.
69 'The Government Must Take Steps to Halt the Ratings Downgrades', *Business Report*, 9 December 2012, based on South African Institute of Race Relations reports.

# 9 Pharmaceutical innovation in the public and private spheres in the twentieth century

*Viviane Quirke*

## Introduction

The growing role played by medicine in the lives of people in the West is in large part the result of pharmaceutical innovation, for over the twentieth century drugs have increasingly complemented, or at times even replaced, other forms of therapy or care. This has been due not only to the effectiveness of the drugs themselves, which have enabled the medical profession to prevent, treat, or cure a wide variety of diseases, but also to the marketing and other business strategies of drug companies, which have helped to shape physicians' and patients' choices, transforming the consumption as well as delivery of healthcare, and contributing to the interweaving of private firms and public bodies that characterizes modern societies. This chapter therefore examines the interaction between the public and private spheres that has underpinned pharmaceutical innovation.[1] To set the scene it begins with an overview of pharmaceutical innovation, before commenting on the public–private interactions underlying it.

## Pharmaceutical growth, the medicalization of society, and the 'Therapeutic Revolution'[2]

One of the most remarkable features of the history of the twentieth century has been the growth of the pharmaceutical industry, and the rapid increase in the consumption of its products, particularly in the West (i.e. in North America and Europe (mainly Germany, France, Italy, Spain, and the UK) and Japan. By the end of the century, worldwide sales by drug companies were valued at around $350 billion, and have continued to rise.[3] By 2014, total global spending on prescription medicines reached over $1 trillion. It is expected to reach $1.2 trillion by 2017, with the major markets (now also joined by China) contributing 59 per cent of the increase.[4]

This trend began towards the end of the nineteenth century, when it was linked to the growth of the middle classes and a general rise in standards of living in the West, and accompanied the 'medicalization' of society: an increasing supply of, demand for, and dependence on medical products and services.[5] It accelerated after the Second World War, when newly established national systems of healthcare created mass markets for drugs, stimulating pharmaceutical innovation within private companies and public research institutions, which underwent a rapid expansion in the second half of the twentieth century. And it is set to continue, according to the most recent IMS predictions.

However, the anticipated rise in drug consumption of $220 billion over the five years between 2012 and 2017 represents in fact an unprecedented drop compared to previous increases. This drop has been attributed to a variety of factors: the recession in developed economies, which has meant more limited funds available for healthcare; the growing patient engagement in healthcare systems; the recent difficulties of the Chinese economy (which has been responsible for a large part of the expansion of drug consumption); and the end of patent coverage for the 'blockbuster drugs',[6] which since the 1970s had made the fortune of the pharmaceutical firms, but have more recently been displaced by cheaper generic alternatives. Nevertheless, new drugs are in the pipeline, and pharmaceutical innovation will endure, even though it appears to be changing in nature, with a novel emphasis on so-called 'orphan drugs', targeting smaller numbers of patients suffering from diseases such as rheumatoid arthritis, hepatitis C, cystic fibrosis, melanoma, and breast or ovarian cancer.[7]

The reasons for the evolution described above have been complex. As well as advances in science, technology, and medicine, there have been important social, economic, and political changes, including the growth of national health systems, the rise in public expectations of health services, and drug safety legislation. The drugs themselves have also played a major role, by providing a stimulus for subsequent scientific and technical improvements, by capturing the public's imagination with tales of 'miracle cures',[8] and by posing a challenge to health departments and regulatory authorities in terms of management and cost. This section focuses on just a few of these discoveries. They were often associated with important events, which had a crucial impact not only on health and medicine, but also on pharmaceutical innovation in the twentieth century. Among them the two world wars and the Cold War and its aftermath stand out. These led to major geopolitical realignments and shifts in the principal sites of drug discovery. I therefore distinguish between five main periods, each associated with specific groups of drugs: up to the start of the First World War; between 1914 and the start of the Second World War; during the war itself; post-war reconstruction and the Cold War; and finally the last 30 years.

### To 1914: From alkaloids to Salvarsan

Medicinal plants have always played a special role in the treatment of disease. Knowledge of their action and the practices associated with their preparation were often the object of secret recipes devised within the confines of the home or workshop. These recipes could also be shared by word of mouth, or disseminated through medical treatises and, later, pharmacopeias.[9]

However, it was not until the beginning of the nineteenth century that the first active principle was successfully extracted from a plant by Friedrich Wilhelm Adam Sertürner, a pharmacist's apprentice in the Prussian city of Paderborn, in 1804. This was the narcotic principle of opium, which was alkaline and formed salts with acids, and was later named morphine.[10] There followed the isolation and identification of many other plant alkaloids, including emetine from the ipecacuanha root for the treatment of dysentery, and quinine from cinchona bark for the treatment of malaria.

Imperial expansion and the prevalence of malaria in various parts of Europe at that time created a stimulus for the large-scale processing of cinchona bark and other plant alkaloids, usually by pharmaceutical wholesale businesses, such as Merck in Darmstadt, Germany. These private companies not only built factories to carry out the manufacture of the drugs, they also developed the chemical expertise required for selecting plant material of suitable quality for their production. The demand for quinine was high, while supplies were scarce. Attempts were therefore made to find cheaper chemical routes to its manufacture, not only within industry, but also within universities. One such attempt, by the young English chemist William Henry Perkin at the Royal College of Chemistry in London (later to become Imperial College), led to the first artificial dye, mauveine or aniline purple, synthesized from benzene, a by-product of the coal tar industry. As for quinine itself, it was not synthesized until 1944. However, synthetic quinine never offered a viable alternative to the many analogues that had, by then, been developed.

The synthetic dyestuffs industry that grew out of Perkin's discovery soon diversified into pharmaceuticals. It became an enterprise of considerable size in Germany, where it benefited from a number of favourable conditions: the strength of scientific teaching and research in German universities, particularly in synthetic organic chemistry; German unification on 18 January 1871 and the new patent law that followed in the same year; the annexation of Alsace-Lorraine, a key industrial region of Northern France ceded to Germany after the Franco-Prussian war. Together, these events formed the basis for the expansion of a powerful German chemical-pharmaceutical industry that would dominate the sector until the 1920s.[11]

Meanwhile, the discovery of synthetic chemicals with anaesthetic properties, such as chloroform, which had been synthesized in the 1830s and was given to Queen Victoria for the birth of the last two of her nine children, kindled the interest of medical practitioners in similar chemicals. It led to a search for other novel compounds with specific pharmacological activities. Among them were hypnotics (such as the barbiturate phenobarbitone, brand name Veronal), antipyretics, and analgesics, the most significant of which was acetylsalicylic acid (better known under the German drug firm Bayer's brand name: Aspirin). Although it had been synthesized in 1853 by the Alsatian chemist Charles Gerhardt, aspirin lay forgotten on the chemists' shelves for almost half a century. When its antipyretic and analgesic properties were finally recognized in 1899, it was probably because of the drug's chemical resemblance to salicylic acid, which is derived from willow bark, a folk remedy used to treat a wide variety of fevers. The actual mechanism of action of aspirin was discovered much later, in 1971, by John (later Sir John) Vane, and novel uses for the compound are still being found today; for instance, the prevention of heart attacks and strokes.[12]

In parallel with these efforts at curing disease, a new approach aiming to protect individuals against infections became established in the last decades of the nineteenth century, but not without some opposition from the public as well as the medical profession.[13] The new approach was named 'vaccination' (from the Latin *vacca*, meaning cow, as in cowpox), by analogy with variolation (from Latin *variola,* meaning smallpox). Variolation had long been practised in countries such as India and China to protect people against smallpox. At the end of the eighteenth century Edward Jenner in England, and a century later Louis Pasteur in France and Robert Koch in Germany, built not only on this ancient tradition, but also (in the case of Pasteur and Koch) on new knowledge about the causative agents of infectious diseases.

Pasteur showed that it was possible to protect birds from fowl cholera, and sheep from anthrax, by inoculating them with attenuated strains of these organisms. He then developed a vaccine against rabies, which was effective even when administered after the patient had been infected. His demonstration on a young Alsatian boy who had been bitten by a rabid dog, and was saved by his new vaccine, made the headlines and caused a sensation.[14] As a result, Pasteur was able to gather enough funds from an international public subscription to create an institute in Paris, which was named after him. Hence the Pasteur Institute was founded in 1888. Its purpose was fourfold: to produce the rabies vaccine, to distribute it in a dispensary, to carry out research into infectious diseases, and to teach microbiology.

The Pasteur Institute provided an inspiration for other medical research institutions elsewhere.[15] In 1891, The Royal Prussian Institute for Infectious Diseases was founded in Berlin by the new Prussian state (it was renamed The Royal Prussian Institute for Infectious Diseases 'Robert Koch' in 1919, and The Robert Koch Institute in 1942). In 1893, the British Institute for Preventive Medicine was created in London by a spontaneous association of scientists. Five years later the institute received a generous benefaction of £250,000 from the Irish philanthropist and businessman Edward Guinness, the First Earl of Iveagh, who sat on the governing body and requested that it be renamed after a British scientist. The name of Joseph Lister, best known for promoting the use of antiseptics in surgery, was chosen.[16] Each of these institutes represented a different variation of the complex – and at times controversial – relationship between vaccine manufacturers, the public, and the state at the beginning of the twentieth century.[17]

An important event in the development of a modern drug industry was the discovery of the diphtheria anti-serum at The Royal Prussian Institute by Emil von Behring and Shibasabuto Kitasato in 1891. It not only stimulated drug companies to produce vaccines and anti-sera in countries such as

Germany, Britain, and the USA, where before long firms like Parke Davis of Detroit became involved in the production of other biologicals, including organ and glandular extracts.[18] It also presented a challenge to governments in terms of public health policy and control of industrially produced medicines, often with very different outcomes in different national contexts.[19]

However, it was in Germany where the chemical capabilities of the dyestuffs industry combined with the bacteriological and immunological expertise of medical research institutes to produce another development that would have a profound and long-term impact on pharmaceutical innovation in the twentieth century. Indeed, it was at the Institute for Experimental Therapy in Frankfurt-am-Main, created with the support of the Prussian state as well as the local chemical industry for one of Koch's former research assistants, Paul Ehrlich, that chemotherapy was 'invented'.[20] Based on Ehrlich's concept of chemo-receptors (groupings of atoms by which chemical substances attach themselves to cells, in the same way as dyes attach themselves selectively to certain tissues, and antibodies to bacterial toxins), it became a reality with the arsenical drug Salvarsan, the most active among hundreds of compounds screened by Ehrlich and his research team in 1909, and marketed by Hoechst AG in 1910.[21] Also known as compound 606, or arsphenamine, Salvarsan was a 'magic bullet' capable of killing the micro-organisms responsible for syphilis, without harming their human host. Even though pharmacologists remained sceptical about Ehrlich's receptor theory, his extensive network of national and international contacts (both academic and industrial) meant that knowledge about Salvarsan spread quickly, and the drug itself was soon used to treat syphilis, not only in Germany but in other countries too.[22] Analogues of the compound were synthesized, beginning with 'Neo-Salvarsan', which was more stable and easier to use than its predecessor. Although arsenical drugs were eventually superseded 40 years later by penicillin, Ehrlich's innovative approach to drug discovery – screening a large number of molecules made according to a theory of drug action, before assessing their efficacy in experimentally infected animals – provided a model for the search for numerous other chemotherapeutic agents throughout the interwar period, and beyond.

### 1914 to 1939: from Salvarsan to the sulphonamides

Shortly after the launch of Salvarsan, the First World War broke out, and it revealed the extent of Germany's monopoly over synthetic remedies. The war interrupted supplies of Salvarsan and other German imported drugs, on which many countries had become reliant, even those with a powerful chemical sector such as Switzerland.[23] On the other hand, the war offered a justification for the abolition of German patent rights in countries at war with Germany. It therefore facilitated the transfer of scientific knowledge and technical knowhow, and created the impetus for the manufacture of synthetic drugs by pharmaceutical firms elsewhere. In Britain, Boots and Burroughs Wellcome & Co. began to acquire the necessary chemical expertise in collaboration with university departments, under the co-ordination of the newly formed Medical Research Committee – later renamed Medical Research Council (MRC) – in government schemes that prefigured the scientific-military-industrial complex of the Second World War.[24]

However, the period that followed the First World War is often considered a low point in the history of drug discovery. Other than a few successes against protozoal (mainly tropical) diseases, with Germanin against sleeping sickness, and Plasmochin and Atebrin against malaria,[25] chemotherapy appeared to have failed to deliver on its early promise. Moreover, it was not until Raymond Ahlquist formulated his dual-receptor theory in 1948, and drugs were developed in the 1960s that blocked the beta-receptors in the heart for the treatment of cardiac arrhythmias and hypertension (such as propranolol, brand name Inderal), that the receptor concept provided a truly fruitful basis for pharmaceutical innovation.[26]

Chemotherapy competed at first unsuccessfully with immunotherapy, at a time when anti-sera proliferated, although often with little effect against infectious diseases such as streptococcal or pneumococcal infections. Nevertheless, the interwar years saw important achievements in the new field of replacement therapy, directed against deficiency diseases caused by a lack of vitamins or hormones in the body. In this field, the most significant developments occurred mainly in Britain and North America, where the strength of the physiological tradition in medicine made up for relative weaknesses in synthetic organic chemistry.

The word 'vitamin' was coined by a Polish chemist, Casimir Funk, when he was a guest worker at the Lister Institute in 1912. The Lister Institute later became involved in a collaborative research programme with the MRC to study rickets in post-war, famine-stricken Vienna. The project led to the identification of the anti-rachitic factor, vitamin D. Other vitamins followed, and by the 1930s most of them had been isolated, their structures worked out, and their chemical synthesis realized. This led some companies like Glaxo, who were baby-food manufacturers and began adding vitamin supplements to infant milk, to enter the pharmaceutical sector.[27]

There were also a number of important breakthroughs in the field of hormones during this period: the isolation of the active principle of the thyroid gland by E.C. Kendall at the Mayo Clinic in Rochester, Minnesota, in 1919; the extraction of the pancreatic hormone insulin, by F. Banting, J.J.R. Macleod, C. Best and J.B. Collip at the University of Toronto in 1922; and the characterization of steroid hormones by a number of different researchers in the 1920s and 1930s. But the discovery of insulin, the lack of which had been shown to cause diabetes mellitus, was perhaps the most significant from the point of view of the history of pharmaceutical innovation.[28] It provided the first example of a potentially fatal disease rendered chronic by a drug, which required skilful management on the part of the patient as well as the physician, and led to the first disease-based patient associations. It had an important role in the development of biological standardization, the evolution of academic–industrial relations,[29] and the internationalization of pharmaceutical innovation, transforming what had initially been a North American network of academic and industrial laboratories into a transatlantic one, involving public and private research institutions not only in the USA and Canada but also in Britain, and then elsewhere in Europe.[30] In certain countries with a limited chemical industry (for example Denmark) it would play a key part in the growth of an indigenous pharmaceutical sector.[31]

Such is the significance of insulin that it remained a focal point for scientific research and pharmaceutical innovation throughout the twentieth century: from the determination of its primary structure by Fred Sanger in Cambridge using sequencing methods in 1955, and the elucidation of its complete 3-D structure by Dorothy Hodgkin in Oxford using X-ray crystallography in 1969, to the development of the first biotechnology drug, Humulin, by the American drug company Eli Lilly using recombinant DNA techniques in 1982.[32]

Meanwhile, the search for chemical agents to treat bacterial infections had continued, especially in the Bayer laboratories, now part of the chemical group IG Farben, where it was modelled on Ehrlich's approach. In 1932, Bayer's director of research in experimental pathology, Gerhard Domagk, carried out experiments on mice infected with streptococci using a red dye, named Prontosil rubrum. He found that the animals treated with the compound survived, while the controls died. Later, Domagk succeeded in curing his own daughter from a streptococcal infection using Prontosil. By 1935, clinical trials were under way, and the results of Domagk's experiments and tests were published.[33]

The study of Prontosil was taken up by numerous centres in Germany and abroad, including the Therapeutic Chemistry Laboratory of the Pasteur Institute in Paris. There, Ernest Fourneau's team, which included a future Director of the Pasteur Institute, Jacques Tréfouël, and future Nobel Prize winner, Daniel Bovet, showed that, contrary to the belief that the power of dyes to destroy bacteria came from their ability to colour their vital elements, Prontosil was broken down in the body, and that the active principle was, in fact, the colourless compound sulphanilamide. Because it had been known for a long time, sulphanilamide could not be patented. Hence, other drugs, all based on the sulphanilamide molecule, soon followed Prontosil. Septoplix was launched in 1936 by Rhône-Poulenc, which had a longstanding collaborative arrangement with Fourneau. M&B 693, which became famous for saving Winston Churchill's life when he contracted pneumonia during the Second World War, was developed in 1937 by the British subsidiary of Rhône-Poulenc, May & Baker.[34]

By effectively breaking Germany's monopoly on synthetic drugs, the discovery of the antibacterial action of sulphanilamide spurred some chemical companies, such as Imperial Chemical Industries (ICI),[35] who would become important players in the history of pharmaceutical innovation during and after the Second World War, to embark on pharmaceutical research.[36] It led them to develop sulphamezathine, for a time the most widely used sulpha-drug in Britain.[37]

### *1939 to 1945: Synthetic anti-malarials, compound E, and penicillin*

At the start of the Second World War, the production of sulpha-drugs was well under way outside Germany. Nevertheless, as had happened in the First World War, supplies of other German synthetic drugs, including Plasmochin and Atebrin, were once again interrupted. When the conflict extended from Europe to the Far East, not only exposing the troops to malaria but cutting off the main source of quinine from Java, it created potential difficulties for the Allied war effort. These difficulties had been anticipated, however, and the search for novel anti-malarials had begun before the Japanese attack on Pearl Harbour in December 1941, resulting in the production of the German drugs and the development of new ones: Paludrine by ICI in 1945, and Chloroquine by Winthrop in 1946.

Soon after Dunkirk, Anglo-American discussions started with a view to setting up Lend-Lease agreements, by which the USA would provide Britain with material support. As a result of these discussions, co-operative research programmes were initiated in order to pool British and American scientific knowledge and technical expertise. Radar and the atom bomb are the most famous of these projects, but there were also collaborative schemes to develop pharmaceutical products: compound E (later known as cortisone), penicillin, as well as synthetic anti-malarials.[38] By 1942, the programme to produce penicillin in large quantities for the treatment of war wounds and other infections, and to find a synthetic route to its manufacture, dominated the Allies' co-operative ventures in pharmaceuticals. Such was the importance of penicillin, which not only saved many lives but also represented one of the more benign aspects of the victorious Allies' scientific–military–industry complex, that it would serve as a blueprint for subsequent collaborative schemes, and become a reference-point for biomedical research projects, in Britain, America, and elsewhere.[39] For this reason, the story of penicillin deserves to be told here in some detail.

The ability of the mould *Penicillium notatum* to inhibit bacterial growth had been known since ancient times.[40] However, it was Alexander Fleming's chance observation in 1928 of the mould's activity against staphylococci, and his subsequent study of the antibacterial substance it secreted, which he named 'penicillin', that laid the foundations for the development of the life-saving drug by Howard Florey's team at the Sir William Dunn School of Pathology in Oxford ten years later.

The declaration of war in 1939 gave special urgency to Florey's multi-disciplinary research programme, which had originally aimed to study micro-organisms with known antibacterial activity, but now focused on penicillin. While Norman Heatley, a biochemist with expertise in micro-methods, focused on the problem of production, Ernst Chain (a Jewish refugee from Germany who acquired refugee status after his arrival in Britain in 1933) worked on the chemistry of the mould, and Florey himself devised a series of biological experiments that would help to establish penicillin as a new kind of chemotherapeutic agent, less toxic than the sulphonamides, but active against staphylococci, against which the sulpha-drugs had little effect.[41] The team's preliminary results were published in *The Lancet* in 1940. However, before the publication of the reports of the first clinical tests, Florey and Heatley flew to the USA, with the British government's blessing, in the hope of getting the large-scale manufacture of penicillin started there. The outcome of this visit, and of the combined British and American efforts that followed, was the mass production of the drug using deep-fermentation methods, which were developed by the North Regional Research Laboratory at Peoria, Illinois, and perfected by various American companies under the aegis of the Office for Scientific Research and Development (OSRD).[42] Penicillin therefore became available in sufficiently large quantities for the D-Day landings, and for the wider public afterwards, although this happened sooner in some countries, where firms were quicker either to take up American licences or to develop deep-fermentation themselves, than in others.[43]

The impact of penicillin on pharmaceutical innovation was immense. The penicillin industry that emerged from the war included newcomers to the pharmaceutical sector from the fermentation industries, whose expertise would contribute to the growth of the new biotechnology in the 1970s,[44] and from countries such as Japan, which would make a significant contribution to pharmaceutical innovation in the second half of the twentieth century.[45] Although deep-fermentation was never completely superseded, the search for a synthetic route eventually led to the first semi-synthetic penicillin, which was active against gram-negative bacteria (unaffected by ordinary penicillin), and was named Penbritin by Beechams in 1959.[46]

Penicillin represented the culmination of the chemotherapeutic approach in medicine.[47] Drug companies that had previously steered clear of chemotherapy, such as the manufacturers of galenicals Allen & Hanburys,[48] now adopted it in their search for novel remedies.[49] So began what has been described as the 'Antibiotic Era'.[50] Penicillin was followed by numerous other antibacterial substances. One of these was streptomycin, which was discovered by Selman Waksman's team at Rutgers University in 1943, and was the first effective chemotherapeutic treatment for one of the great killers of the late nineteenth and early twentieth centuries: tuberculosis.[51] Antibiotics appeared to spell the end of infectious diseases, and opened up a window of opportunity for companies such as ICI to embark on ambitious programmes to tackle chronic diseases.[52] Together with the great vaccination campaigns of the post-war years, it helps to explain the new optimism and faith in modern medicine that reigned in this period,[53] before bacterial resistance became a major problem.[54] At the same time, it put pressure on the new national health systems, leading to an increase in public expectations and a spiralling drugs bill, the legacy of which endures to this day.[55]

The American pharmaceutical sector, and to a lesser degree its British counterpart, had emerged victorious from the war. By contrast, like Germany itself, the German drug industry had been defeated. The links between German industry and Hitler's brutal racial policies led to the dismantling of the almighty IG Farben.[56] German scientists, especially biologists tainted by their association with eugenics, were for a time excluded from the international scientific community. This compounded the effects of emigration of Jewish scientists in the 1930s, which had not only benefited Germany's enemies during the war,[57] but afterwards led to delays in the development of a German school of molecular biology, and to a need on the part of public and private research institutions later to 'catch up' with developments abroad.[58]

But what of countries such as France, which, although allied to Britain, had experienced military defeat and German occupation? France's case suggests that isolation from the Allies' research programmes was in fact favourable to pharmaceutical innovation. The history of the first psychotropic drug (i.e. a drug affecting mood), chlorpromazine, which was discovered by Rhône-Poulenc, illustrates well this twist in our story. Indeed, unaware in 1944 that an American team at Iowa State College had synthesized a series of phenothiazine amines, but found them useless as anti-malarials, Rhône-Poulenc continued with their research. In the process they discovered that, although ineffective against malaria, phenothiazine amines had anti-histaminic properties. Not only did these lead them to promethazine (brand name Phénergan), for the treatment of allergies, but also to compound RP 3276, which later formed the core of the chlorpromazine molecule (marketed as Largactil in Europe and Thorazine in North America). As the Director of Pharmaceutical Research at Rhône-Poulenc, Pierre Viaud, later pointed out, if in 1944 the French had known of the Americans' work, they would probably have abandoned their own.[59]

### 1945 to 1975: From cortisone to cancer chemotherapy

The period following the Second World War, often referred to as the 'Therapeutic Revolution', saw an explosion in the number of new drugs being developed and marketed. Some of them had their origins in wartime projects, but many others were the product of increased investments in pharmaceutical and biomedical research in the aftermath of war, and of the mass-market for drugs created by the new national health services.

The magnitude of this increase has been so great this chapter can do little more than touch on a few of the most significant innovations. These have extended across all pharmacological groups, from antibiotics to drugs for cancer, heart disease and psychiatric illness. The main subject areas discussed here are corticosteroids, chlorpromazine, receptor-blockers, and anti-cancer drugs.

*Cortisone and corticosteroid drugs*

Cortisone had been synthesized from bile acids by Merck during the war using a method devised by Kendall. The dramatic demonstration of the efficacy of the drug against rheumatoid arthritis, made by Philip Hench, a colleague of Kendall, at the Seventh International Congress of Rheumatology in New York in 1949, caused the 'outpouring of steroidal investigations' that has given us many of the drugs we are familiar with today,[60] including the contraceptive pill, which is often thanked (or blamed) for the 'Sexual Revolution' of the 1960s.[61]

By the mid-1950s, the serious side effects brought on by the high dosage of cortisone required to treat rheumatoid arthritis had led to the development of analogues with reduced toxicity and increased physiological activity. Hence, as the use of cortisone in the treatment of rheumatoid arthritis declined, the important part that corticosteroids would play in modern medicine began to emerge.[62] Like cortisone, these drugs seemed a 'panacea' for a number of diseases of unknown cause, but which share the feature of excessive inflammation, such as allergies, acute infections, and autoimmune disorders.[63] By providing a treatment for such a wide range of diseases, corticosteroids transformed the outlook of numerous medical specialties, from rheumatology

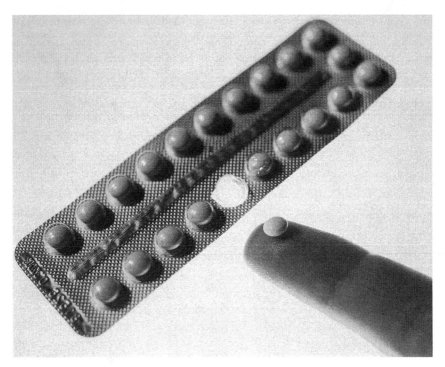

*Figure 9.1* Pack of contraceptive pills – one has been removed and is shown on finger.
© Kate Whitley, The Wellcome Library, London.

to respiratory medicine. Moreover, because cortisone treatment had to be sustained over a long period of time, raising issues of appropriate dosage and long-term patient care, rheumatoid arthritis became the prototype of a chronic illness,[64] and corticosteroids offered companies a helpful angle of attack in the search for drugs against chronic diseases.

Thus, the discovery of cortisone had a great impact not only on medicine, but also on pharmaceutical innovation. Shortages of bile acids or of dollars with which to import intermediates from the USA encouraged some firms, such as Boots, to look for non-steroidal anti-inflammatory drugs (NSAIDs), leading to ibuprofen (Nurofen). Others, such as Glaxo, began searching for alternative sources of raw material and for new means of producing the drug in collaboration with the American drug company Merck, as well as with British academic consultants, and then as part of a wider collaborative scheme devised by the MRC, which eventually led to Betnovate.[65] This second approach also resulted in the development of biosynthetic methods from plant materials by Upjohn, Schering, and Syntex almost simultaneously, using micro-organisms as reagents in a process that would not only 'revolutionize the steroid industry'[66] but also offer yet another pathway to the new biotechnology.[67]

### Chlorpromazine and psychotropic drugs

Like cortisone, chlorpromazine, which has already been referred to earlier, had a considerable effect on pharmaceutical innovation in the second half of the twentieth century. This drug, which calmed disturbed patients until then locked up in mental hospitals, contributed to a new, open-door policy in the treatment of the mentally ill. Thanks to the efforts of the French psychiatrists Jean Delay and Pierre Deniker, to a well-orchestrated marketing campaign on the part of Rhône-Poulenc, and to a receptive audience of medical professionals, the use of chlorpromazine spread rapidly to Britain, Europe, North America, and further afield.[68]

By giving substance to a biochemical understanding of mental disorders, chlorpromazine transformed the practice of psychiatry, and created a new discipline: psychopharmacology.[69] It stimulated the development of other psychotropic drugs, beginning with the tranquilizer Miltown, which was launched onto the American market by Wallace Laboratories in 1955, and was enthusiastically received by patients, leading to a veritable 'Miltown Mania'.[70] Miltown was soon followed by Librium, synthesized by Leo Sternbach in the Nutley (New Jersey) Division of the Swiss pharmaceutical firm Hoffmann-La Roche in 1955, and marketed in 1960. Librium was then succeeded by Valium, which became the most widely prescribed drug in the Western world between 1968 and 1981, tapping into the 'Age of Anxiety'[71] and contributing to what David Healy has described as the 'Antidepressant Era'.[72] However, by the 1970s, concerns had developed about the addictive nature of prescription drugs such as Valium. Their proliferation on the market, the commercial interests linked to their sale, their administration by a sometimes over-zealous medical profession to an ever widening patient-base, including children, and their role in the medicalization of emotions hitherto considered as inherent to the human condition, have since then also caused questions to be raised about their use and abuse.[73]

*Receptor-blockers and stimulants*

Although most of the early psychotropic drugs were developed without any clear understanding of their mechanism of action, the receptors for many of the neurotransmitters present in the brain were later identified. Other areas of research that were to benefit from the study of receptors were cardiovascular, respiratory, and gastric medicine. This happened after the beta-blockers began what has been called the 'Age of the Receptor'.[74]

The first clinically useful beta-blockers were synthesized in ICI's new pharmaceutical laboratories at Alderley Park, in Cheshire, where the British physiologist James (later Sir James) Black arrived in 1958. There he was responsible for the project to find remedies for coronary artery disease, within a wider programme of developing cardiovascular drugs. Applying Ahlquist's theory of alpha- and beta-receptors, which was then just beginning to gain acceptance, Black reasoned that, instead of trying to *increase* the supply of oxygen to the heart, as was being done at the time with nitrites, it might be possible to *reduce* the demand for oxygen by blocking the beta-receptors in the heart. By 1960, Black and his team had developed pronethalol, which was launched under the name Alderlin in 1963. However, because it had been found to cause tumours in mice, it was withdrawn from the market, and replaced by propranolol (Inderal) in 1965. Following extensive trials, propranolol became the favourite treatment for cardiac arrhythmias, as well as for angina. After it had been found by clinicians to reduce blood-pressure, it was also used to treat hypertension.[75]

The success of propranolol, and the large size of the market it targeted, led to an active search by companies in Britain and elsewhere for new beta-blockers, with different properties, for the treatment of various conditions. Although in hypertension the beta-blockers have to some extent been superseded by other drugs, such as the ACE inhibitors, they are still among the most widely used heart drugs today. Moreover, by giving substance to the receptor concept, they prompted a search for further receptor-blockers and stimulants, for use in gastric and respiratory medicine.

An important breakthrough was the development by David (later Sir David) Jack's team at Allen & Hanburys, which had recently become part of Glaxo, of the bronchodilator salbutamol (Ventolin) for the treatment of asthma.[76] In gastroenterology, it was the development by Black, since 1964 in the British subsidiary of SK&F, of the histamine antagonist cimetidine (Tagamet) for the treatment of stomach ulcers that later inspired the development of the bestselling drug Zantac by Glaxo.[77] For his contribution to medicine, in 1988 James Black received the Nobel Prize for Physiology and

Medicine, jointly awarded also to the American biochemists George Hitchings and Gertrude Elion. This was the first time that the prize was awarded to scientists working in the pharmaceutical industry. I will describe Hitchings and Elion's contribution, which was made in the American laboratories of the British company Burroughs Wellcome, further below.

*Anti-cancer agents*

Thanks to the considerable sums of money from private as well as public sources invested in what became known as the 'War on Cancer', this most dreaded disease provided a major focus for pharmaceutical and biomedical innovation, producing some of the most expensive drugs on the market, assessed in global multi-centre trials due to the small numbers of patients suffering from any single type of cancer.[78] However, advances in cancer treatment usually resulted from the convergence of many different areas of therapeutic research, not all of which were initially concerned with cancer. The beginnings of cancer chemotherapy examined in this section occurred in three broadly defined phases. Although they overlapped with one another, each phase represented a change in the style and scale of research: from largely local experimentation (in the 1940s–50s), to national and then international mass-screening programmes (1950s–60s), and finally global multi-centre trials (1960s–70s).[79] In the first phase, the USA – where organized science had been mobilized on a large scale in the Second World War and then the Cold War – provided a fruitful context for the battle against cancer, more especially for the development of chemotherapy.[80]

The origins of this particular form of cancer treatment lay in the Second World War, when renewed fears about chemical gas attacks had led researchers at Yale University, under contract with the OSRD, to examine the pharmacology of nitrogen mustards. These showed the ability to shrink tumours, and were therefore studied on both sides of the Atlantic after the American workers had shared their results with their British colleagues. The outcome of this research was the use of nitrogen mustards as the first effective anti-cancer agents. A search for compounds exhibiting a similar action began, and thereafter chemotherapy became closely associated with the fight against cancer.[81]

A number of other substances were also tried against cancer, including steroid hormones and antibiotics. Following the discovery in the early 1950s of natural sources of steroids in plants such as the Mexican wild yam, and of therapeutic properties in *Rauwolfia serpentina* (Indian snakeroot: for hypertension), and more pertinently here *Catharanthus rosea* (Madagascar periwinkle: for leukaemias and lymphomas), there was renewed interest in plants as a potential source of anti-cancer drugs. They became the object of a vast screening effort led by the National Cancer Institute, in collaboration with the US Department of Agriculture, the product of which was Taxol, derived from the bark of *Taxus braevifolia* (the Pacific Yew tree).[82]

However, a different angle of attack that was to prove fruitful not only against cancer but against other diseases too, in particular disorders of the immune system and viral infections, was the search for anti-metabolites.[83] This search was carried out in a number of laboratories, among them the American laboratories of the British firm Burroughs Wellcome, which hired the biochemist George Hitchings in 1942. The programme on which Hitchings worked was based on his knowledge of folic acid, of its role in the synthesis of nucleic acids, and therefore also in cell growth.[84] In 1944 he was joined by Gertrude Elion, who remained his close collaborator for the rest of his career.[85] Although the team's strategy was primarily led by their ideas about drug action and the anti-metabolites they made,[86] a major impetus for their research was cancer, for Burroughs Wellcome's laboratories in Tuckahoe, near New York City, had an arrangement with a private cancer research institution and treatment centre, the nearby Sloan-Kettering Institute (later the Memorial Sloan-Kettering Cancer Centre), to screen their compounds. By the late 1940s, these pharmacological screens had identified two promising groups of compounds: the purine and pyrimidine analogues.

Elion focused on the purines, which proved the most fruitful part of the programme. It was she who synthesized 6-mercaptopurine, in 1951. Almost at

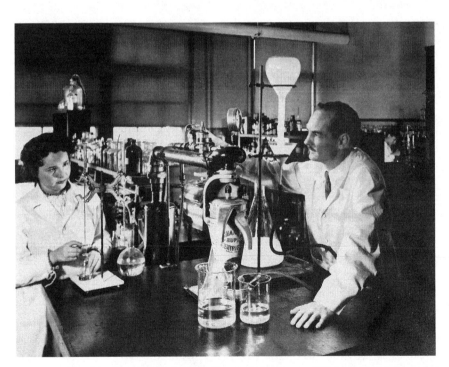

*Figure 9.2* Photograph of Dr Gertrude Elion and Dr George Hitchings in a laboratory, 1948. © The Wellcome Library, London.

once, it became involved in a 'myriad biochemical studies'. As it came to be known, 6-MP was tested in leukaemia patients at the Sloan-Kettering Institute, was approved by the Food and Drug Administration (FDA) in 1953, and launched onto the market as Purinethol. Eventually 6-MP was used in combination with other drugs and radiation treatment, and made childhood leukaemia one of the more curable forms of cancers. One of the first clinically useful chemical derivatives of a component of DNA, 6-MP is often considered a landmark discovery in the history of pharmaceutical innovation. It gave substance to the idea of anti-metabolites, sparking a race for the 'magic bullet' against cancer.[87]

Another reason why 6-MP was important was that it encouraged Hitchings's team to pursue the nucleic acid anti-metabolite route. It was followed by several 'spin-offs': in 1957, a derivative of 6-MP (Imuran), which was longer acting than 6-MP, was used as an immunosuppressant in the first renal transplant patients; in 1966 the purine analogue allopurinol (Zyloprim) was approved by the FDA for the treatment of gout. The team later applied their knowledge of nucleic acid metabolism to the problem of viruses, and developed acyclovir (Zovirax), launched in 1985, to treat the symptoms of herpes infections, shingles, and chickenpox.

### *From 1975 to the present: The (largely unfulfilled?) promises of biotechnology*

By 1975, the pace of innovation had begun to slacken, not only at Burroughs Wellcome, but in other companies too. Many (particularly in the industry)[88] have explained this by the tightening of safety regulations that occurred in the wake of the thalidomide tragedy, which caused babies to be born with deformed or stunted limbs in the early 1960s.[89] Another explanation has been that the easiest drugs were discovered first, often by accident, and that the purposeful search for novel remedies, based on an understanding of the underlying mechanisms of disease, is more difficult and therefore takes much longer.

As the number of blockbuster drugs, which kept pharmaceutical firms in profit in the face of mounting competition and soaring R&D costs, has declined, and the patent period for existing drugs has come to an end, companies have tended to increase their expenditure on marketing rather than research, and turned to mergers and acquisitions as means of achieving economies of scale and scope. However, the proliferation of 'me-too' drugs on the market[90] has led to questions as to whether such measures are conducive to innovation. At a time of growing drug resistance (with new, hospital-acquired infections such as MRSA), and new, emerging infectious diseases, from AIDS to SARS and swine flu,[91] these issues have posed challenges for governments in terms of regulation and policy.

The new biotechnology, which built on the fundamental discoveries in molecular biology of Cohen and Boyer (recombinant DNA) in 1973, and of Milstein and Kohler (hybridoma of monoclonal antibodies) in 1975, has benefited from this dearth of new drugs, tapping into public anxieties about new scourges and the end of the 'Age of Optimism'.[92] Hence, in the 1980s biotechnology became an important focal point for national scientific and industrial policies, with the USA leading the way. However, the extent to which biotechnology has fulfilled its early promise in the field of human healthcare is debatable.[93] Although since the 1990s many new diagnostic technologies, as well as many of the most innovative drugs, have come not from the large R&D laboratories of the pharmaceutical industry but from the much smaller biotech companies, for instance human insulin and the human growth hormone, the true benefits of these, often expensive, new drugs compared with their predecessors are often unclear.

Nevertheless, there is little doubt that a shift has taken place from Big Pharma to Biotech, and has resulted in a change in the nature of pharmaceutical innovation. The advent of the new biotechnology has brought back the individual scientist-entrepreneur, who for much of the twentieth century had been eclipsed by the multi-disciplinary research team. It has led to the growth of what has been termed the 'Bioscience industry', the product of strategic alliances between Big Pharma and Biotech start-ups, which has tended to develop in clusters around top-ranking universities, in North America, then in Europe, and most recently in some countries of the Far East.[94] And at the beginning of the twenty-first century, it continues to promise us new and better medicines, such as gene and stem cell therapies, targeting the individual patient rather than the disease.

In the next section, I examine more closely the collaboration between the public and private sectors that has underpinned the evolution described above, and in turn has been shaped by it.

## Pharmaceutical innovation in public and private: Collaborative relations and blurred boundaries

Collaboration between the public and private sectors has long been understood as playing a key role in pharmaceutical innovation, especially the increase in the rate of drug discovery associated with the second (pharmacological) Therapeutic Revolution.[95] It was therefore often encouraged by governments keen to promote public health as well as to foster strong national pharmaceutical industries, which gained an unprecedented economic, social, and political importance that has endured to this day.

The activities involved in the collaboration between the two sectors varied, depending on where and when it occurred. Although academic–industrial collaboration has attracted much interest from academic historians and industry analysts, to date there has been no systematic study of its evolution. Therefore, what follows is a general overview that is based on the available literature as well as the author's own research. It would benefit from being grounded in both time and space, and being refined with local case studies to a greater extent than is possible here.[96]

## Relations before the Second World War

Formal, organized relations between public research institutions (not only universities, but also other not-for-profit research institutions)[97] and drug companies were relatively rare until the Second World War.[98] Before then, they tended to take place between individuals. The close relations that existed between academic scientists and their colleagues in industry were often based on personal friendships, going back to university days and early laboratory training.[99] The mobility of researchers, particularly chemists and pharmacists, who switched with relative ease between academic and industrial careers, helped to break down the boundaries between the public and private sectors.[100] In countries such as France, the practice of 'cumul' (the joint holding by a single person of different posts in different institutions) also contributed to this blurring of boundaries. Activities occurring at the interface between academia and industry ranged from consultancies, through which academic scientists provided expert advice to firms, to practical research carried out on specific company projects (to develop a new process or drug, for example).[101] A more direct form of academic entrepreneurship also existed, involving the patenting of discoveries or inventions.[102] However, the outright involvement of academic scientists in the foundation of commercial enterprises remained relatively rare until the new biotechnology in the 1980s.

Meanwhile, in industry, a major transformation had occurred to accompany this evolution. Influenced by the example of German chemical firms, the first science-based drug companies began building analytical laboratories to analyse competitors' products as well as test the quality of their own, which were later followed by research laboratories using scientific knowledge and experimental practice to develop new products and processes.[103] These early science-based companies played a crucial role in the development of a modern pharmaceutical sector, not least by providing a model for other firms to follow in order to innovate and compete in the national, and increasingly international, medical marketplace. Usually referring to themselves as 'ethical' drug manufacturers to distinguish themselves from patent drug makers and pill peddlers,[104] they included firms such as Merck, Hoechst, Bayer, and Schering in Germany; Parke Davis, Merck, Smith Kline & French, E.R. Squibb & Sons, and Eli Lilly in the US; Burroughs Wellcome & Co. and Allen & Hanburys in Britain; Poulenc Frères and the Laboratoires Houdé in France.[105] As well as inviting academic colleagues to provide scientific advice or work on particular research projects for a limited period of time, the most 'open' among these science-based firms often encouraged their own researchers to join learned societies, communicate their findings at scientific conferences, and publish.[106]

## After the Second World War

After the Second World War, as the industry came to be dominated by large, international and multi–divisional corporations,[107] academic-industrial relations were institutionalized to a greater extent, involving not only public research institutions and firms, but also government departments, in what has been described as the 'Triple Helix'.[108] In the fields of health and medicine, the postwar period saw the emergence of a biomedical complex (referred to in this way by analogy with the scientific–military–industrial complexes of the Second World War and the Cold War).[109] Although personal ties between individual researchers continued to play an important role within this complex, the practice of collaboration became more formal, with research contracts being drawn up at the institutional level. Industrial sponsorship in the form of grants to finance specific research projects, studentships and laboratories was therefore more common, and benefited hospital as well as university medicine.

For medicine had similarly experienced a radical transformation. From a largely marginal pursuit, research had become a significant component of clinical practice, accelerating a trend that had begun before the Second World War in a number of countries.[110] The term 'biomedicine', which originated in the interwar programmes of public research institutions such as the National Institutes of Health (NIH) in the USA or the MRC in Britain and aimed to legitimize the alignment of clinical medicine with scientific medicine, became more widely used.[111] Symptomatic of this new alignment of clinical medicine with the biological – and later molecular – sciences, clinical trials became the 'gold standard' of experimental practice in medicine, particularly once landmark trials such as the MRC's streptomycin trial had given them their modern form: the randomized controlled trial (RCT).[112] Collaborative relations with hospital clinicians likely to be involved in such trials therefore became increasingly important for firms keen to secure the help and expertise of the arbiters of best medical practice, as well as attract the good will of the gatekeepers to the medical marketplace. At the same time, following the example of American marketing practices, armies of 'detail men' were dispatched to doctors' surgeries and clinics to provide information and samples about company products, while learning about new trends and preferences in therapy.[113] Spurred by wartime developments in operations research and inspired by management science models, which were disseminated to Europe and elsewhere by American firms of management consultants in the 1950s and 1960s,[114] 'scientific marketing' was another feature of the American influence on pharmaceutical firms.[115] This influence was not limited to industry, however; it also extended to charitable, medical, and government organizations.[116]

These new collaborative relations, with the clinic as well as with the state, were not only formalized, they were institutionalized within companies. This happened at first by creating integrated R&D departments, through which the research, marketing, and production functions of firms were combined and co-ordinated. In the aftermath of a series of drug disasters (the elixir of sulphonamide in 1930s USA, Stalinon in 1950s France, thalidomide in 1960s Britain and elsewhere),[117] drug safety legislation was tightened and the pharmaceutical industry became one of the most highly regulated sectors of the economy, resulting in the creation of medical and/or clinical research departments within many companies in the 1950s–60s. These new departments facilitated the internalization of clinical norms and values within the industry, where the traditional product-based approach to drug discovery was gradually replaced by a disease-focused approach, targeting chronic diseases such as rheumatoid arthritis, heart disease, and cancer.[118] What was happening within the industry coincided with medicine beginning to adopt managerial practices and rationalize its operations to become more bureaucratic as part of new, state-sponsored health systems.[119] The convergence between these two trends contributed to an alignment between the aims and agendas of public health authorities and the R&D and marketing activities of pharmaceutical firms, and helped to place drugs at the heart of modern medical practice in an unprecedented and fundamental way, with profound implications both for medicine and for the public at large.[120]

### Since the 1980s

The fundamental discoveries of recombinant DNA and monoclonal antibodies led to the creation of biotechnology start-ups. These appeared first in the USA, where they were facilitated by the massive knowledge-base created by the NIH, by state policies stimulating technology transfer and pharmaceutical innovation in the 1980s (such as the Bay-Dohle Act of 1980 and the Orphan Drug Act of 1983),[121] as well as by the comparatively easy availability of venture capital. Other Western countries followed, spurred on by government initiatives aiming to emulate the American example. Pharmaceutical firms responded cautiously to these initiatives at first. Very few entered the biotechnology business themselves, forming strategic alliances with biotech companies instead.[122] As a result, the academic–industrial interaction in biomedicine became more complex still, and the boundaries between the public and private sectors became even more blurred.[123] For not only was the outright involvement of academic scientists in the foundation of commercial enterprises increasingly frequent in the 1980s, but confronted by the risk-averse nature of much of Big Pharma, governments found themselves obliged to invest public money in new companies. An example of a part-private, part-public enterprise was the British start-up Celltech (now UCB Celltech), created under Thatcher in 1980 with funding from the National Enterprise Board.[124]

Since the 1970s, economic recession and budgetary constraints have also led Western governments to encourage academic researchers to consider the practical applications of their research, and collaborate closely with the private sector in order to find funding that is no longer available from the public purse.[125] However, such pressures have tended to exacerbate earlier anxieties about the risks of contamination of the ideals of 'pure science',[126] and existing concerns over undue corporate influence and potential conflicts of interest in medicine and the biomedical sciences.[127] The dilemmas and ambiguities of patenting and intellectual property rights (particularly concerning substances of natural and human origin, such as hormones, stem cells, and genes)[128] have compounded the effects of unethical practices such as the ghost writing of clinical trial reports, not to mention drug disasters that the companies responsible tried to conceal,[129] and have given the industry and their collaborators an especially bad press.[130]

However, against this background of anxieties, ambiguities, and potential conflicts of interests, consumers of medicines have shown a remarkable resilience. Indeed, not only have they regained hope and faith in the curative powers of medicine after each crisis of confidence that has affected modern medical practice, but they have remained far from passive in the face of professional power and corporate influence. There has been a long tradition of self-medication, which is all too often neglected in studies of pharmaceutical innovation. The resort to home remedies, over-the-counter drugs, and complementary therapies, and more recently the use of the internet as a source of prescription medicines and a site for exchanging recipes, all testify to the enduring inventiveness and relative independence of users of pharmaceutical products. The birth of the healthcare consumer movement in the 1950s, and the growing influence of patient activism and disease-based associations, which often demand better or more targeted pharmaceutical innovation,[131] suggest that despite longstanding attempts to curb this inventiveness and control this independence through prescription or regulation, or indeed to shape it through advertising, cultural traditions and attitudes to drugs have endured across time periods, spanning the long twentieth century.[132] Histories of pharmaceutical innovation, in addition to focusing on change, therefore also need to take into account continuities, which requires considering the active role played by the users of such products.[133]

Like other contributions to this volume, therefore, this chapter suggests that, in relation to medicine and health, a dual definition of public and private is required. More specifically in relation to pharmaceutical innovation, it means: 1. publicly funded research institutions vs private for-profit companies; 2. the public face of drug consumption vs the private use of drugs by consumers.

## Conclusion

Continuities in the demand and use of drugs as well as discontinuities in the production and supply of pharmaceutical products raise questions about the causes of the evolution described above. They have been complex, involving a multitude of actors, and including fundamental socio-economic and political changes, transformations in science, technology, and medicine, and the drugs themselves. The pivotal role played by drugs in the history of pharmaceutical innovation has not only been due to their therapeutic efficacy, but also their cost effectiveness, helping to avoid (although sometimes – as in the case of organ transplants – facilitating) other expensive medical procedures, enabling shorter hospitalization times, and allowing care in the community, rather than in institutions. The experience of developing and consuming the most innovative among them – i.e. the most likely to make a difference to people's health and well being, such as diphtheria anti-serum, Salvarsan, insulin, penicillin, cortisone, propranolol, and 6-MP, to name but a few – therefore set precedents for other drugs. Hence, the practices adopted by their users, the doctors, researchers, and policy makers, in particular the collaborative practices that bound them together, served as models for subsequent drugs. Thus, drugs have functioned as 'boundary objects', helping to bridge the gap, and contributing to the interweaving between the two spheres of the public and the private, which we have come to understand as underpinning pharmaceutical innovation. However, I hope this chapter has shown that this understanding is historically contingent, and is therefore worthy of historical study. In particular, historians need to consider both the extent to which the two spheres are 'actors' categories that have served mainly the interests of publicly supported biomedical science, and the extent to which the collaboration between them has suited the public health agendas and managerial ambitions of the modern state.

## Further reading

The field of science and technology studies (STS) has produced a number of seminal studies on 'boundary work' and 'boundary objects', for example: Susan Star and James Griesemer, 'Institutional Ecology, "Translations", and Boundary Objects: Amateurs and Professionals in Berkeley's Museum of Vertebrate Zoology, 1907–1939', *Social Studies of Science*, 19 (1989): 387–420; Thomas Gieryn, 'Boundary Work and the Demarcation of Science from Non-science: Strains and Interests in Professional Ideologies of Scientists', *American Sociological Review*, 48 (1983): 781–95; Stephen Shapin, 'Discipline and Bounding', *History of Science*, 30 (1992): 33–69; Joan Fujimura, 'Crafting Science: Standardized Packages, Boundary Objects, and "Translations"', in Andrew Pickering (ed.), *Science as Practice and Culture* (Chicago: Chicago University Press, 1992), 168–211; Ilana Löwy, 'The Strength of Loose Concepts: Boundary Objects, Federative Experimental Strategies and Discipline Growth: The Case of Immunology', *History of Science*, 30 (1992): 371–96; Steven Epstein, 'The Construction of Lay Expertise: AIDS Activism and the Forging of New Credibility in the Reform of Clinical Trials', *Science, Technology and Human Values*, 20 (1995): 408–37; Brigitte Gorm Hansen, 'Beyond the Boundary: Science, Industry, and Managing Symbiosis', *Bulletin of Science Technology and Society*, 31 (2011): 493–505, and other articles in this issue.

On the role of academic–industrial collaborations in bridging such boundaries, see: John Swann, *Academic Scientists and the Pharmaceutical Industry: Cooperative Research in Twentieth-century America* (Baltimore: The Johns Hopkins University Press, 1988); Jonathan Liebenau, 'The MRC and the Pharmaceutical Industry: The Model of Insulin', in Joan Austoker and Linda

Bryder (eds), *Historical Perspectives on the Role of the Medical Research Council* (Oxford: Oxford University Press, 1989), 163–80; Jonathan Liebenau and Michael Robson, 'L'Institut Pasteur et l'industrie pharmaceutique', in Michel Morange (ed.), *L'Institut Pasteur: Contributions à son histoire* (Paris: Presses Universitaires de France, 1991), 52–61; Trevor Jones, 'The Value of Academia/Industry Links in R&D', in S.R. Walker (ed.), *Creating the Right Environment for Drug Discovery* (Lancaster: Quay Publishing, 1991), 77–84; Nelly Oudshoorn, 'United We Stand: The Pharmaceutical Industry, Laboratory and Clinic in the Development of Sex Hormones into Scientific Drugs, 1920–1940', *Science, Technology and Human Values*, 18 (1993): 5–24; Jordan Goodman, 'Can It Ever Be Pure Science? Pharmaceuticals, the Pharmaceutical Industry and Biomedical Research in the Twentieth-Century', in Jean-Paul Gaudillière and Ilana Löwy (eds), *The Invisible Industrialist: Manufactures and the Production of Scientific Knowledge* (Basingstoke: Macmillan, 1998), 143–65, and other contributions to this volume; Nicholas Rasmussen, 'The Moral Economy of the Drug Company–Medical Scientist Collaboration in Interwar America', *Social Studies of Science*, 34 (2004): 161–85; Jay Chin-Dusting *et al.*, 'Finding Improved Medicines: The Role of Academic Industrial Collaborations', *Nature Reviews Drug Discovery*, 5 (2005): 891–7; Viviane Quirke, *Collaboration in the Pharmaceutical Industry: Changing Relationships in Britain and France* (Abingdon and New York: Routledge, 2008); Dominique Tobbell, 'Allied against Reform: Pharmaceutical Industry–Academic Physician Relations in the United States, 1945–1970', *Bulletin of the History of Medicine*, 82 (2008): 878–912.

While there are numerous histories of pharmaceutical companies, histories of national pharmaceutical industries are less plentiful, although their number has risen in recent years. To name but a few: Paul Starr, *The Social Transformation of American Medicine: The Rise of a Sovereign Profession and the Making of a Vast Industry* (New York: Basic Books, 1982); Jonathan Liebenau, *Medical Science and Medical Industry: The Formation of the American Pharmaceutical Industry* (Baltimore: The Johns Hopkins University Press, 1987); various contributions in Jonathan Liebenau, Greg Higby and Elaine Stroud (eds), *Pill Peddlers: Essays on the History of the Pharmaceutical Industry* (Madison, WI: American Institute of the History of Pharmacy, 1990); Michèle Ruffat, *175 Ans d'industrie pharmaceutique française: Histoire de Synhélabo* (Paris: La Découverte, 1996); Sophie Chauveau, *L'Invention pharmaceutique: La pharmacie entre l'Etat et la société* (Paris: Institut d'Edition Sanofi-Synthélabo, 1999); David Chandler, *Shaping the Industrial Century: The Remarkable Story of the Evolution of the Modern Chemical and Pharmaceutical Industries* (Cambridge, MA: MIT Press, 2005); Viviane Quirke and Judy Slinn (eds), *Perspectives on Twentieth-century Pharmaceuticals* (Oxford: Peter Lang, 2010); Viviane Quirke (ed.), 'Pharmaceutical Styles of Thinking and Doing: French and British Spheres of Influence in the Nineteenth and Early-Twentieth Centuries', special issue, *Pharmacy in History*, 52 (2010): 134–47.

As to pharmaceutical innovation, while it has received much attention from historians of science, technology and medicine, because of its significance for business and policy it has also interested business analysis: David Schwartzman, *Innovation in the Pharmaceutical Industry* (Baltimore: The Johns Hopkins University Press, 1976); Jeremy Howells and Ian Neary, *Intervention and Technological Innovation* (Basingstoke: Macmillan, 1988); Luigi Orsenigo, *The Emergence of Biotechnology: Institutions and Markets in Industrial Innovation* (London: Pinter, 1989); Robert Ballance, Helmut Forstner and János Pogány (eds), *The World's Pharmaceutical Industries: An International Perspective on Innovation, Competition and Policy* (Aldershot: Edward Elgar, 1992); Alfonso Gambardella, *Science and Innovation: The US Pharmaceutical Industry during the 1980s* (Cambridge: Cambridge University Press, 1995); Ralph Landau, Basil Achilladelis and Alexander Scriabine (eds), *Pharmaceutical Innovation* (Philadelphia: Chemical Heritage Press, 1999); M. McKelvey, *Evolutionary Innovations: The Business of Biotechnology* (Oxford: Oxford University Press, 1996); Rebecca Henderson, Luigi Orsenigo and Gary Pisano, 'The Pharmaceutical Industry and the Revolution in Molecular Biology: Interactions Among Scientific, Institutional and Organizational Change', in David Mowery and Robert Nelson (eds), *Sources of Industrial Leadership* (Cambridge: Cambridge University Press, 1999); Marriana Mazzucato and Giovanni Dosi (eds), *Knowledge Accumulation and Industry Evolution: The Case of Pharma Biotech* (Cambridge: Cambridge University Press, 2006); Frank Sloan and Chee-Ruey Hsieh (eds), *Pharmaceutical Innovation: Incentives, Competition, and Cost-Benefit Analysis in International Perspective* (Cambridge: Cambridge University Press, 2007); Oliver Gassmann, Gerrit Reepmeyer and Maximilian von Zedwitz (eds), *Leading Pharmaceutical Innovation: Trends and Drivers for Growth in the Pharmaceutical Industry* (Berlin: Springer, 2nd edn, 2008).

## Notes

1 While most people would agree that pharmaceutical innovation is desirable, there are many debates as to what it actually is, and how best to achieve it. At its most simple, a pharmaceutical innovation can be either incremental, substantial, or radical depending on the gravity of the unmet healthcare need it addresses, and on its effectiveness in meeting that need. Steven Morgan, Ruth Lopert and Devon Greyson, 'Toward a Definition of Pharmaceutical Innovation', *Open Medicine*, 2 (2008): 4–7 (5).

2 The expression 'Therapeutic Revolution' was coined by the American historian of medicine Charles Rosenberg in his classic essay entitled 'The Therapeutic Revolution: Medicine, Meaning and Social Change in Nineteenth-Century America', *Perspectives in Biology and Medicine*, 20 (1977): 485–506. It has since been used to refer to the pharmacological revolution of the mid-twentieth century (i.e. the explosion in the number of drug treatments for a wide variety of ailments), and more recently to the behavioural turn in certain fields of medicine, in particular those relating to mental health (see J.V. Basmanjian, 'The Third Therapeutic Revolution: Behavioural Medicine', *Applied Psychophysiology Biofeedback*, 24 (2) (1999): 107–16.

3 IMS Health 2000.

4 The IMS Institute for Healthcare Informatics report: *Global Use of Medicines: Outlook to 2017*, www.imshealth.com/portal/site/imshealth/menuitem.762a961826aa d98f53c753c71ad8c22a/?vgnextoid=9f819e464e832410VgnVCM10000076192ca2RCRD& vgnextchannel=a64de5fda6370410VgnVCM10000076192ca2RCRD&vgnextfmt=default (accessed 9 April 2014).

5 Medicalization is usually understood as the process by which human conditions come to be considered medical problems, and therefore become the subject of medical study, diagnosis, prevention, or treatment. The factors driving this process include new hypotheses or evidence about these conditions; changing social attitudes or economic circumstances; and, last but not least, the development of new treatments and medications. Ivan Illich, 'The Medicalization of Life', *Journal of Medical Ethics,* 1 (2) (July 1975): 73–7; Peter Conrad, *The Medicalization of Society: On the Transformation of Human Conditions into Medical Disorders* (Baltimore: The Johns Hopkins University Press, 2007).

6 Blockbuster drugs usually treat common conditions such as high blood pressure or cholesterol, diabetes, asthma, and certain forms of cancer, and are capable of generating more than $1Bn for the company making them.

7 See video clips of IMS Institute Executive Director Murray Aitken's analysis of trends, in *Global Use of Medicines* (n. 2).

8 See for example Toine Pieters, *Interferon: The Science and Selling of a Miracle Drug* (Abingdon and New York: Routledge, 2005). See also John Lesch, *The First Miracle Drugs: How the Sulfa Drugs Transformed Medicine* (Oxford: Oxford University Press, 2007).

9 See various contributions in Louise Hill Curth (ed.), *From Physick to Pharmacology: Five Hundred Years of British Drug Retailing* (Aldershot: Ashgate, 2006).

10 Walter Sneader, *Drug Discovery: The Evolution of Modern Medicines* (Chichester: John Wiley & Sons, 1985), 2, 6–7.

11 John Beer, *The Emergence of the German Dye Industry* (Urbana: University of Illinois Press, 1959).

12 Diarmuid Jeffreys, *The Remarkable Story of a Wonder Drug: Aspirin* (London: Bloomsbury, 2004).

13 See for example: Dorothy Porter and Roy Porter, 'The Politics of Prevention: Anti-vaccinationism and Public Health in Nineteenth-Century England', *Medical History,* 32 (1988): 231–252; Nadja Durbach, *Bodily Matters: The Anti-vaccination Movement in England, 1853–1907* (Durham, NC: Duke University Press, 2004); Mark Largent, *Vaccine: The Debate in Modern America* (Baltimore: The Johns Hopkins University Press, 2012). See also Alysa Levene's contribution to this volume.

14 Gerald Geison, *The Private Science of Louis Pasteur* (Princeton, NJ: Princeton University Press, 1995).

15 William Bynum, *Science and the Practice of Medicine in the Nineteenth Century* (Cambridge: Cambridge University Press, 1994), 152–7.

16 Harriet Chick, Margaret Hume and Marjorie Macfarlane, *War on Disease: A History of the Lister Institute* (London: Deutsch, 1971).

17 For a comparison of the Pasteur and Koch Institutes, especially in terms of their different relations to the public and the state, see Paul Weindling, 'Scientific Elites and Laboratory Organisation in *fin de siècle* Paris and Berlin: The Pasteur Institute and Robert Koch's Institute for Infectious Diseases Compared', in Andrew Cunningham and Perry Williams (eds), *The Laboratory Revolution in Medicine* (Cambridge: Cambridge University Press, 1992), 170–88; for a comparison of the Pasteur and Lister Institutes in terms of their different relationships with the private sector see Viviane Quirke, *Collaboration in the Pharmaceutical Industry: Changing Relationships in Britain and France* (Abingdon and New York: Routledge, 2008), esp. Ch. 1.

18 Jonathan Liebenau, 'Ethical Business: The Formation of the Pharmaceutical Industry in Britain, Germany and the US before 1914', in Richard Davenport-Hines and Geoffrey Jones (eds), *The End of Insularity: Essays in Comparative Business History* (London: Cass, 1988), 117–29.

19 Jonathan Simon and Axel Hüntelmann, 'Two Models of Production and Regulation: The Diphtheria Serum in Germany and France', in Viviane Quirke and Judy Slinn (eds), *Perspectives on Twentieth-Century Pharmaceuticals* (Oxford: Peter Lang, 2010), 37–61; see also various contributions in Christoph Gradmann and Jonathan Simon (eds), *Evaluating and Standardizing Therapeutic Agents 1890–1950* (Basingstoke: Palgrave Macmillan, 2010).

20 Jonathan Liebenau, 'Paul Ehrlich as a Commercial Scientist and Research Administrator', *Medical History*, 34 (1990): 65–78.

21 John Parascandola, 'The Theoretical Basis of Paul Ehrlich's Chemotherapy', *Journal of the History of Medicine*, 36 (1981): 19–43; Arthur Silverstein, *Paul Ehrlich's Receptor Immunology: The Magnificent Obsession* (San Diego and London: Academic Press, 2002); Cay-Rüdiger Prüll, 'Part of a Scientific Master Plan? Paul Ehrlich and the Origins of his Receptor Concept', *Medical History*, 47 (2003): 332–56.

22 Axel Hüntelmann, 'Making Salvarsan: Experimental Therapy and the Development and Marketing of Salvarsan at the Crossroads of Science, Clinical Medicine, Industry and Public Health', in Jean-Paul Gaudillière and Volker Hess (eds), *Ways of Regulating Drugs in the Nineteenth and Twentieth Centuries* (Houndmills, Basingstoke and New York: Palgrave Macmillan, 2013), 43–65.

23 Renate Riedl, 'A Brief History of the Pharmaceutical Industry in Basel', in Jonathan Liebenau, Gregory Higby and Elaine Stroud (eds), *Pill Peddlers: Essays on the History of the Pharmaceutical Industry* (Madison, WI: American Institute of the History of Pharmacy, 1990), 49–72.

24 Judy Slinn, 'Research and Development in the UK Pharmaceutical Industry from the Nineteenth Century to the 1960s', in Miculáš Teich and Roy Porter (eds), *Drugs and Narcotics in History* (Cambridge: Cambridge University Press, 1996), 168–86.

25 On the development of these drugs see Marion Hulverscheidt, 'The Scientist-Entrepreneur or Financing in Pharmaceutical Research: A Portrait of the Malariologist Werner Schulemann, 1888–1975', in Quirke and Slinn (eds), *Perspectives*, 121–48.

26 Viviane Quirke, 'Putting Theory into Practice: James Black, Receptor Theory, and the Development of the Beta-blockers at ICI', *Medical History*, 50 (2006): 69–92; Cay-Rüdiger Prüll, 'Scientists, Doctors and Drug Development: The History of Raymond P. Ahlquist's Receptor Theory, 1948–1988', in Quirke and Slinn (eds), *Perspectives*, 149–84.

27 Richard Davenport-Hines and Judy Slinn, *Glaxo: A History to 1962* (Cambridge: Cambridge University Press, 1992); Edgar Jones, *The Business of Medicine* (London: Profile Books, 2001).

28 Michael Bliss, *The Discovery of Insulin* (Toronto: McClelland & Stewart, 1982).

29 Jonathan Liebenau, 'The MRC and the Pharmaceutical Industry: The Model of Insulin', in Joan Austoker and Linda Bryder (eds), *Historical Perspectives on the Role of the Medical Research Council* (Oxford: Oxford University Press, 1989), 163–80.

30 Christiane Sinding, 'Making the Unit of Insulin: Standards, Clinical Work, and Industry, 1920–1925', *Bulletin of the History of Medicine*, 76 (2002): 231–70.

31 Helge Kragh, 'The Take-off Phase of Danish Chemical Industry, ca 1910–1940', in Anthony Travis, Harm Schröter, Ernst Homburg and Peter Morris (eds), *Determinants in the Evolution of the European Chemical Industry, 1900–1939: New Technologies, Political Frameworks, Markets and Companies* (Dordrecht: Kluwer Academic, 1998), 321–39.

32 J.D.H. Homan and J. Tepstra, 'Insulin', in M.J. Parnham and J. Bruinvels (eds), *Discoveries in Pharmacology, Volume 2: Haemodynamics, Hormones and Inflammation* (Amsterdam: Elsevier, 1984), 431–60.

33 John Lesch, 'Chemistry and Biomedicine in an Industrial Setting: The Invention of the Sulfa Drugs', in Seymour Mauskopf (ed.), *Chemical Sciences in the Modern World* (Philadelphia: University of Pennsylvania Press, 1999), 158–215; John Lesch, *The First Miracle Drugs*.

34 Judy Slinn, *A History of May & Baker, 1834–1984* (Cambridge: Hobsons, 1984), 124–5.

35 In 1993 ICI spun off its pharmaceutical and agrochemicals divisions to form Zeneca, which in 1999 merged with the Swedish drug company Astra to create AstraZeneca.

36 Carol Kennedy, *ICI: The Company That Changed Our Lives* (London: Hutchinson, 1986), Ch. 8.

37 William Reader, *Imperial Chemical Industries: A History, Volume 2: The First Quarter-Century, 1926–52* (London: Oxford University Press, 1975), 458.

38 Nicholas Rasmussen, 'Steroids in Arms: Science, Government, Industry and the Hormones of the Adrenal Cortex in the United States, 1930–1950', *Medical History*, 46 (2002): 299–324.

39 Quirke, *Collaboration*, Chs 3–6.

40 John Crellin, 'Antibiosis in the Nineteenth Century', in John Parascandola (ed.), *The History of Antibiotics: A Symposium* (Madison, WI: American Institute of the History of Pharmacy, 1980), 5–13.

41 Quirke, *Collaboration*, Ch. 3. For their work on penicillin, Florey and Chain shared the Nobel Prize for Physiology or Medicine with Fleming in 1945.

42 Gladys Hobby, *Penicillin: Meeting the Challenge* (Yale: Yale University Press, 1985).

43 On the case of Spain, see María Jesús Santesmases, 'Distributing Penicillin: The Clinic, the Hero and Industrial Production in Spain, 1943–1952', in Quirke and Slinn (eds), *Perspectives*, 90–117.

44 Robert Bud, *The Uses of Life: A History of Biotechnology* (Cambridge: Cambridge University Press, 1993).

45 Yukimasa Yasigawa, 'Early History of Antibiotics in Japan', in Parascandola (ed.), *The History of Antibiotics*, 69–90.

46 H.G. (Leslie) Lazell, *From Pills to Penicillin: The Beechams Story* (London: Heinemann, 1975).

47 Margaret Goldsmith, *The Road to Penicillin: A History of Chemotherapy* (London: Lindsay Drummond, 1946).

48 Remedies made from herbs or vegetables, as opposed to mineral or chemical drugs, and prepared according to Galen's formulas.

49 Geoffrey Tweedale, *At the Sign of the Plough: 275 Years of Allen & Hanburys and the British Pharmaceutical Industry, 1715–1990* (London: Murray, 1990).

50 Carl Moberg and Zerwin Cohn, *Launching the Antibiotic Era: Personal Accounts of the Discovery and Use of the First Antibiotics* (New York: Rockefeller University Press, 1990).

51 Selman Waksman, *The Conquest of Tuberculosis* (London: Cambridge University Press, 1964); on the introduction of streptomycin in Britain, see Alan Yoshioka, 'Streptomycin in Postwar Britain: A Cultural History of a Miracle Drug', in Marijke Gijswijt-Hofstra, Godelieve van Heteren and E.M. (Tilli) Tansey (eds), *Biographies of Remedies: Drugs, Medicines and Contraceptives in Dutch and Anglo-American Healing Cultures* (Amsterdam: Rodopi, 2002), 203–27.

52 Viviane Quirke, 'From Evidence to Market: Alfred Spinks's 1953 Survey of New Fields for Pharmacological Research, and the Origins of ICI's Cardiovascular Research Programme', in Kelly Loughlin and Virginia Berridge (eds), *Medicine,*

*the Market and the Mass Media: Producing Health in the Twentieth Century* (London: Routledge, 2005), 146–71.

53 James Le Fanu, *The Rise and Fall of Modern Medicine* (London: Abacus, 2000); Druin Burch, *Taking the Medicine: A Short History of Medicine's Beautiful Idea, and Our Difficulty Swallowing It* (London: Chatto & Windus, 2009).

54 E.M. (Tilli) Tansey and Lois Reynolds (eds), *Wellcome Witnesses to Twentieth Century Medicine: Volume 6, Post Penicillin Antibiotics: From Acceptance to Resistance?* (London: Wellcome Trust, 2000), 59; Robert Bud, *Penicillin: Triumph and Tragedy* (Oxford: Oxford University Press, 2007).

55 These issues were explored by the Irish-born journalist Brian Inglis, *Drugs, Doctors and Disease: A Survey of the Pharmaceutical Industry* (London: Andre Deutsch, 1965). See also Brian Inglis, *Private Conscience, Public Morality* (London: Andre Deutsch, 1964).

56 Peter Hayes, *Industry and Ideology: IG Farben in the Nazi Era* (Cambridge: Cambridge University Press, 1987).

57 Lady Jean Medawar, *Hitler's Gift: Scientists Who Fled Nazi Germany* (London: Piatkus, 2001).

58 Ute Deichmann, 'Emigration, Isolation and the Slow Start of Molecular Biology in Germany', in Soraya de Chadarevian and Bruno Strasser (eds), 'Molecular Biology in Post-war Europe', *Studies in History and Philosophy of Biology and Biomedical Sciences*, 30 (2002): 449–71.

59 Viviane Quirke, 'War and Change in the Pharmaceutical Industry: A Comparative Study of Britain and France in the Twentieth Century', in Sophie Chauveau (ed.), 'Industries du médicament et du vivant', *Enterprises et Histoire*, 36 (2004): 64–83.

60 William F. Johns, *Steroids* (London: Butterworths, 1973), preface; see also David Cantor, 'Cortisone and the Politics of Drama, 1949–1955', in John Pickstone (ed.), *Medical Innovations in Historical Perspective* (Basingstoke: Macmillan, 1993), 165–84.

61 Elizabeth Watkins, *On the Pill: A Social History of Contraceptives, 1950–1970* (Baltimore: The Johns Hopkins University Press, 1998); Lara V. Marks, *Sexual Chemistry: A History of the Contraceptive Pill* (New Haven and London: Yale University Press, 2001).

62 Leo Slater, 'Industry and Academy: The Synthesis of Steroids', *Historical Studies in the Physical and Biological Sciences*, 30 (2000): 443–79 (469).

63 Jacob Karsh and Geza Heteny, 'A Historical Review of Rheumatoid Arthritis Treatment: 1948–1952', *Seminars in Rheumatism and Arthritis*, 27 (1997): 57–65 (63).

64 Karl Harpuder, 'Basic Medical Principles in the Treatment of the Chronically Ill Patient', *Journal of Chronic Diseases*, 4 (1956): 170–6 (175).

65 Viviane Quirke, 'Making *British* Cortisone: Glaxo and the Development of Corticosteroid Drugs in the UK in the 1950s and 1960s', *Studies in History and Philosophy of Biology and Biomedical Sciences*, 36 (2005): 645–74.

66 S.A. Szpilfogel, 'Adrenalcortical Steroids and Their Synthetic Analogues', in Parnham and Bruinvels (eds), *Discoveries in Pharmacology, Volume 2*, 253–84 (279).

67 Arthur Kornberg, *The Golden Helix: Inside the Biotech Ventures* (Sausalito, CA: University Science Books, 1995).

68 Judith Swazey, *Chlorpromazine in Psychiatry: A Study of Therapeutic Innovation* (Cambridge, MA: MIT Press, 1974). On the dissemination of chlorpromazine to the Low Countries, see Toine Pieters and Benoît Majerus, 'The Introduction of Chlorpromazine in Belgium and the Netherlands (1951–1968): Tango between Old and New Treatment Features', *Studies in History and Philosophy of Biological and Biomedical Science*, 42 (2011): 443–52. See also other articles in this issue.

69 E.M. (Tilli) Tansey, '"They Used to Call it Psychiatry": Aspects of the Development and Impact of Psychopharmacology', in Marijke Gijswijt-Hofstra and Roy Porter (eds), *Cultures of Psychiatry and Mental Health Care in Postwar Britain and the Netherlands* (Amsterdam: Rodopi, 1998), 79–101.

188    *Pharmaceutical innovation in the twentieth century*

70 Andrea Tone, 'Tranquilizers on Trial: Psychopharmacology in the Age of Anxiety', in Andrea Tone and Elizabeth Siegel Watkins (eds), *Medicating Modern America: Prescription Drugs in History* (New York and London: New York University Press, 2007), 156–79; Andrea Tone, *The Age of Anxiety: A History of America's Turbulent Affair with Tranquilizers* (New York: Basic Books, 2009).
71 The expression, coined by the Anglo-American poet Wystan H. Auden, referred to man's anxious search for identity in an increasingly industrialized world, and coincided with the onset of the Cold War. Wystan H. Auden, *The Age of Anxiety: A Baroque Eclogue* (London: Faber, 1st UK edn, 1948).
72 David Healy, *The Antidepressant Era* (Cambridge, MA: Harvard University Press, 1997).
73 David Healy, *Let Them Eat Prozac: The Unhealthy Relationship between the Pharmaceutical Industry and Depression* (New York and London: New York University Press, 2004); Joanna Moncrieff, *The Myth of the Chemical Cure: A Critique of Psychiatric Drug Treatment* (Basingstoke and New York: Palgrave Macmillan, revised edn, 2009). See also Jörg Blech, *Inventing Disease and Pushing Pills: Pharmaceutical Companies and the Medicalisation of Normal Life* (London and New York: Routledge, Engl. trans., 2006).
74 A.W. Cuthbert, 'Men, Molecules and Machines', *Trends in Pharmacological Sciences*, Inaugural issue 3, (1979): 1–3.
75 Quirke, 'Putting Theory into Practice'.
76 Mark Jackson, *Asthma: The Biography* (Oxford and New York: Oxford University Press, 2009), 186–8; see also Jones, *The Business of Medicine*, 329–32.
77 Jackson, *Asthma*, 249–54, 334–6.
78 James Patterson, *The Dread Disease: Cancer and Modern American Culture* (Harvard, MA and London: Harvard University Press, 1987); Peter Keating and Alberto Cambrosio, 'Cancer Clinical Trials: The Emergence and Development of a New Style of Practice', in David Cantor (ed.), 'Cancer in the Twentieth Century', *Bulletin for the History of Medicine*, 81 (2007): 197–223; Siddhartha Mukherjee, *The Emperor of All Maladies: A Biography of Cancer* (London: Fourth Estate, 2011).
79 Le Fanu, *The Rise and Fall*, Ch. 10; see also Viviane Quirke, 'Targeting the American Market for Medicines: ICI and Rhône-Poulenc Compared, c. 1950s–1970s', *The Bulletin for the History of Medicine* (Dec. 2014, forthcoming).
80 Robert Bud, 'Strategy in American Cancer Research after World War II: A Case Study', *Social Studies of Science*, 8 (1978): 425–59; Gerald Kutcher, *Contested Medicine: Cancer Research and the Military* (Chicago and London: University of Chicago Press, 2009). On the Soviet side of the Cold War cancer story see Nikolai Krementsov, *The Cure: A Story of Cancer and Politics from the Annals of the Cold War* (Chicago and London: University of Chicago Press, 2002).
81 B.A. Chabner and T.G. Roberts Jr, 'Chemotherapy and the War on Cancer', *Nature Reviews Cancer*, 5 (Jan. 2005): 65–72.
82 Jordan Goodman and Vivien Walsh, *The Story of Taxol: Nature and Politics in the Pursuit of an Anti-cancer Drug* (Cambridge: Cambridge University Press, 2001), Ch. 1.
83 Anti-metabolites are substances that closely resemble essential metabolites and compete with, or replace, the metabolite in physiological reactions.
84 K.H. George, 'George H. Hitchings, 1905– : American Pharmacologist', in Emily J. McMurray *et al.* (eds), *Notable Twentieth Century Scientists*, Vol. 2 (Detroit, MI: Gale Research, 1995), 933–4.
85 L. Marshall, 'Gertrude Belle Elion, 1918– : American Biochemist', in Emily J. McMurray *et al.* (eds), *Notable Twentieth Century Scientists*, Vol. 1 (Detroit, MI: Gale Research, 1995): 583–4.
86 George Hitchings, 'Chemotherapy and Comparative Biochemistry', G.H.A. Clowes Memorial Lecture, *Cancer Research*, 29 (1969): 1895–1903.

87 Alfredo Giner-Sorolla, 'The Excitement of a Suspense Story, the Beauty of a Poem: The Work of Hitchings and Elion', *Trends in Pharmacological Sciences*, 9 (Dec. 1988): 437–8.

88 Nicholas E.J. Wells, *Pharmaceutical Innovation: Recent Trends, Future Prospects* (London: Office of Health Economics (OHE), 1983).

89 Robert Nilsson and Henning Sjöström, *Thalidomide and the Power of the Drug Companies* (Harmondsworth: Penguin, 1972); Arthur Daemmrich, 'A Tale of Two Experts: Thalidomide and Political Engagement in the United States and West Germany', *Social History of Medicine*, 15 (2002): 137–58; Rock Brynner and Trent Stephens, *Dark Remedy: The Impact of Thalidomide and Its Revival as a Vital Medicine* (London: Basic Books, 2001).

90 These are slight variations of already existing drugs.

91 Virginia Berridge and Philip Strong (eds), *AIDS and Contemporary History* (Cambridge: Cambridge University Press, pbk edn, 2000).

92 Le Fanu, *The Rise and Fall*, Part 2.

93 Gary Pisano, *Science Business: The Promise, the Reality, and the Future of Biotech* (Boston, MA: Harvard Business School Press, 2006).

94 For an example of a biotech cluster see Anne-Laure Saives *et al.*, 'Knowledge Creation Dynamics and the Growth of Biotech Firms in Quebec', in Quirke and Slinn (eds), *Perspectives*, 435–66.

95 For an analysis of how such an understanding evolved, see Quirke, *Collaboration*.

96 The seminal text is John Swann, *Academic Scientists and the Pharmaceutical Industry: Cooperative Research in Twentieth-Century America* (Baltimore: The Johns Hopkins University Press, 1988). For other key texts see further reading.

97 Such as the Royal Prussian (later Robert Koch) Institute in Germany, the Pasteur Institute and then also the CNRS, INH and INSERM in France, the MRC in Britain, and NIH in the US. These institutions were in principle not-for-profit, although the sale of vaccines and other remedies did generate profits that were usually re-invested internally in order to help fund research. See Quirke, *Collaboration*, Ch. 1.

98 Elsewhere I have suggested that such arrangements at the institutional level were perhaps more prevalent before the Second World War in countries such as Britain or France. Quirke, *Collaboration*, 5.

99 Ibid., Ch. 1. See also Rolv Peter Amdam, 'Professional Networks and the Introduction of Research in the British and Norwegian Pharmaceutical Industry in the Interwar Years', *History and Technology*, 13 (1996): 101–114; Viviane Quirke, 'Foreign Influences, National Styles, and the Creation of a Modern Pharmaceutical Industry in Britain and France', in Viviane Quirke (ed.), 'Pharmaceutical Styles of Thinking and Doing: French and British Spheres of Influence in the Nineteenth and Early-Twentieth Centuries', *Pharmacy in History*, 52 (2010): 134–47.

100 Quirke, *Collaboration*, Ch. 2. More specifically on British chemists, see Gerrylynn Roberts, 'Dealing with Issues at the Academic–Industry Interface in Interwar Britain: UCL and ICI', *Science and Public Policy*, 24 (1997): 29–35; Robin Mackie and Gerrylynn Roberts, 'Career Patterns in the British Chemical Profession in the Twentieth Century', in David Mitch, John Brown and Marco van Leeuwen (eds), *Origins of the Modern Career* (Aldershot: Ashgate, 2004), 317–36. On French pharmacists: Marika Blondel-Mégrelis, 'La Pharmacie en France 1900–1950, points de repères', in Claude Debru, Jean Gayon and Jean-François Picard (eds), *Les Sciences biologiques et médicales en France 1920–1950* (Paris: CNRS Editions, 1994), 283–96.

101 See John Swann's typology of roles, which is based on the American drug company Eli Lilly's own typology from the 1920s–30s, in Swann, *Academic Scientists and the Pharmaceutical Industry*. See also Quirke, *Collaboration*, Ch. 2.

102  See articles in the special issue of *History and Technology*, 24 (2008); see also
     Graham Dutfield, *Intellectual Property Rights and the Life Science Industries:
     Past, Present and Future* (New Jersey etc.: World Scientific, 2nd edn, 2008).
103  Georg Meyer-Thurow, 'The Industrialisation of Invention: A Case Study from
     the German Chemical Industry', *Isis*, 73 (1982): 363–81; Ernst Homburg,
     'The Emergence of Research Laboratories in the Dyestuffs Industry, 1870–1900',
     *British Journal of the History of Science*, 25 (1992): 91–111.
104  Jonathan Liebenau, 'Industrial R&D in Pharmaceutical Firms in the Early
     Twentieth Century', *Business History*, 26 (1984): 329–46; Liebenau, 'Ethical
     Business'; Amdam, 'Professional Networks'; Slinn, 'Research and Develop-
     ment'. See also Frank Huisman, 'Struggling for the Market: Strategies of Dutch
     Pharmaceutical Companies, 1880–1940', in Quirke and Slinn (eds), *Perspectives*,
     63–89.
105  While there are numerous histories of pharmaceutical companies, histories of
     national pharmaceutical industries are less plentiful, although their number has
     risen in recent years. See further reading.
106  Because of its alleged role in fostering high levels of social, economic, and poli-
     tical performance, 'open innovation' has become a field of study in its own right.
     Jan Fagerberg, David Mowery and Richard Nelson (eds), *The Oxford Handbook
     of Innovation* (Oxford and New York: Oxford University Press, 2005), esp. Part
     IV; more specifically on open innovation: Henry Chesbrough, Wim Vanhaverbeke
     and Joel West (eds), *Open Innovation: Researching a New Paradigm* (Oxford and
     New York: Oxford University Press, 2006).
107  On the growth of large, American-style multi-divisional corporations in the post-
     war period see David Chandler, *Shaping the Industrial Century: The Remarkable
     Story of the Evolution of the Modern Chemical and Pharmaceutical Industries*
     (Cambridge, MA: MIT Press, 2005).
108  Terry Shinn, 'The Triple Helix and the New Production of Knowledge', *Social
     Science Information*, 19 (1980): 607–40.
109  Viviane Quirke and Jean-Paul Gaudillière, 'The Era of Biomedicine: Science,
     Medicine and Health in Britain and France, ca 1945–65', in Viviane Quirke and
     Jean-Paul Gaudillière (eds), special issue of *Medical History*, 52 (2008): 441–52.
110  For Britain see Christopher Booth, 'Clinical Research', in William Bynum and
     Roy Porter (eds), *Companion Encyclopedia of the History of Medicine* (London
     and New York: Routledge, 1990), Vol. 1, 205–9; Christopher Lawrence, 'Clinical
     Research', in John Krige and Dominique Pestre (eds), *Science in the Twentieth
     Century* (Amsterdam: Harwood Academic, 1997), 439–60; Steve Sturdy, 'Medical
     Chemistry and Clinical Medicine: Academics and the Scientisation of Medical
     Practice in Britain, 1900–1925', in Ilana Löwy (ed.), *Medicine and Change: His-
     torical and Sociological Studies of Medical Innovation* (Montrouge: John Libbey
     Eurotext, and Paris: INSERM, 1993), 371–93; for a recent revisiting of the sci-
     ence/medicine debate see Steve Sturdy, 'Looking for Trouble: Medical Science
     and Clinical Practice in the Historiography of Modern Medicine', *Social History
     of Medicine*, 24 (2011): 739–57.
111  On the USA: Victoria Harden, *Inventing the NIH: Federal Biomedical Research
     Policy, 1887–1937* (Baltimore and London: The Johns Hopkins University Press,
     1986); Adele Clarke, Laura Mamo and Jennifer Fosket, *Biomedicalization:
     Technoscience, Health, and Illness in the US* (Durham, NC: Duke University
     Press, 2010). On the UK: Joan Austoker, 'Walter Morley Fletcher and the Origins
     of a Basic Biomedical Research Policy', in Austoker and Bryder (eds), *Historical
     Perspectives*, 23–33; Quirke and Gaudillière, 'The Era of Biomedicine' and other
     articles in special issue, *Medical History*, 52 (2008).
112  Lise Wilkinson, 'Sir Austin Bradford Hill: Medical Statistics and the Quantitative
     Approach to Disease', *Addiction*, 92 (1997): 657–66; Alan Yoshioka, 'Use of

Randomisation in the Medical Research Council's Clinical Trial of Streptomycin in Pulmonary Tuberculosis in the 1940s', *British Medical Journal*, 317 (1998): 1220–3. In methodological terms, however, the streptomycin trial had been preceded by a less celebrated trial, that of the – largely ineffective – treatment for the common cold, patulin: Iain Chalmers and Mike Clarke, 'The 1944 Patulin Trial: The First Properly Conducted Multicentre Trial Conducted under the Aegis of the British Medical Research Council', *International Journal of Epidemiology*, 32 (2004): 253–60. On their later incarnation, the cancer trial, see Keating and Cambrosio, 'Cancer Clinical Trials'.

113 Some companies, such as the British firm S.M. Burroughs & Co. (later renamed Burroughs Wellcome & Co., and later still the Wellcome Foundation), which was created in the last decades of the nineteenth century by two American pharmacists Silas Burroughs and Henry Wellcome, had started using 'detail men' long before the Second World War. See Roy Church, 'The British Market for Medicine in the Late Nineteenth Century: The Innovative Impact of S.M. Burroughs & Co.', *Medical History*, 49 (2005): 281–98.

114 On the history of management consultant firms see Christopher McKenna, *The World's Newest Profession: Management Consulting in the Twentieth Century* (Cambridge: Cambridge University Press, 2006); Matthias Kipping and Timothy Clark (eds), *The Oxford Handbook of Management Consulting* (Oxford and New York: Oxford University Press, 2013); Matthias Kipping and Ove Bjarnar (eds), *The Americanisation of European Business: The Marshall Plan and the Transfer of US Management Models* (London and New York: Routledge, 2014); also Duff McDonald, *The Firm: The Inside Story of McKinsey, the World's Most Controversial Management Consultancy* (London: Simon & Schuster: 2013).

115 More specifically on marketing science/scientific marketing see special issue of the *Journal of Marketing*, fall 1983. On the American influence on the industry see Viviane Quirke, 'Anglo-American Relations and the Co-production of American "Hegemony" in Pharmaceuticals', in Hubert Bonin and Ferry de Goey (eds), *American Firms in Europe* (Geneva: Droz, 2009), 363–84.

116 On the impact of operations research on medicine, see Norman Bailey, 'Operational Research in Medicine', *Operational Research Quarterly (1950–1952)*, 3 (1952): 24–30; see also Daniel Fox, 'The Administration of the Marshall Plan and British Health Policy', *Journal of Policy History*, 16 (2004): 191–211.

117 On the elixir of sulphanilamide disaster see John Swann, 'Pharmaceutical Regulation before and after the Food and Drug Cosmetic Act', in Ira R. Berry (ed.), *The Pharmaceutical Regulatory Process* (New York: Marcel Dekker, 2005), 1–46; on Stalinon see Christian Bonah, 'Professional, Industrial and Juridical Regulation of Drugs: The 1953 Stalinon Case and Pharmaceutical Reform in Postwar France', in Gaudillière and Hess (eds), *Ways of Regulating Drugs*, 245–69; Viviane Quirke, 'Thalidomide, Drug Safety Regulation and the British Pharmaceutical Industry: The Case of Imperial Chemical Industries', in Gaudillière and Hess (eds), *Ways of Regulating Drugs*, 151–80.

118 Quirke, 'From Evidence to Market', in Berridge and Loughlin (eds), *Medicine, the Market and the Mass Media*; Viviane Quirke, 'Standardizing R&D in the Second Half of the Twentieth Century: ICI's Nolvadex Development Programme in Historical and Comparative Perspective', in Christian Bonah, Christophe Masutti, Anne Rasmussen and Jonathan Simon (eds), *Harmonizing Drugs: Standards in Twentieth-Century Pharmaceutical History* (Paris: Eds Glyphe, 2009), 105–32.

119 On the history of the British National Health Service, which became the archetype of a socialist, technocratic, and bureaucratic national health system, see Charles Webster, *The Health Services since the War: Volume 1, Problems of Health Care* (London: HMSO, 1988); Charles Webster, *The National Health*

*Service: A Political History* (Oxford: Oxford University Press, 2nd edn, 2002); see also John Stewart, 'The Political Economy of the British National Health Service, 1945–1975: Opportunities and Constraints?', in Quirke and Gaudillière (eds), 'The Era of Biomedicine', 453–70.

120 Jeremy Greene, *Prescribing by Numbers: Drugs and the Definition of Disease* (Baltimore: The Johns Hopkins University Press, 2007), 3–4.

121 In the USA, the patenting of discoveries made in the public sector was encouraged by the Bay-Dohle Act of 1980, which is often credited with re-invigorating pharmaceutical innovation there, and inspiring similar measures elsewhere. Ashley Stevens, 'The Enactment of Bay-Dohle', *Journal of Technology Transfer*, 29 (2004): 93–9. As to the Orphan Drug Act of 1983, it included tax incentives, clinical and R&D subsidies, fast-track drug approval and other rights for products developed for rare conditions, i.e. those affecting fewer than 200,000 people. The Act enabled small companies, particularly biotech companies, to carve out a slice of the drug market. See Mariana Mazzucato, *The Entrepreneurial State: Debunking Public vs Private Sector Myths* (London, New York and Delhi: Anthem Press, 2014), 81–3.

122 Louis Galambos and Jeff Sturchio, 'Pharmaceutical Firms and the Transition to Biotechnology: A Study in Strategic Innovation', *Business History Review*, 72 (1998): 250–78. For an example of a traditional pharmaceutical firm that successfully adapted to the advent of biotechnology, see Beat Bächi, 'Producing Ascorbic Acid: How Microbes Transformed the Pharmaceutical Company Hoffmann-La Roche, 1933–1953', in Quirke and Slinn, *Perspectives*, 367–92; Michael Bürgi and Bruno Strasser, 'Pharma in Transition: New Approaches to Drug Development at F. Hoffmann-La Roche & Co., 1960–1980', in ibid., 393–434.

123 For a discussion of the 'public' vs 'private' debate in biotechnology see various contributions in Arnold Thackray (ed.), *Private Science: Biotechnology and the Rise of the Molecular Sciences* (Philadelphia: University of Pennsylvania Press, 1998).

124 Robert Bud, 'From Applied Microbiology to Biotechnology: Science, Medicine, and Industrial Renewal', *Notes and Records of the Royal Society*, 64 (2010): 17–29; see also other articles in this issue.

125 This has been the case in a number of countries ruled by different political parties but facing similar economic and budgetary constraints, for instance Britain under Thatcher's conservative, and France under Mitterrand's socialist government, which set up a scheme called 'Valorisation à la Recherche' in the 1980s.

126 For a discussion in the American case, see Kelly Moore, 'Organizing Integrity: American Science and the Creation of Public Interest Organizations', *American Journal of Sociology*, 101 (1996): 1592–1627.

127 Marc Rodwin, *Conflicts of Interest and the Future of Medicine: The United States, France, and Japan* (Oxford and New York: Oxford University Press, 2011).

128 See for example articles in special issue of *History and Technology*, 24 (2008); Dutfield, *Intellectual Property Rights and the Life Science Industries*.

129 On ghost writing and other similar practices see David Healy and Dinah Cattell, 'Interface between Authorship, Industry and Science in the Domain of Therapeutics', *British Journal of Psychiatry*, 183 (2003): 22–7; Sergio Sismondo, 'Ghosts in the Machine: Publication Planning in the Medical Sciences', *Social Studies of Science*, 39 (2009): 171–98; Alastair Matheson, 'Corporate Science and the Husbandry of Scientific and Medical Knowledge by the Pharmaceutical Industry', *Biosocieties*, 3 (2008): 355–82; Joseph S. Ross, Kevin Hill, David Egilman and Harlan Krumholz, 'Guest Authorship and Ghostwriting in Publications Related to Rofecoxib: A Case Study of Industry Documents from Rofecoxib Litigation', *Journal of the American Medical Association*, 299 (2008): 1800–12.

130 For an early critical assessment of the drug industry see Tom Mahoney, *The Merchants of Life: An Account of the American Pharmaceutical Industry* (New York: Harper, 1959). See also James Crawford, *Kill or Cure? The Role of the Pharmaceutical Industry in Society* (London: Arc Print, 1988); Lisa Marsa, *Prescription for Profit: How the Pharmaceutical Industry Bankrolled the Unlikely Marriage between Science and Business* (New York: Scribner, 1997); Jacky Law, *Big Pharma: How the World's Biggest Drug Companies Control Illness* (London: Constable, 2006); Jennifer Moran and Ces Guerra, *Pill Pushers: A Big Pharma Battle for Market Share* (Charleston, SC: BookSurge Publishers, 2007).

131 Much of the literature on patient activism has tended to focus on American breast cancer activism, which pre-dated AIDS activism and often influenced patient activism elsewhere. Baron Lerner, *The Breast Cancer Wars: Fear, Hope and the Pursuit of a Cure in Twentieth-Century America* (Oxford and New York: Oxford University Press, 2001); Karen M. Kedrowski and Marilyn S. Sarow, *Cancer Activism: Gender, Media and Public Policy* (Urban and Chicago: University of Illinois Press, 2007); Steven Epstein, *Impure Science: AIDS, Activism and the Politics of Knowledge* (Berkeley: University of California Press, 1996); on the relationship between pharmaceutical innovation, AIDS activism and regulatory reform: Donna Messner, 'AZT and Drug Regulatory Reform in the Late Twentieth-Century US', in Gaudillière and Hess (eds), *Ways of Regulating*, 228–44. See also Dominique Tobbell, 'Charitable Innovations: The Political Economy of Thalassemia Research and Drug Development in the United States, 1960–2000', in Quirke and Slinn (eds), *Perspectives*, 302–37; Alex Mold, 'Repositioning the Patient: Patient Organisations, Consumerism and Autonomy in Britain during the 1960s and 1970s', *Bulletin of the History of Medicine*, 87 (2013): 225–49.

132 See for example Nicolas Rasmussen, *On Speed: The Many Lives of Amphetamine* (New York and London: New York University Press, 2008); Manon Niquette and William Buxton, 'Relieving Twentieth-Century Excesses: The Socialization of Antacid and Laxative Uses Through Advertising', in Quirke and Slinn (eds), *Perspectives,* 257–81; David Herzberg, 'Blockbusters and Controlled Substances: Miltown, Quaalude, and Consumer Demand for Drugs in Postwar America', *Studies in History and Philosophy of Biological and Biomedical Sciences*, 42 (2011): 415–26.

133 Roy Porter, 'The Patient's View: Doing Medical History from Below', *Theory and Society*, 14 (1985): 175–98; Nelly Oudshoorn and Trevor Pinch (eds), *How Users Matter: The Co-construction of Users and Technologies* (Cambridge, MA and London: MIT Press, 2003), esp. Chs 5–8, 10.

# 10 International health between public and private in the twentieth century

*Paul Weindling*

## Introduction: The case for international health

The cataclysmic upheavals of war, revolution, social conflict and genocide that convulsed the twentieth century found a response in the founding of international health organisations. There was a need to go beyond the nation state to provide relief and care for the wounded and sick in war, prevent the spread of epidemics, give support to refugees, and improve overall levels of health. State medical administrations and private philanthropies recognised common interests to promote health and prevent infections, as well as wider humanitarian agendas.

The later nineteenth century was characterised by private philanthropic committees and state sanitary conventions. These became transformed in the course of the twentieth century into large-scale international agencies, although the private/state dichotomy persisted. Some medical and humanitarian visionaries nurtured hopes of a world state, or at least a set of international health agencies, whereas others insisted that independent charitable and non-governmental agencies should be extended and developed to cope with sickness and distress. A range of pressures accumulated for the formation of international health organisations.[1] These regulated medical matters between states, across whole regions, and on a global basis, and provided relief to the diseased, famished and oppressed. They functioned as multilateral organisations, through the League of Nations in the interwar period and the United Nations after 1945. Others were 'non-governmental': they were empowered by a sense that the humanitarian issues were best dealt with by organisations acting beyond the state and the multilateral framework. Here, ideas of charity moved from the local and parochial to the plutocratic and the global.

At their most limited, international health agencies continued the sanitary controls of the nineteenth century, imposing quarantines and closing borders to exclude disease carriers. During the early twentieth century public health became increasingly interventive, moving toward sanitary surveillance of whole communities. There was a shift from the limited liberal state, in which most health-related matters were essentially in the private sphere, to organisational forms complementing new and ever more comprehensive welfare states. This chapter investigates diverse models of public and private medicine at an increasingly structured international level. In part these organisations reflected the strategic aspirations of their founders, and in part they were responses to hitherto unprecedented mass migration, socio-economic upheavals, two world wars resulting in devastation and population displacements, and the Cold War.

Dedicated health evangelicals were often political misfits, and took to the international sphere to overcome national strictures. Between the wars a new generation of international health experts offered visionary solutions to medical problems. Some experts were avowed internationalists, who were critical of imperialist nations and saw the dangers of nationalist extremists. There is a long history of global health volunteers, who were committed health internationalists and set out to develop a new international health landscape.[2] The new League of Nations Health Organisation (LNHO) attracted dynamic experts, not least its charismatic Polish director Ludwik Rajchman and the innovative Croatian health reformer Andrija Štampar. Such figures became embroiled with representatives of powerful member states, notably the doggedly restrictionist British representative George Buchanan, who opposed transnational initiatives. By way of contrast, the British nutritionist John Boyd Orr saw the international route as a way to critique inadequacies of social provision and their dietary implications in the UK.[3] Political conflicts over fascism caused further polarisation between experts and national representatives, and resulted in organisational crisis during the Second World War. A brief but vigorous few years of laying new human rights foundations occurred. The resulting conventions formed the basis for a new system of health organisations under the mantle of the United Nations. But this innovative phase did not last, and internationalism became politically suspect during the Cold War.

The Geneva based International Committee of the Red Cross (ICRC), founded in 1863, was a legacy of nineteenth-century battlefield slaughter, providing private and voluntary medical assistance and nursing within an internationally regulated military framework.[4] National Red Cross organisations were federated within the international structure overseen by the ICRC. The Red Cross performed well in the First World War, assuring care for the wounded, and successfully extending its remit to ensuring humane conditions for prisoners of war. Yet the emergence of welfare states, and the changing nature of war, meant the Red Cross was faced by immense challenges in the new century – not least responsibility to civilians facing the devastation of total war culminating in genocide, which characterised the Second World War, matters where the ICRC's responses were limited and inadequate.

Forms of private funding varied between the plutocratic and the populist: corporate donors established high-prestige and high-profile organisations, and expansive medical charities drummed up mass donations. Whole sectors of medical research, notably cancer, became supported by new mass philanthropies. Multilateral state organisations and plutocratic foundations were similarly innovative organisational forms. The new wave of highly dynamic corporate foundations at the start of the twentieth century came with the inauguration of the Rockefeller Foundation in 1913, and their durability was shown at the close of the century by the way the Bill and Melinda Gates Foundation for tackling global health was launched in 1994. Both foundations developed global agendas but encountered criticism on the basis of the sources of their wealth.[5] Intricate links came to be established between commerce and medical charities, well demonstrated by the emergence of the Wellcome Foundation Ltd, which ploughed profits back into the Wellcome Trust (established in 1936) for pharmaceutical and physiological research as well as support for medical history and archaeology.[6] There continued to be religious foundations such as Caritas, Christian Aid and Quaker philanthropic initiatives, some based on missionary work. The clinic of Albert Schweitzer at Lambaréné in French Equatorial Africa represented an internationally renowned model of the religiously dedicated physician. Other organisations were sustained by public appeals, such as Oxfam (from 1942) and Doctors without Borders (from 1971), to provide healthcare and medical training. Doctors and medical researchers could themselves become refugees: the Academic Assistance Council was founded in 1933, and is now CARA, the Council for At-risk Academics, many of its former grantees making major discoveries in medical research.[7] One approach was defensive and minimalist, in that such organisations had a restricted role of emergency relief. But another was expansive in terms of promoting positive and long-term solutions. In the health sphere, efforts were made to promote medical improvements in states where medical provision was defective, and social infrastructure (such as clean water) and large-scale measures had to be supplied.

## Epidemiology and organisation

At times of epidemic crisis there was a need to regulate borders and harbours, passengers and trade for pathogens and pests. New national hygiene institutes provided diagnosis, disinfection and vaccines. Renowned institutions such as the Pasteur Institute (founded in Paris by public donations in 1887) and the Robert Koch Institute (founded in Berlin in 1891 by the Prussian State) established international reputations through visiting foreign researchers. The Pasteur Institute spawned an international network of overseas institutes, and the Hamburg Institute of Tropical Medicine, founded in 1900 after the cholera epidemic of 1892, established influence in Latin America.[8]

The Rockefeller Foundation was based in New York with strong commitments to raise standards in American medicine and public health; yet its mission was global. The opening of its archives to historians since the 1980s has paved the way for a variety of interpretations of the Foundation's history.[9] Some historians have stressed the motivating ideals of humanitarianism linked to Christian notions of philanthropy (the Rockefellers were Baptists).[10] By way of contrast, others highlighted the extensive exploitation of corporate capitalism, whether within the US or internationally (the Rockefellers had mining, iron and steel, and oil investments). Hookworm eradication (an early priority of the Rockefeller Foundation) can thus be interpreted as being due either to a benign interest in sanitation and education, or an employer's interest in a healthy workforce. A further set of interpretations postulated that power, in terms of decision making on programmes in science and medicine, lay with an expert managerial group that was seeking to promote its own agendas. For example, the Rockefeller Foundation programme officer Alan Gregg had strong commitments to 'molecular medicine' and to extending its precepts to studies of behaviour.[11] The diverse interpretations of the Rockefeller Foundation can be applied to other organisations, notably to the less wealthy but expert-driven Milbank Memorial Fund.[12] These foundations offered important resources to multilateral organisations, notably the LNHO, in terms of expertise and funding, as well as to disease control strategies. Central state hygiene institutes became pivotal in newly sovereign interwar states. The Rockefeller Foundation supported (somewhat paradoxically, for an organisation committed to non-state funding) a series of central state institutes in Eastern and southeastern European countries from the Baltic to the Black Sea.[13]

Public health functioned at local, provincial, national and international levels, and strategies varied between the bacteriological, sanitary, eugenic and educational. New arenas of activity were deemed necessary. Beyond the emerging welfare states, administrators and experts developed a new international sphere both in multilateral organisations and with the support of corporate philanthropies and new mass public associations. Alcohol, tuberculosis and sexually transmitted diseases emerged as pressing issues both nationally and internationally, prompting the founding of national and then federated international organisations. Infant mortality was looked on as a medical and humanitarian problem open to interventive measures. The scientisation of medicine meant that strategic aims concerning population and disease changed over the century. At the start of the century there was still an entrenched minimalism that held that public health was merely a matter of epidemic control of pathogenic microbes. But as the twentieth century unfolded, there emerged new techniques in combating viral diseases, and new vaccines and drugs such as the sulphonamides and penicillin. These brought about more effective means of combating infectious diseases, but also required more powerful organisational forms of delivery.[14]

Beyond the political upheavals, there were changing morbidity, mortality and fertility patterns; life expectancy increased but families became smaller, with a shift from large families with high mortality. These interconnected changes have come to be known as the 'demographic transition'. Among the features of this process was female education, and consequent delay of marriage and having children. These socio-cultural changes associated with the spread of mass culture and consumption contributed to the decline in the birth rate. The type of disease being encountered also changed. The epidemics of cholera and plague that punctuated nineteenth-century history diminished markedly. Typhus, a louse-borne disease, was absent from Germany and Western Europe by 1900 due to improved personal hygiene in terms of washing of bodies and clothing. Typhus, however, remained endemic in Eastern Europe, becoming a major threat to invading military forces without acquired immunity from childhood infection.[15] The great shock was the global influenza pandemic of 1918–19, as the viral aetiology of flu defeated the scientists of the era.[16] The cataclysmic influenza pandemic was in many ways a unique catastrophe and stood in contrast to post-First World War typhus control and delousing measures, and starvation relief. There was an organisational and political shift to intervention at the point of distress. No longer was mass migration the solution to starvation and disease; instead, gigantic international relief measures were mounted to shift medical supplies and food surpluses to the epicentres of distress. This represented a novel modern means of tackling medical crises: the hope was not to contain the spread of a disease but to tackle its causes at root.

Infectious diseases such as diphtheria could be prevented thanks to the new antitoxin therapy for diphtheria, which was successfully pioneered in Paris and Berlin in the 1890s.[17] The twentieth century saw a series of new vaccines and ultimately the eradication of smallpox. Immunisation was introduced for TB. Public campaigns on avoiding sexually transmitted infections and seeking treatment, and barrier contraceptives – and ultimately penicillin – were meant to keep syphilis in check. Chronic diseases such as cancer and heart disease – especially from the mid-1930s – increased. These changes, conceptualised by Abdel Omran as 'the epidemiologic transition', can be seen as essential attributes of modernisation.[18]

Eugenicists in the 1890s, notably Francis Galton in Britain and Alfred Ploetz in Germany, presciently foresaw these changes in epidemiology and reproduction. They welcomed lower infant mortality but contemplated the trend toward lower birth rates and smaller families with dismay, as a decline in national vitality. Galton pioneered marriage certificates to certify good health without traces of syphilis or other sexually transmitted diseases prior to marriage. Health examinations before marriage were promoted, on a voluntary basis by eugenicists and feminists alike and as a matter of national legislation, and in international associations, to combat sexually transmitted diseases.[19] Eugenicists' ideas rapidly internationalised. The first societies in Germany (1905) and Britain (1907) were international in scope, and London hosted a major international eugenics congress in 1912. The societies then became more national in scope, often collaborating with the newly founded ministries of health. The interwar period also saw an International Federation of Eugenic Organisations, although the Nazi extremism meant its ultimate demise.[20]

## 1900–1914

The century dawned with unprecedented migration from Eastern and Southern Europe to the United States to escape persecution (with the Russian anti-Jewish pogroms from the 1880s), and destitution. The Ellis Island immigrant screening station at New York, quarantine stations before departure of the migrants so there should be no epidemics on board ships, and disinfection at borders provided elaborate public health screening for infections as part of highly organised migration. What began as permissive processing of migrants became ever more restrictive in terms of mass migration. The free movement of populations was to become increasingly inhibited under the impetus of concerns to exclude the sick and subnormal as a potential burden on society. Racial and eugenic elements became increasingly prominent, with quotas restricting the immigration of impoverished Southern and Eastern Europeans, and Irish, and by the 1930s Jewish refugees. At the same time as countries developed welfare legislation for sickness, accidents and old age pensions, there was also exclusion, with aliens' acts and migration quotas. The emergence of welfare state systems had its corollary in exclusive regulation of migration. Dealing with medical disasters at their point of origin was a way of stemming migration and any epidemic threats, and did not burden the emergent state welfare systems.

International health before the First World War was limited to conventions and treaties between countries to halt the spread of contagious diseases. International sanitary conferences held since 1851 dealt with preventive measures, notably quarantine and disinfection.[21] The sanitary conferences led to the establishment of the Office for International Public Health in 1907, regarded as very much a French initiative. This office pursued an administrative and regulatory role, clinging on in Nazi-dominated Europe until the end of the Second World War.

State policy was essentially negative: to safeguard the nation's health by halting the spread of infectious, epidemic diseases, both domestically and from overseas. An International Sanitary Bureau was founded in 1902, and this became the Pan-American Health Organization (PAHO) based in Washington DC.[22] The US Public Health Service took a preventive role at the Ellis Island immigration station, where inspectors weeded out carriers of infectious diseases such as typhoid and granuloma eye infection, and, increasingly, those deemed mentally and physically unfit.[23]

The period 1890–1914 saw the emergence of the new type of corporate foundation, with an immensely wealthy single donor, trustees and executive staff, in contrast to a medical research institute sustained by mass donations (such as the Pasteur Institute) or state agencies (such as Koch's institute). The new central laboratories acted as centres for research as well as strategic management for campaigns to contain and eradicate disease outbreaks. The Pasteur Institute in France (founded through charitable donations in 1888) and Robert Koch's Prussian Institute for Infectious Diseases (founded in 1891) were national as well as international centres for research and training.

The trinity of John D. Rockefeller Senior and Junior and their visionary mentor Frederick Gates were mesmerised by the French and German development of diphtheria antitoxin at the new scientific powerhouses of the

Pasteur and Koch institutes, as this showed the immense potential of financing an institute for pure medical research. They established the Rockefeller Institute for Medical Research in 1901, thereby implanting the model of a research institution with outstanding facilities into the United States. The intention was that their institute should make major medical discoveries to improve human health.

Wealthy individuals commenced in the twentieth century to support medical research. A motive was the realisation that hand-outs to the poor were condemned as costly and unproductive, merely exacerbating the problem of chronic poverty. In Britain Henry Wellcome was an example of a noted medical philanthropist. The field of charity saw new collective endeavours. The chemist and medical researcher Louis Pasteur used the discovery of rabies vaccine to mount a public appeal for the new Pasteur Institute, opening in 1888. Donations ranging from the very large to those of just a few francs were received. It was funded mainly by private donations; the state contributed indirectly by support for the training of military medical researchers.

The Rockefeller Foundation's International Health Commission (from 1913) and Board (from 1916) extended the evangelising anti-hookworm campaigns to Latin America and the Pacific. It then tackled malaria, yellow fever, yaws and schistosomiasis. Rockefeller Foundation officers saw with some satisfaction the displacement of British, French and German medical influence, which they condemned as scientifically too narrow. Providing that the Foundation could maintain distance between itself and the US State Department on the one side, and recipient states on the other, its activities appeared purely altruistic. In practice it was hard not to stray from the straight and narrow path of non-involvement, not least because social stability was deemed a prerequisite for funding. Ultimately, however, foundations considered that endowments to consolidate and raise standards in medical research and teaching would benefit world civilisation rather than national or sectional economic interests.

Tensions persisted between a microbe-hunting approach and one that aimed to improve social conditions and regulate behaviour. Eugenicists realised the importance of a population based approach, and argued that therapy for an individual could harm both the present population and future generations. Eugenicists formed international networks and associations. At first the Racial Hygiene Society, founded in Berlin in 1905, was international in scope without any reference to its being a 'German' society. The Eugenics Education Society, founded in London in 1907, had branches in Australia and New Zealand. In the interwar period the stage was held by an International Federation of Eugenics Organisations, which contributed something to the transfer of expertise, but was also an arena of conflict as Nazi-oriented eugenicists and their international sympathizers gained control.

Corporate foundations such as the Rockefeller Foundation and Milbank Memorial Fund supported research on the causes of sickness, and monitored 'the demographic transition' from infectious to chronic degenerative diseases, and from extended families with several children to families with one or two children. These private foundations, although US based, had a wider global outreach. The period from the mid-1890s to 1914 saw the founding of national and international associations to combat alcoholism, infant mortality, tuberculosis and sexually transmitted diseases. These combined demands for changes in lifestyle with providing resources such as sanatoria beds. These prestigious philanthropies were run by a mix of doctors and the socially notable in patriotic national associations.

The twentieth century saw the founding, expansion and consolidation of welfare states. Germany led the way with its model health insurance scheme of 1881 that was extended to family dependants by 1914. Prime Minister Lloyd George's National Insurance Act of 1911 for medical and unemployment benefits was less comprehensive than the German model but still notable for covering an extending range of occupations. Ideas regarding maternity insurance arose, notably in France, and opened the way for family allowances in the interwar period. While a significant boost to private medicine, the regulatory system and the sickness funds were socially regulated, non-profit, corporate institutions. On the public side, the rise of public health continued to be shaped by bacteriology and models of environmental health. This meant that physicians were to attend to personal health, but environmental and wider social issues were left to state authorities. This division was to be challenged by the war.

### The First World War and its aftermath

The First World War saw medical problems of infectious disease, starvation and plunging birth rates. A response came with ideas of state responsibility for family health and new ministries for health as service providers. The first was a Ministry for Public Health in Austria in 1917. The chapter by Marius Turda outlines developments in Central Europe. Great Britain instigated a Ministry of Health in 1920. The founding of new states in Europe based on national self-determination meant also the state's recognition of its responsibility for the family. Here the Weimar constitution was notable, as was the new Soviet Union. The Soviet model of 'Red Medicine' exercised a fascination for health internationalists. The Rockefeller Foundation representatives visited Soviet laboratories and provided some modest funding for scientific literature.[24]

The mass starvation resulting from the war resulted in new international relief measures. The forthright Eglantyne Jebb, who founded the Save the Children Fund in 1919, criticised Britain's blockade of food supplies to Austria-Hungary and Germany during the First World War.[25] She caused an immense stir by drawing attention to child starvation and resulting illness. Jebb courageously called for assistance for starving children in Germany and Austria. This marked the origins of the Save the Children Fund, which organised relief in Vienna to counter childhood malnutrition. Despite the revolution, Herbert

Hoover's American Relief Administration provided massive relief for the sick and famished in communist Russia; Save the Children, the Hamburg Institute of Tropical Diseases, and the Quakers also mounted major relief missions.[26] This situation set a new organisational form and strategy for disease and hunger relief: state and non-governmental organisations all followed this newly interventive model of providing relief at the point of distress rather than allowing mass migration. As state welfare systems became ever more elaborate, countries closed their borders to migrants.

Different organisations scrambled for a share in the new landscape of international health. The American Red Cross became an ambitious player between 1918 and the early 1920s. The banker Henry Davison allied with President Woodrow Wilson to promote a scheme for the Red Cross to assume responsibility for welfare as opposed to wartime emergency relief. They supported a League of Red Cross Societies seeking a civilian welfare role, in contrast to the Geneva based and Swiss staffed International Committee of the Red Cross that prioritised protection for military prisoners. A meeting at Cannes in 1919 set out an agenda for a voluntaristic scheme for international health in a new peacetime federation. The ICRC pointed out that the meeting excluded the Central Powers, which had lost the war, but on whose territories the social need was immense.[27] In the event, the American retreat into isolationism undermined the new peacetime strategy, and a multi-state scheme was to emerge through the League of Nations.

The founding of states on the basis of national self-determination triggered massive population transfers. The Norwegian explorer Fridtjof Nansen oversaw massive population exchanges between Greece and the newly sovereign Turkey. This set the pattern for expulsions and transfers of ethnic groups. The  trend to ethnic homogeneity continued to pose profound problems for minorities and the socially marginal.

## The interwar period

The League's Health Committee developed into the LNHO.[28] Although US foreign policy was isolationist in the 1920s, US foundations were perversely at their most interventionist in working within state administrations and exerting pressure for the development of public health policies and institutions. Post-war animosities continued with a blockade against Germany's participation in international medical conferences.[29] Despite this, the LNHO made early efforts to include Germany in its health committees, such as for malaria. Germany became a full member of the League in 1926, but Hitler cancelled all LNHO participation in 1933.

The League of Nations initiatives developed from an Epidemic Commission in 1920. The League's Health Organisation continued to provide services for epidemic prevention. Its Singapore office re-inforced its capacity for epidemic early warning on a global basis. The next step was the LNHO developing a standardisation programme on a biological basis. Its ambitious

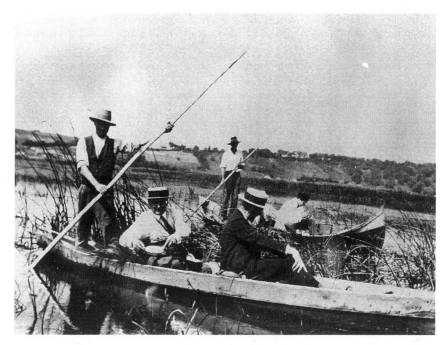

*Figure 10.1* Members of the Malaria Commission of the League of Nations collecting larvae on the Danube Delta, 1929. © The Wellcome Library, London.

entry into social provision was indicated by country surveys of health that allowed members to assert their identities as modern states. The Rockefeller Foundation supported public health systems in Central Europe.[30]

The International Labour Office (ILO), founded in 1919, marked a successful venture into industrial and rural health. It collated legislation and laboratory literature for newly recognised occupational health hazards such as silicosis and asbestosis. Its organisation had not only member states but also employers and worker representation. This meant an extension of sickness insurance to family dependants, as well as improvements in maternity provision, not least in response to persistently high rates of maternal mortality.[31]

The interwar period saw the rise of innovative schemes of preventive medicine and social medicine. At an international level there were innovative fusions of the public and private, as with the Rockefeller support of the LNHO, and on the private side the League of Red Cross Societies represented a new attempt to bring the caring ethos of the Red Cross into civil society. The Milbank Memorial Fund made important innovations in primary healthcare in such arenas as the United States, Eastern Europe and China. International organisations such as the LNHO had a significant impact in terms of the standardisation of vaccines and assay techniques such as the Wassermann test for syphilis. Supplementary funding from the Rockefeller Foundation contributed to meetings and study tours of public health experts.

On occasions such funding meant that Latin American public health officials would tour North America and Europe. While the author Louis Destouches (alias Céline) debunked such initiatives, the idea was that they should internationalise public health and promote and disseminate best practice at an expert level.[32] The Rockefeller Foundation offered public health fellowships and – a noted innovation – fellowships for public health nurses. These were signs of the emergence of expert knowledge underpinning a new generation of international health workers.

Sickness insurance allowed for access to medical practitioners and clinics such as public sanatoria for tuberculosis. There were also innovative new forms of dispensary clinics, including multifunctional health centres. Examples were the ambulatory (walk-in) clinics in Berlin providing medical care on a socialised basis rather than through individual physicians, the Finsbury Health Centre in London, and the village co-operative clinics known as *Zadrugas* in the newly united Yugoslavia. Dedicated to family health, health centres as integrated providers of multiple forms of healthcare well demonstrated health and wellbeing as central social values.

A twin process occurred: the more social security and public health were extended, the greater became the barriers to immigration. The spectre of the immigrant or refugee as a burden on state public health provision was constant. In Britain each refugee required deposits from a guarantor to ensure that the refugee would not become a burden on public assistance. Here public provision forced the development of a private sphere of charitable assistance. In the United States the antagonism to migrants taking employment and lowering wages meant borders remained sealed to all but a few migrants under the quota system. This meant that during the 1930s there was immense resistance to absorbing refugees from Nazi persecution.

The Rockefeller Foundation pursued a dual approach involving both a central laboratory researching new cures – such as for malaria and yellow fever – and sanitary measures in the field – such as drainage schemes and personal protection such as mosquito nets. The International Health Board (later Division) of the Rockefeller Foundation became a major force on the landscape of international health, not least in Latin America and South East Asia.[33] Its laboratory in New York supported research in virology. The Rockefeller Foundation had a special organisation for medicine in China. The risk of deprived populations being used as experimental cohorts for testing drugs and vaccines increased. The Tuskegee experiment on the non-treatment of syphilis and the deliberate infection by the US Public Health Service of 700 Guatemalans during the period 1946 to 1948 well illustrates such medical exploitation.[34]

Health experts assisted by a growing army of social workers and public health nurses began to intervene in the hitherto private spheres of reproduction and the family. The LNHO remained indifferent to eugenics, but the ILO under Albert Thomas certainly recognised the potential of birth control, as advocated by the American feminist Margaret Sanger. Public health became part of efforts to promote what was called 'positive health' in terms of life-style and reproductive behaviour, seeking to rationalise behaviour and consumption on medical grounds. Conversely, the private came increasingly to shape public measures involving corporate foundations and philanthropic ventures. There was also a combining of the academic with the entrepreneurial: this can be seen in the introduction of new vaccines and drugs, conducting diagnostic tests such as the Wassermann test for syphilis, and products such as vitamin fortified foods. The LNHO offered international standardisation of vaccines and pharmaceutical products. The Polish-Jewish bacteriologist Ludwik Fleck critically examined reasons for divergent scientific outcomes of standardisation and diagnostic tests.[35]

On the primary healthcare side, private healthcare was supplemented by state and philanthropic clinics, such as for infant welfare and tuberculosis prevention. These identified personal behaviour, domestic arrangements, sexuality and reproduction, and consumption of alcohol and food as matters of public interest. The Rockefeller Foundation found corporate systems of public health clinics, staffed by nurses, to be more efficient for healthcare delivery. Although certain programme officers of the Rockefeller Foundation and the Milbank Memorial Fund favoured public systems of medicine, the boards of these foundations could not condone anything appearing to be socialised. Whether dispensary clinics could offer treatment was a matter of controversy: on the one hand the professional representative organisations opposed therapy in such public clinics, and on the other it was a matter of public interest that individuals and families who could not otherwise afford healthcare should be offered treatment. The physician straddled both public and private.

A counterpart to these community clinics was how the LNHO selected urban and rural districts where multiple health indicators were analysed in the 1930s. There were studies of the interactions of working and domestic living conditions. These complemented pioneering studies on unemployment and sickness, as carried out by Marie and Gustav Jahoda in Marienthal in Austria, and subsequently in South Wales.[36] There were efforts to transfer best practice, albeit culturally adapted. This can be seen in the local healer concept from Croatia becoming the barefoot doctor in Ting Hsien in China. The Milbank and Rockefeller Foundations supported the Ting Hsien experiment in mass health movements in China, regarding this as the logical extension of the international motives underpinning health demonstration unit schemes in New York.[37]

The development of welfare schemes was accompanied by draconian persecution in authoritarian states, notably fascist Italy and Nazi Germany. Here schemes were generous for those deemed of suitable quality for the corporate state, but those who were racially or politically undesirable were excluded from entitlements and from citizenship. The 1930s saw increasingly desperate efforts to migrate on the part of refugees from National Socialism, while the United States and Canada steadfastly maintained highly restrictive immigration quotas: although refugees did find their way to locations such as the UK, Palestine and Shanghai, many others perished in the Holocaust.

## Second World War and post-war

The Second World War unleashed a massive crisis in international health. The International Committee of the Red Cross tragically failed to protect civilian populations under enemy occupation. The Nazis pursued policies of racial extermination in camps and in occupied territories with impunity. The refugee Polish-Jewish lawyer Raphael Lemkin had drawn attention to the vulnerability of ethnic minorities; he first used the term 'genocide' in 1944 to describe the physical and cultural extermination of whole peoples, notably the Jews and the gypsies (or Sinti and Roma).[38] Genocide exposed the vulnerability of the person to public collectivities.

The older generation of health organisations retained a shadowy existence. A much reduced LNHO clung on in neutral but isolated Geneva, and the ILO moved to Montreal. The Nazis planned German-dominated networks for international health. Despite the relative success of the LNHO in the interwar period, the supporting political principles of collective security and arbitration were deemed bankrupt. Instead, a new set of international organisations began to formulate plans and policies for what was hoped would be a post-war world based on social justice and international collaboration for reconstruction, resettlement of displaced persons, and to raise levels of health. The new United Nations set about establishing the new framework for international health. A starting point was the Atlantic Charter of 14 August 1941. There followed the planning and founding of a new range of international organisations, based on ideas of human rights and respect for national sovereignty. At first, the Allies could claim leadership given the war-torn conditions of a shattered Europe. But by 1948 the leadership became paralysed, as the Cold War took hold.

The UN instigated an ambitious agency for relief through UNRRA (the United Nations Relief and Rehabilitation Agency).[39] It deployed new medical weapons for radical strategies of disease eradication – with DDT for malaria, or penicillin against infections. The expectation was not just disease containment but a wholesale eradication of the pathogens. The new technologies posed problems as to their most appropriate organisational form: were these to be internationally produced and patent free, or were they (like penicillin manufactured by UNRRA in Italy) to be delivered by the industrial system of one or another of the Allies?

To remedy the chaos of displaced persons, forced migration and war casualties, there were a few liminal years of idealism and visionary experts between 1945 and 1948. The Nuremberg Trials showed the extent of the Nazi system of destruction, invoking the novel concept of 'crimes against humanity'. The Doctors Trial concluded in August 1947 with a judicial declaration on the need for voluntary consent in medical research. There was a new sense of the importance of universalist human rights protecting the integrity and health of the person. The UN Declaration on Human Rights, promulgated on 10 December 1948, was a landmark. Article 25 stated:

(1) Everyone has the right to a standard of living adequate for the health and wellbeing of himself and of his family, including food, clothing, housing and medical care and necessary social services, and the right to security in the event of unemployment, sickness, disability, widowhood, old age or other lack of livelihood in circumstances beyond his control.
(2) Motherhood and childhood are entitled to special care and assistance. All children, whether born in or out of wedlock, shall enjoy the same social protection.[40]

The UN Human Rights Division sought compensation for victims of medical experiments.[41] The UN's Economic and Social Council had an agenda of women's rights, and the protection of minorities. The UN Convention on the Prevention and Punishment of the Crime of Genocide, authored by Raphael Lemkin, marked another such landmark. UNESCO set about tackling the iniquities of the idea of race, leading to a series of momentous (but contradictory) statements on race. Even so, eugenic methods of prevention avoided scrutiny, and in Scandinavia coerced sterilisation continued until the mid-1960s; mothers deemed to be failing were a particular target.

The years immediately after the war represented an era of fluidity in terms of manifold professional and organisational possibilities – and evident human need. The western zones of Germany were flooded by expelled ethnic Germans and, a new administrative category, displaced persons. Some looked to a new era of rational expert leadership through international agencies. The only League of Nations agency to survive was the ILO. Here, its unique tripartite model of employer and worker representation along with the state gave the organisation greater durability. At the international level the new landscape of the World Health Organization (WHO), UNESCO (directed at first by the mercurial biologist Julian Huxley with the historian of Chinese science Joseph Needham as assistant director) show the significance of multilateral organisations. The nutritionist John Boyd Orr directed the FAO (Food and Agriculture Organization).

One contrast between the interwar and post-1945 periods is the greater attention paid to mental health in the latter. While having interwar roots, the appointment of an expert in 'mental hygiene' in the shape of Brock Chisholm as Director General of WHO marked this change. UNESCO developed a dynamic interest in mental health, along with psychology and educational provision. In part, the employment of figures such as the peripatetic psychiatrist John Thompson until 1954/5 to develop the German programme for therapy for a war-ravaged generation made this possible.[42]

The Rockefeller Foundation was interventive in war-ravaged Europe and Asia. WHO was established in 1948 for 'the attainment by all peoples of the highest possible level of health'. The United Nations established UNICEF (the United Nations Children's Fund) for child medical and food relief in December 1946. The former LNHO Director Ludwik Rajchman drew on residual funds of UNRRA to make the agency permanent as the United

Nations Children's Fund in 1953.[43] Article 24 of the UN Convention on Refugees of 1951 stated that refugees should have the same entitlement to medical care as the host country's citizens. This symbolised the transition from a military to an internationalist and civilian ethos well.

## Cold War medicine

By 1948 the Cold War divisions had begun to harden. The World Medical Association (WMA) (an organisation of national physicians' associations) successfully fought social medicine in the United States; together with the British Medical Association, it unsuccessfully resisted the founding of the National Health Service in 1948; and it fought with partial success in Europe where the not-for-profit insurance model remained pre-eminent. More problematic was German participation in the WMA, with its representative Hans Joachim Sewering having been implicated in Nazi euthanasia.[44] The WHO and WMA collaborated amicably on the regulation of medical research, as both organisations recognised that the dangers of the unregulated nightmare of Nazi experimental medicine could happen again. This can be seen in the WMA's Declaration of Helsinki of 1963 on the ethics of consent in medical research.

In other respects the Cold War gripped international agencies ever more tightly. The US State Department made determined efforts to screen internationally based staff and to control appointments.[45] The Rockefeller Foundation was terrified about its having funded left-wing biologists such as the biochemist John Desmond Bernal.[46] After 1951 the Rockefeller Foundation terminated its International Health Division. This can be seen as a response to the Cold War.[47] Yet the foundation continued social and community based initiatives, such as for social medicine in South Africa. A host of newly independent countries having emerged from decolonisation, combined with compliant support from the Warsaw Pact countries, provided the Soviet Union with opportunities to assert power over WHO and UNESCO policies by the 1960s. International tensions contributed to bureaucratic inertia, and deflected energies to bilateral programmes. Beyond the ideological divide, a divide persisted between technical approaches based on drugs and vaccines, and the focus on lifestyle and social conditions. Saturation programmes with penicillin against syphilis, such as in Yugoslavia, appeared to offer the prospects of eliminating this medical scourge. The US Federal government began to invest massively in scientific and medical research. There were strategic interests underpinning this, such as with massive studies of radiation fall out and the effects on malformations.[48] Scientists became accustomed to large-scale funds from state agencies. A competitive situation developed, with the US and its NATO allies rivalling the Soviet Union in medicine and science more generally. Recipient countries recognised how to play off competing donors against each other.

There remained profound differences in organisational strategies of international health agencies. International health initiatives can broadly be grouped into two strategies. The first comprises low-cost technologies that have a wide impact on the health of populations. Immunisation programmes are an out-standing example, although, as polio illustrates, they face intractable problems of political and cultural animosities. Smallpox offers the sole example of a successful eradication programme.[49] Polio and cholera immunisation programmes had limited these diseases. Birth control programmes for barrier contraceptives and the pill continue to be opposed on religious grounds.[50]

The other approach is community based. We see this with a plethora of NGOs arising after the Second World War. Oxfam and Médecins sans Fron-tières/Doctors Without Borders are noted examples.[51] WHO itself promoted education, especially for females, and clean water. The 'Health for All by the Year 2000' strategy – launched at Alma Ata in 1978 – exemplifies this new focus on primary healthcare. Indeed, one can even see communities of researchers shaping WHO mental health policy from the 1970s.[52]

The WHO had complex problems of funding and organisation to contend with. Disillusion with its lack of relevance for industrial countries and inabil-ity to deliver in the developing countries meant a preference for NGOs and bilateral schemes (such as USAID).[53] The World Bank Strategy of 'Investing in Health' gained increasing influence as a way of curing problems of defec-tive infrastructure.

By 2000 the WHO strategy was focused on tobacco and malaria. New UN task-specific organisations have appeared on the scene as UNAIDS, reflecting a situation of disenchantment with the omni-competence of WHO. In the twenty-first century chronic non-infectious diseases have been an increasing focus of attention. On the private side the Bill and Melinda Gates Foundation has represented a major initiative to tackle a range of infectious diseases.

Global contraception has proved controversial. Sterilisation in Indian states to meet set targets, for nominal rewards such as transistor radios, was a noted human rights abuse. The Cold War saw a rapid diminution of explicit eugenics and instead a shift to issues of population and development. The Rockefeller Foundation established the Population Council that in turn made efforts to permeate the UN and shape policy on birth control.[54] The idea of a 'population explosion', particularly in the Far East, was the pretext for draconian policies of intervention. Coercive policies imposed on economically poor populations could result in infections (from poorly fitted IUDs), or the pill could have problematic side-effects.[55]

The recognition of HIV/AIDS during the early 1980s (but with origins probably in the instabilities of Equatorial Africa during the late 1950s and 1960s) re-inforced the importance of barrier contraception and highlighted the dangers of casual penetrative sex. Demands for a policing approach clashed with enlightened ideas of human rights. Princess Diana showed the world the need to de-stigmatise AIDS sufferers. The initial stigma gave way to new ideas of the need to protect children and other vulnerable groups. The first World AIDS Day was held in 1988. In part, preventing AIDS was a matter of public education on transmission, prevention and the need to de-stigmatise the disease. In part, AIDS prevention and control was a matter of making therapies involving relatively costly pharmaceuticals available to some of the poorest countries in the world.

The second half of the twentieth century saw a rise in public medical provision in the context of welfare states. The German sickness insurance system, one that is mainly not for profit, has proved to be resilient – even in contexts such as the former East Germany. Although costly, it has been effective in delivering a market-led demand for high quality healthcare. The problems are control of costs and regulation of contracting physicians. The model has only suited relatively wealthy countries, leaving the rest of the world under-provided. Despite the interest of the Rockefeller Foundation and American experts in social medicine, a health insurance scheme only came to fruition late in the USA, in the twenty-first century.

The strengthening of welfare states and the emergence of regional blocs such as the European Union has a corollational politics of migrant exclusion and the stress on relief in situ provided by NGOs. The fall of the Iron Curtain and collapse of dictatorial regimes has caused population pressures for migration. These have coincided with new agendas of 'global health', posited in opposition to public health and state-specific interests. The idea was to improve health irrespective of any national priorities.[56] Anne-Emanuelle Birn has critically assessed the increasingly prominent role of private funding, as tied to corporate interests, and the neglect of socio-economic deprivation as a factor in disease.[57] Tensions arise between the corporate interests of the donors and the agendas of humanitarian health workers in the field. Humanitarianism has itself been a matter of critical discussion, in terms of whether it is genuinely disinterested or merely represents an attempt to make foreign commercial interests acceptable. To protect against such invasive exploitation of the body, new ideas of informed consent and patient rights arose. These were set against increasing concerns with the cost of healthcare in such areas as heart disease and cancer.

In conclusion, the ideal of world health exercised great power throughout the twentieth century, but the role of states, corporate philanthropies and experts resulted in organisational diversity. Accountability has been problematic: member countries rightfully wish to see appropriate expenditure, while experts seek to avoid political strictures on necessary expenditures. Multilateral state organisations associated with the League of Nations and then the United Nations have a creditable record of achievement. But often governments prefer bilateral relations between donor and any recipient as more amenable to control. Any notion of a sharp public/private dichotomy is questionable, as state-funded multilateral organisations (notably LNHO and then WHO) often appreciate the flexibility from supplementary private funding. States have supported the delivery of overseas relief to stem tides of potential refugees. Corporate foundations are a fundamental feature of the century's innovations, while public generosity remains unabated in supporting medical charities and medical relief organisations. The delivery of healthcare has taken a multitude of forms with diverse forms of social arrangements often involving the voluntary sector. One can conclude that the state and private sectors have continued to co-exist in the international sphere, but have found a series of new forms of complementarity and partnership in relation to a changing landscape of epidemiological and demographic problems.

## Further reading

The publications, statistics and reports of international organisations are an immense and readily accessible resource. Sinclair Lewis's *Arrowsmith* is an evocative novel, published in 1925, featuring international health. The Rockefeller Foundation is by far the best studied organisation, and the model for a variety of interpretative frameworks. A basic set of studies of the international organisations of the interwar period is provided in Paul Weindling (ed.), *International Health Organisations and Movements 1918–1939* (Cambridge: Cambridge University Press, 1995). Iris Borowy, *Coming to Terms with World Health: The League of Nations Health Organisation* (Berlin: Peter Lang, 2009) provides a comprehensive account of the LNHO. Jessica Reinisch is developing the study of UNRRA in the immediate post-war period; see her '"We Shall Rebuild Anew a Powerful Nation": UNRRA, Internationalism and National Reconstruction in Poland', *Journal of Contemporary History* 43(2008) 451–76. Holdings of the International Tracing Service offer a major resource for studies of Displaced Persons; see www.its-arolsen.org/en/homepage/index.html (accessed 16 May 2014). For the post-1945 period, see Sanjoy Battacharya, *Expunging Variola: The Control and Eradication of Smallpox in India, 1947–1977* (New Delhi & London: Orient Longman India and Sangam Books, 2006). Wider aspects of WHO have yet to find definitive historical treatment; see www.who.int/kms/initiatives/ghh_bibliography.pdf (accessed 16 May 2014).

## Notes

1 Mark Mazower, *Governing the World: The History of an Idea* (Harmondsworth: Penguin, 2012).
2 Anne-Emanuelle Birn and Theodor Brown (eds), *Comrades in Health: US Health Internationalists, Abroad and at Home* (Rutgers: Rutgers University Press, 2013); Paul Weindling (ed.), *International Health Organisations and Movements 1918–1939* (Cambridge: Cambridge University Press, 1995).
3 Charles Webster, 'Healthy or Hungry Thirties?', *History Workshop Journal*, 13 (1982): 110–29.
4 Caroline Moorehead, *Dunant's Dream: War, Switzerland and the History of the Red Cross* (London: HarperCollins, 1998).
5 Anne-Emanuelle Birn, 'Gates's Grandest Challenge: Transcending Technology as Public Health Ideology', *The Lancet*, 366, 9484 (2005): 514–19.
6 Frances Larson, *An Infinity of Things: How Sir Henry Wellcome Collected the World* (Oxford: Oxford University Press, 2009).
7 Shula Marks, Paul Weindling and Laura Wintour, *In Defence of Learning: The Plight, Persecution and Placement of Academic Refugees 1933–1980s* (Oxford: Oxford University Press for the British Academy, 2011).

8  Paul Weindling, 'Scientific Elites and Laboratory Organization in *fin de siècle* Paris and Berlin: The Pasteur Institute and Robert Koch's Institute for Infectious Diseases Compared', in Andrew Cunningham and Perry Williams (eds), *The Laboratory Revolution in Medicine* (Cambridge: Cambridge University Press, 1992), 170–88.

9  Howard Berliner, *A System of Scientific Medicine: Philanthropic Foundations in the Flexner Era* (New York: Tavistock Publications, 1985); Richard E. Brown, *Rockefeller Medicine Men: Medicine and Capitalism in America* (Berkeley: University of California Press, 1979).

10  John Ettling, *The Germ of Laziness: Rockefeller Philanthropy and Public Health in the New South* (Cambridge, MA: Harvard University Press, 1981).

11  William H. Schneider, 'The Model American Foundation Officer: Alan Gregg and the Rockefeller Foundation Medical Divisions', *Minerva*, 41 (2003): 155–66.

12  Paul Weindling, 'From Moral Exhortation to Socialised Primary Care: The New Public Health and the Healthy Life, 1918–45', in E. Rodriguez Ocana (ed.), *The Politics of the Healthy Life: An International Perspective* (Sheffield: European Association for the History of Medicine and Health, 2002), 113–30.

13  Paul Weindling, 'Public Health and Political Stabilisation: Rockefeller Funding in Interwar Central/Eastern Europe', *Minerva*, 31 (1993): 253–67.

14  Paul Weindling (ed.), *International Health Organisations and Movements 1918–1939*, Cambridge Monographs in the History of Medicine (Cambridge: Cambridge University Press, 1995).

15  Paul Weindling, *Epidemics and Genocide in Eastern Europe, 1890–1945* (Oxford: Oxford University Press, 2000).

16  Alfred W. Crosby, *America's Forgotten Pandemic: The Influenza of 1918* (Cambridge: Cambridge University Press, 2nd edn, 2003); Nancy K. Bristow, *American Pandemic: The Lost Worlds of the 1918 Influenza Epidemic* (Oxford: Oxford University Press, 2012).

17  Weindling, 'Scientific Elites in *fin de siècle* Paris and Berlin', 170–88; Weindling, 'Children's Hospitals and Diphtheria Wards in *fin de siècle* Paris, London and Berlin', in Roger Cooter (ed.), *In the Name of the Child* (London and New York: Routledge, 1992), 124–45; Weindling, 'From Medical Research to Clinical Practice: Serum Therapy for Diphtheria in the 1890s', in John Pickstone (ed.), *Medical Innovations in Historical Perspective* (London and Basingstoke: Macmillan, 1992), 72–83, 222–4.

18  Abdel Omran, 'The Epidemiological Transition: A Theory of the Epidemiology of Population Change', *The Millbank Quarterly*, 83, 4 (2005): 731–57. Reprinted from *The Millbank Memorial Fund Quarterly*, 49, 1 (2005 [1971]): 509–38.

19  Paul Weindling, 'The Politics of International Co-ordination to Combat Sexually Transmitted Diseases, 1900–1980s', in Virginia Berridge and Philip Strong (eds), *AIDS and Contemporary History* (Cambridge: Cambridge University Press, 1993), 93–107.

20  Stefan Kuehl, *For the Betterment of the Race: The Rise and Fall of the International Movement for Eugenics and Racial Hygiene* (Basingstoke: Palgrave, 2013).

21  Norman Howard-Jones, *The Scientific Background of the International Sanitary Conferences, 1851–1938* (Geneva: World Health Organization, 1974); http://whqlibdoc.who.int/publications/1975/14549_eng.pdf (accessed 9 May 2014); http://ocp.hul.harvard.edu/ contagion/sanitaryconferences.html (accessed 9 May 2014)

22  Marcos Cueto, *The Value of Health: A History of the Pan American Health Organisation* (Rochester, NY: Rochester University Press, 2009).

23  Amy L. Fairchild, *Science at the Borders: Immigrant Medical Inspection and the Shaping of the Modern Industrial Labor Force* (Baltimore: The Johns Hopkins University Press, 2003).

24  Nikolai Krementsov and Susan Solomon, 'Giving and Taking across Borders: The Rockefeller Foundation and Soviet Russia, 1919–1928', *Minerva*, 39 (2001):

265–98; Susan Solomon, 'Through a Glass Darkly: The Rockefeller Foundation's International Health Board and Soviet Public Health', *Studies in the History and Philosophy of the Biomedical Sciences*, 31 (2000): 409–18.

25 Clare Mulley, *The Woman Who Saved the Children: A Biography of Eglantyne Jebb* (London: Oneworld Publications, 2009).

26 Benjamin M. Weissmann, *Herbert Hoover and Famine Relief to Soviet Russia 1921–23* (Stanford, CA: Hoover Press, 1974); Bertrand M. Patenaude, *The Big Show in Bololand* (Stanford, CA: Stanford University Press, 2002).

27 League of Red Cross Societies, *Proceedings of the Medical Conference Held at the Invitation of the Committee of Red Cross Societies Cannes, France April 1 to 11, 1919* (Geneva: LRCS, 1919).

28 Iris Borowy, *Coming to Terms with World Health: The League of Nations Health Organisation* (Berlin: Peter Lang, 2009).

29 Brigitte Schroeder-Gudehus, *Les scientifiques et la paix* (Montreal: Presses de l'Université de Montreal, 1978).

30 Paul Weindling, 'Public Health and Political Stabilisation: Rockefeller Funding in Interwar Central/Eastern Europe', *Minerva*, 31 (1993): 253–67. See also Marius Turda in this volume.

31 Sandrine Kott and Joëlle Droux (eds), *Globalizing Social Rights: The ILO and beyond* (London: Palgrave Macmillan, 2013).

32 Louis-Ferdinand Céline, *Semmelweis et autres écrits médicaux*. Édition de Jean-Pierre Dauphin et Henri Godard Collection Cahiers Céline (n° 3) (Paris: Gallimard, 1977).

33 Anne-Emanuelle Birn, *Marriage of Convenience: Rockefeller International Health and Revolutionary Mexico* (Rochester, NY: University of Rochester Press, pbk edn, 2012).

34 Susan M. Reverby, *Examining Tuskegee: The Infamous Syphilis Study and its Legacy* (Chapel Hill: University of North Carolina Press, 2009); http://en.wikipedia.org/wiki/Guatemala_syphilis_experiment (accessed 16 May 2014).

35 Pauline Mazumdar, 'In the Silence of the Laboratory: The League of Nations Standardises Syphilis Tests', *Social History of* Medicine, 16 (2003): 43–459.

36 Marie Jahoda, Paul Lazarsfeld and Hans Zeisel, *Marienthal: The Sociography of an Unemployed Community* (New Brunswick: Transaction Publishers, 2002). Her study of South Wales is Christian Fleck (ed.), *Marie Jahoda: Arbeitslose bei der Arbeit. Die Nachfolgeuntersuchung zu 'Marienthal' aus dem Jahr 1938* (Frankfurt am Main: Campus, 1989).

37 Paul Weindling, 'From Moral Exhortation to Socialised Primary Care: The New Public Health and the Healthy Life, 1918–45', in Esteban Rodriguez Ocana (ed.), *The Politics of the Healthy Life: An International Perspective* (Sheffield: European Association for the History of Medicine and Health, 2002), 113–30; Paul Weindling, 'Social Medicine at the League of Nations Health Organisation and International Labour Office Compared', in Weindling (ed.), *International Health Organisations*, 134–53.

38 Samantha Power, *A Problem from Hell: America and the Age of Genocide* (New York: Basic Books, 2002).

39 Jessica Reinisch, 'Auntie UNRRA at the Crossroads', in Rana Mitter and Matthew Hilton (eds), 'Transnationalism and Contemporary Global History', *Past and Present Supplement*, 218, 8 (2013): 70–97.

40 UN Declaration on Human Rights, Article 25, 10 December 1948.

41 Paul Weindling, *Victims and Survivors of Nazi Human Experiments: Science and Suffering in the Holocaust* (London: Bloomsbury, 2014); John Peters Humphrey, *Human Rights and the United Nations: A Great Adventure* (New York: Transnational Publishers, 1984).

42 Paul Weindling, *John W. Thompson, Psychiatrist in the Shadow of the Holocaust* (Rochester, NY: Rochester University Press, 2010).

43 Maggie Black, *Children First: The Story of UNICEF, Past and Present* (Oxford: Oxford University Press, 1996).

44 http://en.wikipedia.org/wiki/Hans_Joachim_Sewering (accessed 16 May 2014).

45 Anne-Emanuelle Birn and Theodore Brown (eds), *Comrades in Health: US Health Internationalists, Abroad and at Home* (New Brunswick: Rutgers University Press, 2013).

46 Paul Weindling, 'From Disease Prevention to Population Control: The Realignment of Rockefeller Foundation Policies 1920s–1950s', in Helke Rausch and John Krige (eds), *American Foundations and the Coproduction of World Order in the Twentieth Century*, Schriftenreihe der FRIAS School of History (Göttingen: Vandenhoeck & Ruprecht, 2012), 125–45.

47 Ibid.

48 Susan M. Lindee, *Suffering Made Real: American Science and the Survivors at Hiroshima* (Chicago: University of Chicago Press, 1994).

49 Sanjoy Battacharya, *Expunging Variola: The Control and Eradication of Smallpox in India, 1947–1977* (New Delhi and London: Orient Longman India and Sangam Books, 2006).

50 *The First Ten Years of the World Health Organization* (Geneva: WHO 1958); *The Second Ten Years of the World Health Organization 1958–1967* (Geneva: WHO, 1968); *Four Decades of Achievement: Highlights of the Work of the WHO* (Geneva, WHO: 1988).

51 Rene Fox, 'Medical Humanitarianism and Human Rights: Reflections on Doctors without Borders and Doctors of the World', *Social Science and Medicine*, 41, 12 (1995): 1607–16.

52 Steve Sturdy, Richard Freeman and Jennifer Smith-Merry, 'Making Knowledge for International Policy: WHO Europe and Mental Health Policy, 1970–2008', *Social History of Medicine*, 26, 3 (2013): 532–554.

53 Javed Siddiqi, *World Health and World Politics: The World Health Organisation and the UN System* (London: Hurst, 1995).

54 Richard Symonds and Michael Carder, *The United Nations and the Population Question 1945–1970* (London: Chatto & Windus for Sussex University Press, 1973); Stanley P. Johnson, *World Population and the United Nations: Challenge and Response* (Cambridge: Cambridge University Press, 1987).

55 Matthew Connelly, *Fatal Misconception: The Struggle to Control World Population* (Cambridge, MA: The Belknap Press of Harvard, 2009); Lara V. Marks, *Sexual Chemistry: A History of the Contraceptive Pill* (New Haven, CT: Yale University Press, 2001).

56 Theodor Brown, Marcos Cueto and Elizabeth Fee, 'The World Health Organization and the Transition from "International" to "Global" Public Health', *American Journal of Public Health*, 96, 1 (2006): 62–72.

57 Anne-Emanuelle Birn, 'Philanthrocapitalism, Past and Present: The Rockefeller Foundation, the Gates Foundation, and the Setting(s) of the International/Global Health Agenda', *Hypothesis*, 12, 1 (forthcoming).

# Bibliography

Abel, E. (2011) '"In the Last Stages of Irremediable Disease": American Hospitals and Dying Patients before World War II', *Bulletin of the History of Medicine*, 85: 29–56.

Aisenberg, A. R. (1999) *Contagion: Disease, Government, and the 'Social Question' in Nineteenth-Century France*, Stanford, CA: Stanford University Press.

Althammer, B. (2006) 'Functions and Developments of the *Arbeitshaus* in Germany: Brauweiler Workhouse in the Nineteenth and Early Twentieth Centuries', in A. Gestrich and L. Raphael (eds), *Being Poor in Modern Europe: Historical Perspectives 1800–1940*, Oxford: Peter Lang, 273–98.

Amdam, R. P. (1996) 'Professional Networks and the Introduction of Research in the British and Norwegian Pharmaceutical Industry in the Interwar Years', *History and Technology*, 13: 101–14.

Andrews, J., Briggs, A., Porter, R., Tucker, P. and Waddington, K. (1997) *The History of Bethlem*, Abingdon: Routledge.

Antonakopoulos, G. (2012) 'The Royal Medical Council of Greece, 1834–1922', in M. Turda (ed.), 'Private and Public Medical Traditions in Greece and the Balkans', *Deltos: Journal of the History of Hellenic Medicine*: 33–6.

Apple, R. D. (2006) '"Training the Baby": Mothers' Responses to Advice Literature in the First Half of the Twentieth Century', in B. Beatty, R. D. Cahan and J. Grant (eds), *When Science Encounters the Child: Education, Parenting and Child Welfare in Twentieth Century America*, New York: Teachers College Press, 195–214.

Ash, M. G. and Surman, J. (eds) (2012) *The Nationalization of Scientific Knowledge in the Habsburg Empire, 1848–1918*, Basingstoke: Palgrave Macmillan.

Attlee, C. (1948) 'The New Social Services and the Citizen', *BBC Home Service*, 4 July, www.bbc.co.uk/archive/nhs/5147.shtml.

Auden, W. H. (1948) *The Age of Anxiety: A Baroque Eclogue*, 1st UK edn, London: Faber.

Austoker, J. (1989) 'Walter Morley Fletcher and the Origins of a Basic Biomedical Research Policy', in J. Austoker and L. Bryder (eds), *Historical Perspectives on the Role of the Medical Research Council*, Oxford: Oxford University Press, 23–33.

Austoker, J. and Bryder, L. (eds) (1989) *Historical Perspectives on the Role of the Medical Research Council*, Oxford: Oxford University Press.

Ayliffe, G. A. J. and English, M. P. (2003) *Hospital Infection: From Miasmas to MRSA*, Cambridge: Cambridge University Press.

Baader, G., Hofer, V. and Mayer, T. (2008) *Eugenik in Österreich: Biopolitische Strukturen von 1900–1945*, Vienna: Czernin Verlag.

Bächi, B. (2010) 'Producing Ascorbic Acid: How Microbes Transformed the Pharmaceutical Company Hoffmann-La Roche, 1933–1953', in V. Quirke and J. Slinn (eds), *Perspectives on Twentieth-Century Pharmaceuticals*, Oxford: Peter Lang, 367–92.

Bailey, N. (1952) 'Operational Research in Medicine', *Operational Research Quarterly (1950–1952)*, 3: 24–30.

Baldwin, P. (1990) *The Politics of Social Solidarity and the Bourgeois Basis of the European Welfare State, 1875–1975*, Cambridge: Cambridge University Press.

Balińska, M. A. (1996) 'The National Institute of Hygiene and Public Health in Poland, 1918–1939', *Social History of Medicine*, 9, 3: 427–45.

Balińska, M. A. (1995) 'Assistance and Not Mere Relief: The Epidemic Commission of the League of Nations, 1920–1923', in Weindling (ed.), *International Health Organisations and Movements 1918–1939*, Cambridge: Cambridge University Press, 99–100.

Ballance, R., Forstner, H. and Pogány, J. (eds) (1992), *The World's Pharmaceutical Industries: An International Perspective on Innovation, Competition and Policy*, Aldershot: Edward Elgar.

Banu, G. (1927) 'Biologia satelor', *Arhiva pentru ştiinţă şi reformă socială* 7, 1–2: 87–121.

——(1931) 'Organizarea igienei sociale în Ungaria', *Revista de igienă socială*, 1, 9: 800–9.

Bărbulescu, C. (2002) 'Tema degenerării rasei în literatura medicală din România la sfârşitul secolului al XIX-lea', in Nicolae Bocşan, Sorin Mitu and Toader Nicoară (eds), *Identitate şi alteritate. Studii de istorie politică şi culturală*, Vol. 3, Cluj: Presa Universitară Clujeană, 2002, 273–90.

Bărbulescu, C. and Ciupală, A. (eds), (2012) *Medicine, Hygiene and Society from the Eighteenth to the Twentieth Centuries*, Cluj-Napoca: Ed. Mega.

Barras, V. and Bernheim, J. (1990) 'The History of Law and Psychiatry in Europe', in R. Bluglass and P. Bowden (eds), *Principles and Practice of Forensic Psychiatry*, Edinburgh: Churchill Livingstone, 103–16.

Barrington, R. (2000) *Health, Medicine and Politics in Ireland 1900–1970*, Dublin: Institute of Public Administration.

Barrow, L. (2002) 'In the Beginning Was the Lymph: The Hollowing of Stational Vaccination in England and Wales, 1840–98', in S. Sturdy (ed.), *Medicine, Health and the Public Sphere in Britain, 1600–2000*, London and New York: Routledge, 205–23.

Bashford, A. and Levine, P. (eds) (2010) *The Oxford Handbook of the History of Eugenics*, New York: Oxford University Press.

Basmanjian, J. V. (1999) 'The Third Therapeutic Revolution: Behavioural Medicine', *Applied Psychophysiology Biofeedback*, 24, 2: 107–16.

Battacharya, S. (2006) *Expunging Variola: The Control and Eradication of Smallpox in India, 1947–1977*, New Delhi and London: Orient Longman India and Sangam Books.

Bazalgette, J. W. (1865) *On the Main Drainage of London, and the Interception of the Sewage from the River Thames*, London: William Clowes & Sons.

Beccalossi, C. (2012) *Female Sexual Inversion: Same-Sex Desires in Italian and British Sexology, c. 1870–1920*, Basingstoke: Palgrave Macmillan.

Beck, I. F. (1948) *The Almoner: A Brief Account of Medical Social Service in Great Britain*, London: Council of the Institute of Almoners.

Beer, J. (1959) *The Emergence of the German Dye Industry.* Urbana: University of Illinois Press.

Behlmer, G. K. (1982) *Child Abuse and Moral Reform in England, 1870–1908*, Stanford, CA: Stanford University Press.

Bell, E. M. (1961) *The Story of Hospital Almoners: The Birth of a Profession*, London: Faber & Faber.

Berliner, H. (1985) *A System of Scientific Medicine: Philanthropic Foundations in the Flexner Era*, New York: Tavistock.

Berridge, V. and Strong, P. (eds) (2000), *AIDS and Contemporary History* Cambridge: Cambridge University Press (pbk edn).

Bertrand M. Patenaude (2002) *The Big Show in Bololand*, Stanford, CA: Stanford University Press.

Betteridge, T. (ed.) (2002) *Sodomy in Early Modern Europe*, Manchester: Manchester University Press.

Bevan, A. 'National Health Service Bill', Second Reading Debate, 30 April 1946, *House of Commons Debates*, Vol. 422, cols. 45, 49.

Birn, A-E. (2005) 'Gates's Grandest Challenge: Transcending Technology as Public Health Ideology', *The Lancet*, 366, 9484: 514–19.

——(2012) *Marriage of Convenience: Rockefeller International Health and Revolutionary Mexico*, Rochester, NY: University of Rochester Press (pbk edn).

——(2013) 'Philanthrocapitalism, Past and Present: The Rockefeller Foundation, the Gates Foundation, and the Setting(s) of the International/Global Health Agenda', *Hypothesis*, 12: 1.

——(2014) 'Philanthrocapitalism, past and present: The Rockefeller Foundation, the Gates Foundation, and the setting(s) of the International/ Global Health Agenda', *Hypothesis*, 12(1): e6, doi:10.5779/hypothesis. v10i1.229

Birn, A-E. and Brown, T. (eds) (2013) *Comrades in Health: US Health Internationalists, Abroad and at Home*, New Brunswick, NJ: Rutgers University Press.

Black, M. (1996) *Children First: The Story of UNICEF, Past and Present*, Oxford: Oxford University Press.

Blech, J. (2006) *Inventing Disease and Pushing Pills: Pharmaceutical Companies and the Medicalisation of Normal Life*, London and New York: Routledge.

Bliss, M. (1982) *The Discovery of Insulin*, Toronto: McClelland & Stewart.

Blondel-Mégrelis, M. (1994) 'La Pharmacie en France 1900–1950, points de repères', in Claude Debru, Jean Gayon and Jean-François Picard (eds), *Les Sciences biologiques et médicales en France 1920–1950*, Paris: CNRS Editions, 283–96.

Bokor, Z. (2013) *Testtörténetek. A nemzet és a nemi betegségek medikalizálása a két világháború közötti Kolozsváron*, Kolozsvár: Nemzeti Kisebbségkutató Intézet.

Bonah, C. (2013) 'Professional, Industrial and Juridical Regulation of Drugs: The 1953 Stalinon Case and Pharmaceutical Reform in Postwar France', in J.-P. Gaudillière and V. Hess (eds), *Ways of Regulating Drugs in the Nineteenth and Twentieth Centuries*, Houndmills, Basingstoke and New York: Palgrave Macmillan, 245–69.

Booth, C. (1990) 'Clinical Research', in W. Bynum and R. Porter (eds), *Companion Encyclopedia of the History of Medicine*, Vol. 1, London and New York: Routledge, 205–9.

Borowy, I. (2009) *Coming to Terms with World Health: The League of Nations Health Organisation*, Berlin: Peter Lang.

Borowy, I. and Gruner, W. D. (eds) (2005) *Facing Illness in Troubled Times: Health in Europe in the Interwar Years, 1918–1939*, Bern: Peter Lang.

Borowy, I. and Hardy, A. (eds) (2008) *Of Medicine and Men: Biographies and Ideas in European Social Medicine between the World Wars*, Bern: Peter Lang.

Borsay, A. and Shapely, P. (eds) (2007) *Medicine, Charity and Mutual Aid: The Consumption of Health and Welfare in Britain, c. 1550–1950*, Aldershot, Hants: Ashgate.

Borsay, A. and Dale, P. (2012) *Disabled Children: Contested Caring, 1850–1979*, London: Pickering & Chatto.

Bremmer, J. (ed.) (1989) *From Sappho to De Sade: Moments in the History of Sexuality*, London and New York: Routledge.

Brigden, P. (2007) 'Voluntary Failure, the Middle Classes, and the Nationalisation of the British Voluntary Hospitals, 1900–1946', in B. Harris and P. Bridgen (eds), *Charity and Mutual Aid in Europe and North America since 1800*, London: Routledge, 220–6.

Brown, R. E. (1979) *Rockefeller Medicine Men: Medicine and Capitalism in America*, Berkeley: University of California Press.

Brown, T., Cueto, M. and Fee, E. (2006) 'The World Health Organization and the Transition from "International" to "Global" Public Health', *American Journal of Public Health*, 96, 1: 62–72.

Browne, S. G. (1979) 'The Contribution of Medical Missionaries to Tropical Medicine', *Transactions of the Royal Society of Tropical Medicine and Hygiene*, 73: 357–60.

Brynner, R. and Stephens, T. (2001) *Dark Remedy: The Impact of Thalidomide and Its Revival as a Vital Medicine*, London: Basic Books.

Bud, R. (1978) 'Strategy in American Cancer Research after World War II: A Case Study', *Social Studies of Science*, 8: 425–59.

——(1993) *The Uses of Life: A History of Biotechnology*, Cambridge: Cambridge University Press.

——(2007) *Penicillin: Triumph and Tragedy*, Oxford: Oxford University Press.

——(2010) 'From Applied Microbiology to Biotechnology: Science, Medicine, and Industrial Renewal', *Notes and Records of the Royal Society*, 64: 17–29.

Buhlungi, S., Daniel, J., Southall, R. and Lutchman J. (eds) (2007) *State of the Nation: South Africa 2007*, Cape Town: HSRC Press.

Buklijas, T. and Lafferton, E. (eds) (2007) 'Science, Medicine and Nationalism in the Habsburg Empire from the 1840s to 1918', *Studies in the History and Philosophy of Science*, Part C, 38, 4.

Bullough, V. L. (1974) 'Homosexuality and the Medical Model', *Journal of Homosexuality*, 1: 99–110.

Bulmuş, B. (2012) *Plague, Quarantines and Geopolitics in the Ottoman Empire*, Edinburgh: Edinburgh University Press.

Burch, D. (2009) *Taking the Medicine: A Short History of Medicine's Beautiful Idea, and Our Difficulty Swallowing It*, London: Chatto & Windus.

Bürgi, M. and Strasser, B. 'Pharma in Transition: New Approaches to Drug Development at F. Hoffmann-La Roche & Co., 1960–1980' (2010), in V. Quirke and J. Slinn (eds), *Perspectives on Twentieth-Century Pharmaceuticals*, Oxford: Peter Lang, 393–434.

Bynum, W. F. (1994) *Science and the Practice of Medicine in the Nineteenth Century*, Cambridge: Cambridge University Press, 152–7.

Bynum, W. F., Hardy, A., Jacyna, S., Lawrence, C. and Tansey, E. M. (Tilli) (eds) (2006) *The Western Medical Tradition: 1800 to 2000*, Cambridge: Cambridge University Press.

Cadogan, W. (1748) *An Essay upon Nursing and the Management of Children from Their Birth to Three Years of Age*, London J. Roberts.

Caiger, F. F. (1910–11) 'Cubicle Isolation: Its Value and Limitations', *Public Health*, 24: 336–7.

Campbell, C. (2003) *'Letting Them Die': Why HIV/AIDS Prevention Programmes Fail*, Oxford: James Currey.

Cantor, D. (1993) 'Cortisone and the Politics of Drama, 1949–1955', in J. Pickstone (ed.), *Medical Innovations in Historical Perspective*, Basingstoke: Macmillan, 165–84.

Čapka, F. (2011) 'Gustav Kabrhel: The Founder of the Czech Public Health Science and His Contribution to the "School and Health" Issues', *School and Health*, 21: 19–23.

Cassedy, J. H. (1991) *Medicine in America: A Short History*, Baltimore, MD and London: The John Hopkins University Press.

Catanesi, R., Rocca, G., Candelli, C., Solarino, B. and Carabellese, F. (2012) 'Death by Starvation: Seeking a Forensic Psychiatric Understanding of a Case of Fatal Child Maltreatment by the Parent', *Forensic Science International*, 223: e13–e17.

Céline, L.-F. (1977) *Semmelweis et autres écrits médicaux*. Édition de Jean-Pierre Dauphin et Henri Godard Collection Cahiers Céline (n° 3), Paris: Gallimard.

Chabner, B. A. and Roberts Jr, T. G. (2005) 'Chemotherapy and the War on Cancer', *Nature Reviews Cancer*, 5 (Jan.): 65–72.

Chalmers, I. and Clarke, M. (2004) 'The 1944 Patulin Trial: The First Properly Conducted Multicentre Trial Conducted under the Aegis of the British Medical Research Council', *International Journal of Epidemiology*, 32: 253–60.

Chandler, D. (2005) *Shaping the Industrial Century: The Remarkable Story of the Evolution of the Modern Chemical and Pharmaceutical Industries*, Cambridge, MA: MIT Press.

Chanock, M. (1985) *Law, Custom and Social Order: The Colonial Experience in Malawi and Zambia*, Cambridge: Cambridge University Press.

Chapin, C. V. (1901) *Municipal Sanitation in the United States*, Providence, RI: Snow & Farnham.

Chauveau, S. (1999) *L'Invention pharmaceutique: La pharmacie entre l'Etat et la société*, Paris: Institut d'Edition Sanofi-Synthélabo.

Chesbrough, H., Vanhaverbeke, W. and West, J. (eds) (2006), *Open Innovation: Researching a New Paradigm*, Oxford and New York: Oxford University Press.

Chick, H., Hume, M. and Macfarlane, M. (1971) *War on Disease: A History of the Lister Institute*, London: Deutsch.

Chin-Dusting, J., Mizrahi, J., Jennings, G. and Fitzgerald D. (2005) 'Finding Improved Medicines: The Role of Academic Industrial Collaborations', *Nature Reviews Drug Discovery*, 5: 891–7.

Church, R. (2005) 'The British Market for Medicine in the Late Nineteenth Century: The Innovative Impact of S. M. Burroughs & Co.', *Medical History*, 49: 281–98.

Clarke, A., Mamo, L. and Fosket, J. (2010) *Biomedicalization: Technoscience, Health, and Illness in the US*, Durham, NC: Duke University Press.

Clement, P. F. (1985) *Welfare and the Poor in the Nineteenth Century City: Philadelphia 1800–1854*, Cranbury, NJ: Associated University Presses.

Colaizzi, J. (1989) *Homicidal Insanity, 1800–1985*, Tuscaloosa and London: University of Alabama Press.

Colón, A. R. with Colón, P. A. (1999) *Nurturing Children: A History of Pediatrics*, Westport, CT: Greenwood Press.

Conn, M. (2012) 'Sexual Science and Sexual Forensics in 1920s Germany: Albert Moll as (S)expert', *Medical History*, 56: 201–16.

Connelly, M. (2009) *Fatal Misconception: The Struggle to Control World Population*, Cambridge, MA: The Belknap Press of Harvard.

Conrad, P. (2007) *The Medicalization of Society: On the Transformation of Human Conditions into Medical Disorders*, Baltimore, MD: The Johns Hopkins University Press.

Cooter, R. (ed.) (1992) *In The Name of the Child: Health and Welfare, 1880–1940*, London and New York: Routledge.

Corbin, A. (1996) *The Foul and the Fragrant: Odour and the Social Imagination*, London: Papermac.

Crawford, J. (1988) *Kill or Cure? The Role of the Pharmaceutical Industry in Society*, London: Arc Print.

Crellin, J. (1980) 'Antibiosis in the Nineteenth Century', in John Parascandola (ed.), *The History of Antibiotics: A Symposium*, Madison, WI: American Institute of the History of Pharmacy.

Crosby, A. W. (2012) *America's Forgotten Pandemic: The Influenza of 1918*, Cambridge: Cambridge University Press.

Crossman, V. (2013) *Poverty and the Poor Law in Ireland 1850–1914*, Liverpool: Liverpool University Press.

Crozier, I. D. (2001) 'The Medical Construction of Homosexuality and Its Relation to the Law in Nineteenth-Century England', *Medical History*, 45: 61–82.

Cueto, M. (2009) *The Value of Health: A History of the Pan American Health Organisation*, Rochester: Rochester University Press.

Cullen, L. (2012) 'The First Lady Almoner: The Appointment, Position, and Findings of Miss Mary Stewart at the Royal Free Hospital, 1895–99', *Journal of the History of Medicine and Allied Sciences*, 68, 4: 551–82.

Cunliffe, E. (2011) *Murder, Medicine and Motherhood*, Oxford: Hart Publishing.

Cunningham, A. and Williams, P. (eds) (1992) *The Laboratory Revolution in Medicine*, Cambridge: Cambridge University Press.

Curth, L. H. (ed.) (2006) *From Physick to Pharmacology: Five Hundred Years of British Drug Retailing*, Aldershot: Ashgate.

Curtis, H. (2007) *Faith in the Great Physician: Suffering and Divine Healing in American Culture, 1860–1900*, Baltimore, MD: The Johns Hopkins University Press.

Cuthbert, A. W. (1979) 'Men, Molecules and Machines', *Trends in Pharmacological Sciences*, inaugural issue 3: 1–3.

Cutler, T. (2007) 'A Double Irony? The Politics of National Health Service Expenditure in the 1950s', in M. Gorsky and S. Sheard (eds), *Financing Medicine: The British Experience since 1750*, London: Routledge, 201–20.

Daemmrich, A. (2002) 'A Tale of Two Experts: Thalidomide and Political Engagement in the United States and West Germany', *Social History of Medicine*, 15: 137–58.

Daniel, A. E. (2007) 'Care of the Mentally Ill in Prisons: Challenges and Solutions', *Journal of the American Academy of Psychiatry and the Law*, 35: 406–10.

Darling, E. (2007) *Re-forming Britain: Narratives of Modernity before Reconstruction*, London: Routledge.

Daunton, M. (1983) *House and Home in the Victorian City: Working-Class Housing, 1850–1914*, London: Edward Arnold.

Davenport-Hines, R. and Slinn, J. (1992) *Glaxo: A History to 1962*, Cambridge: Cambridge University Press.

Davidson, R. and Davis, G. (2012) *The Sexual State: Sexuality and Scottish Governance, 1950–80*, Edinburgh: Edinburgh University Press.

De Courcy Meade, T. (1900) 'Conference of Engineers and Surveyors to County and Other Sanitary Authorities', *Journal of the Sanitary Institute*, 21: 496–9.

Deichmann, U. (2002) 'Emigration, Isolation and the Slow Start of Molecular Biology in Germany', in S. de Chadarevian and B. Strasser (eds), 'Molecular Biology in Post-war Europe', *Studies in History and Philosophy of Biology and Biomedical Sciences*, 30: 449–71.

'Demographic Problems of Southeastern Europe', *Population Index*, 7, 2 (1941): 84–92.

de Swaan, A. (1988) *In Care of the State: Health Care, Education and Welfare in Europe and the USA in the Modern Era*, Cambridge: Polity Press.

Digby, A. (2005) 'Early Black Doctors in South Africa', *Journal of African History*, 46, 3: 427–54.

——(2006) *Diversity and Division in Medicine: Health Care in South Africa from the 1800s*, Oxford and Bern: Peter Lang.

——(2006) 'The Economic and Medical Significance of the British National Health Insurance Act, 1911', in M. Gorsky and S. Sheard (eds), *Financing Medicine: The British Experience since 1750*, London: Routledge, 182–98.

——(2011) 'The Mid-level Health Worker in South Africa: The In-between Condition of the "Middle"', in R. Johnson and A. Khalid (eds), *Public Health in the British Empire: Intermediaries, Subordinates, and Public Health Practice, 1850–1960*, Routledge: London.

——(2012) 'Evidence, Encounters and Effects of South Africa's Reforming Gluckman National Health Services Commission, 1942–1944', *South African Historical Journal*, May: 187–205.

——(2012) '"The Bandwagon of Golden Opportunities"?: Healthcare in South Africa's Bantustan Periphery', *South African Historical Journal*, 64, 4: 827–51.

——(2013) 'Black Doctors and Discrimination under South Africa's Apartheid Regime', *Medical History*, 57, 2: 269–90.

Digby, A. and Sweet, H. (2012) 'Social Medicine and Medical Pluralism: The Valley Trust and Botha's Hill Health Centre, South Africa, 1940s to 2000s', *Social History of Medicine*, 25: 425–45.

Digby, A., Ernst, W. and Mukharji, P. (eds) (2010) *Crossing Colonial Historiographies: Histories of Colonial and Indigenous Medicines in Transnational Perspective*, Newcastle upon Tyne: Cambridge Scholars Publishing.

Digby, A., Phillips, H., Deacon, H. and Thomson, K. (2008) *At the Heart of Healing: Groote Schuur Hospital, 1938–2008*, Johannesburg: Jacana.

Dinan, S. (2006) *Women and Poor Relief in Seventeenth-Century France: The Early History of the Daughters of Charity*, Farnham: Ashgate.

Donovan, J. M. (1991) 'Infanticide and the Juries in France, 1825–1913', *Journal of Family History*, 16: 157–76.

Downs, J. (2012) *Sick from Freedom: African-American Illness and Suffering during the Civil War and Reconstruction*, Oxford: Oxford University Press.

Drenkhahn, K. (2013) 'Secure Preventive Detention in Germany: Incapacitation or Treatment Intervention?', *Behavioral Sciences and the Law*, 31: 312–27.

Dressing, H. and Salize, H.-J. (2009) 'Pathways to Psychiatric Care in European Prison Systems', *Behavioral Sciences and the Law*, 27: 801–10.

Dressing, H., Salize, H.-J. and Gordon, H. (2007) 'Legal Frameworks and Key Concepts Regulating Diversion and Treatment of Mentally Disordered Offenders in European Union Member States', *European Psychiatry*, 22: 427–32.

Drysdale, C. R. (1896) 'The Royal Commission on Vaccination', *British Medical Journal*, 2, 1864: 786.

Dupree, M. (2011) 'Central Policy and Local Independence: Integration, Health Centres and the National Health Service in Scotland, 1948–1990', in M. Freeman, E. Gordon and K. Maglen (eds), *Medicine, Law and Public Policy in Scotland, c. 1850–1990*, Dundee: Dundee University Press, 180–202.

Durbach, N. (2000) '"They Might as Well Brand Us": Working Class Resistance to Compulsory Vaccination in Victorian England', *The Society for the Social History of Medicine*, 13: 45–62.

——(2004) *Bodily Matters: The Anti-vaccination Movement in England, 1853–1907*, Durham, NC: Duke University Press.

Dutfield, G. (2008) *Intellectual Property Rights and the Life Science Industries: Past, Present and Future*, New Jersey etc.: World Scientific.

Dutton, P. (2007) *Differential Diagnoses: A Comparative History of Health Care Problems and Solutions in the United States and France*, Ithaca, NY: Cornell University Press.

Dynes, W. R. (ed.) (1990) *Encyclopedia of Homosexuality*, London: St James Press, www.williamapercy.com/wiki/index.php?title=Encyclopedia_of_Homosexuality.

'Editorial', South African Health Review (Durban: Health Systems Trust, 1998), 1.

Eigen, J. P. (1991) 'Delusion in the Courtroom: The Role of Partial Insanity in Early Forensic Testimony', *Medical History*, 35: 25–49.

——(1995) *Witnessing Insanity: Madness and Mad-doctors in the English Court*, New Haven and London: Yale University Press.

Elias, N. (1978) *The Civilizing Process, Volume One: The History of Manners*, Oxford: Blackwell Publishing.

——(1982) *The Civilizing Process, Vol. 2: State Formation and Civilization*, Oxford: Blackwell.

Engel, J. (2006) *Poor People's Medicine: Medicaid and American Charity Care since 1965*, Durham, NC: Duke University Press.

Engstrom, E. J. (2003) *Clinical Psychiatry in Imperial Germany: A History of Psychiatric Practice*, Ithaca and London: Cornell University Press.

——(2014) 'Topographies of Forensic Practice in Imperial Germany', *International Journal of Law and Psychiatry*, 37: 63–70.

Epstein, S. (1995) 'The Construction of Lay Expertise: AIDS Activism and the Forging of New Credibility in the Reform of Clinical Trials', *Science, Technology and Human Values*, 20: 408–37.

——(1996) *Impure Science: AIDS, Activism and the Politics of Knowledge*, Berkeley: University of California Press.

Esping-Andersen, G. (1990) *The Three Worlds of Welfare Capitalism*, Cambridge: Polity Press.

Ettling, J. (1981) *The Germ of Laziness: Rockefeller Philanthropy and Public Health in the New South*, Cambridge, MA: Harvard University Press.

Evans, M. and Shisana, O. (2012) 'Gender Differences in Public Perceptions on National Health Insurance', *South African Medical Journal*, 12: 918–24.

Evans, R. (1982) *The Fabrication of Virtue: English Prison Architecture, 1750–1840*, Cambridge: Cambridge University Press.

Eveleigh, D. J. (2006) *Bogs, Baths and Basins: The Story of Domestic Sanitation*, Stroud: Sutton Publishing.

Ewing, C. P. (2008) *Insanity: Murder, Madness and the Law*, Oxford: Oxford University Press.

Fagerberg, J., Mowery, D. and Nelson, R. (eds) (2005), *The Oxford Handbook of Innovation*, Oxford and New York: Oxford University Press.

Fairchild, A. L. (2003) *Science at the Borders: Immigrant Medical Inspection and the Shaping of the Modern Industrial Labor Force*, Baltimore, MD: The Johns Hopkins University Press.

Fazel, S. and Seewald, K. (2012) 'Severe Mental Illness in 33,588 Prisoners Worldwide: Systematic Review and Meta-regression Analysis', *British Journal of Psychiatry*, 200: 364–73.

Feinstein, C. H. (2005) *An Economic History of South Africa: Conquest, Discrimination and Development*, Cambridge: Cambridge University Press.

Ferguson, H. (1992) 'Cleveland in History: The Abused Child and Child Protection', in Cooter, R. (ed.), *In The Name of the Child: Health and Welfare, 1880–1940*, London and New York: Routledge, 146–73.

Finlayson, G. (1994) *Citizen, State and Social Welfare in Britain*, Oxford: Clarendon Press.

Fleck, C. (ed.) (1989) *Marie Jahoda: Arbeitslose bei der Arbeit. Die Nachfolgeuntersuchung zu 'Marienthal' aus dem Jahr 1938*, Frankfurt am Main: Campus.

Flint, K. (2008) *Healing Traditions: African Medicine, Cultural Exchange and Competition in South Africa, 1820–1948*, Athens: Ohio University Press.

Foot, M. (1973) *Aneurin Bevan: A Biography, Vol. 2, 1945–1960*, London: Davis-Poynter.

Forrester, A., Ozdural, S., Muthukumaraswamy, A. and Carroll, A. (2008) 'The Evolution of Mental Disorder as a Legal Category in England and Wales', *Journal of Forensic Psychiatry and Psychology*, 19: 543–60.

Foucault, M. (1965) *Madness and Civilization: A History of Insanity in the Age of Reason*, London: Tavistock.

——(1991) *Discipline and Punish: The Birth of the Prison*, London: Penguin Books.

——(1963) *Naissance de la clinique – une archéologie du regard médical*, Paris: PUF; English edition, (1994) *The Birth of the Clinic: An Archaeology of Medical Perception*, New York: Vintage.

Fowler, N. (2008) *A Political Suicide: The Conservatives' Voyage into the Wilderness*, London: Politico's.

Fox, D. (2004) 'The Administration of the Marshall Plan and British Health Policy', *Journal of Policy History* 16: 191–211.

Fox, R. (1995) 'Medical Humanitarianism and Human Rights: Reflections on Doctors without Borders and Doctors of the World', *Social Science and Medicine*, 41, 12: 1607–16.

Freeden, M. (1978) *The New Liberalism: An Ideology of Social Reform* Oxford: Clarendon Press, 237.

Freeman, R. (2008) 'A National Health Service, by Comparison', *Social History of Medicine*, 21, 3: 503–20.

Frohman, L. (2008) 'Breakup of the Poor Laws – German Style: Progressivism and the Origins of the Welfare State 1900–1918', *Comparative Studies in Society and History*, 50: 981–1009.

Fujimura, J. (1992) 'Crafting Science: Standardized Packages, Boundary Objects, and "Translations"', in A. Pickering (ed.), *Science as Practice and Culture*, Chicago: Chicago University Press, 168–211.

Galambos L. and Sturchio, J. (1998) 'Pharmaceutical Firms and the Transition to Biotechnology: A Study in Strategic Innovation', *Business History Review*, 72: 250–78.

Gallup, G. H. (ed.) (1976) *The Gallup International Public Opinion Polls: Great Britain, 1937–1975*, New York: Random House.

Gambardella, A. (1995) *Science and Innovation: The US Pharmaceutical Industry during the 1980s*, Cambridge: Cambridge University Press.

Gassmann, O., Reepmeyer, G. and von Zedwitz, M. (eds) (2008), *Leading Pharmaceutical Innovation: Trends and Drivers for Growth in the Pharmaceutical Industry*, 2nd edn, Berlin: Springer.

Gaudillière, J.-P. and Hess, V. (eds) (2013) *Ways of Regulating Drugs in the Nineteenth and Twentieth Centuries*, Houndmills, Basingstoke and New York: Palgrave Macmillan.

Geary, L. (2011) 'The Medical Profession, Health Care and the Poor Law in Nineteenth Century Ireland', in Virginia Crossman and Peter Gray (eds), *Poverty and Welfare in Ireland, 1838–1948*, Dublin: Irish Academic Press, 189–206.

Geison, G. (1995) *The Private Science of Louis Pasteur*, Princeton, NJ: Princeton University Press.

Gemzell, C. A. (2002) 'The Welfare State: Britain and Denmark', in J. Sevaldsen, C. Bjørn and B. Bjørke (eds), *Britain and Denmark: Political, Economic and Cultural Relations in the Nineteenth and Twentieth Centuries*, Copenhagen: Odsell, 123–44.

George, K. H. (1995) 'George H. Hitchings, 1905– : American Pharmacologist', *Notable Twentieth Century Scientists*, Vol. 2, Detroit, MI: Gale Research, 933–4.

Georgescu, T. (2010) 'Ethnic Minorities and the Eugenic Promise: The Transylvanian Saxon Experiment with National Renewal in Inter-war Romania', *European Review of History*, 17, 6: 861–80.

Gerhard, W. P. (1908) *Modern Baths and Bath Houses*, New York: John Wiley and Sons.

Geschiere, P. (1997) *The Modernity of Witchcraft: Politics and the Occult in Post-colonial Africa*, Charlottesville: University Press of Virginia.

Gestrich, A. (2013) 'Trajectories of German Settlement Regulations: The Prussian Rhine Province, 1815–1914', in S. King and A. Winter (eds) *Migration, Settlement and Belonging*, New York and Oxford: Berghahn, 254–8.

Gestrich, A., Hurren, E. and King, S. (eds) (2012) *Poverty and Sickness in Modern Europe: Narratives of the Sick Poor, 1780–1938*, London: Continuum.

Gieryn, T. (1983) 'Boundary Work and the Demarcation of Science from Non-science: Strains and Interests in Professional Ideologies of Scientists', *American Sociological Review*, 48: 781–95.

Gijswijt-Hofstra, M. and Marland, H. (eds) (2003) *Cultures of Child Health in Britain and the Netherlands in the Twentieth Century*, Amsterdam: Rodopi.

Gijswijt-Hofstra, M., van Heteren G. and Tansey, E. M. (Tilli) (eds) (2002) *Biographies of Remedies: Drugs, Medicines and Contraceptives in Dutch and Anglo-American Healing Cultures*, Amsterdam: Rodopi.

Gilbert, A. N. (1981) 'Conceptions of Homosexuality and Sodomy in Western History', in S. J. Licata and R. P. Petersen (eds), *Historical Perspectives on Homosexuality*, New York: The Haworth Press, 57–68.

Gilbert, B. B. (1966) *The Evolution of National Insurance in Great Britain: The Origins of the Welfare State*, London: Michael Joseph.

Gillett, M. C. (1987) *The Army Medical Department, 1818–1865*, Washington, DC: Centre of Military History.

Giner-Sorolla, A. (1988) 'The Excitement of a Suspense Story, the Beauty of a Poem: The Work of Hitchings and Elion', *Trends in Pharmacological Sciences*, 9 (Dec.): 437–8.

Gleason, M. (2013) *Small Matters: Canadian Children in Sickness and Health*, Montreal and Kingston: McGill-Queen's University Press.

Golan, T. (2004) *Laws of Men and Laws of Nature: The History of Scientific Expert Testimony in England and America*, Cambridge, MA and London: Harvard University Press.

Goldsmith, M. (1946) *The Road to Penicillin: A History of Chemotherapy*, London: Lindsay Drummond.

Goldstein, J. (2001) *Console and Classify: The French Psychiatric Profession in the Nineteenth Century*, rev. edn, Cambridge: Cambridge University Press.

Goodman, J. (1998) 'Can It Ever Be Pure Science? Pharmaceuticals, the Pharmaceutical Industry and Biomedical Research in the Twentieth-Century', in J.-P. Gaudillière and I. Löwy (eds), *The Invisible Industrialist: Manufactures and the Production of Scientific Knowledge*, Basingstoke: Macmillan, 143–65.

Goodman, J. and Walsh, V. (2001) *The Story of Taxol: Nature and Politics in the Pursuit of an Anti-cancer Drug*, Cambridge: Cambridge University Press.

Gorsky, M. (2008) 'The British National Health Service 1948–2008: A Review of the Historiography', *Social History of Medicine* 21, 3: 437–60.

Gorsky, M. and Mohan, J. (2005) 'Hospital Contributory Schemes and the NHS Debates: The Rejection of Social Insurance in the British Welfare State?', *Twentieth Century British History*, 16, 2: 170–92.

Gorsky, M., Powell, M. and Mohan, J. (2002) 'British Voluntary Hospitals and the Public Sphere: Contribution and Participation before the National Health Service', in S. Sturdy (ed.), *Medicine, Health and the Public Sphere in Britain, 1600–2000*, London: Routledge.

Gosling, G. C. (2011) 'Charity and Change in the Mixed Economy of Healthcare in Bristol, 1918–1948', unpublished PhD thesis, Oxford Brookes University.

Goubert, J.-P. (1986) *The Conquest of Water: The Advent of Health in the Industrial Age*, Oxford: Polity Press.

Gradmann, C. and Simon, J. (eds) (2010), *Evaluating and Standardizing Therapeutic Agents 1890–1950*, Houndsmill, Basingstoke: Palgrave Macmillan.

Greene, J. (2007) *Prescribing by Numbers: Drugs and the Definition of Disease*, Baltimore, MD: The Johns Hopkins University Press.

Griscom, J. H. (1845) *Sanitary Condition of the Labouring Population of New York, with Suggestions for Its Improvement*, New York: Harper & Brothers, 41.

Gutton, J.-P. (1971) *La Société et les pauvres: L'Exemple de la généralité de Lyon 1534–1789*, Paris: Les Belles Lettres.

Habermas, J. (1999) *The Structural Transformation of the Public Sphere: An Inquiry into a Category of Bourgeois Society*, Oxford: Polity Press.

Hall, L. (2001) 'The Archives of the Pioneer Health Centre, Peckham, in the Wellcome Library', *Social History of Medicine*, 14, 3, 525–38.

Hall, P. (1975) 'The Development of Health Centres', in P. Hall, H. Land, R. Parker and A. Webb (eds), *Change, Choice and Conflict in Social Policy*, London: Heinemann.

Haller Jr, J. (2009) *The History of American Homeopathy: From Rational Medicine to Holistic Health Care*, New Brunswick, NJ: Rutgers University Press.

Halliday, S. (1999) *The Great Stink of London: Sir Joseph Bazalgette and the Cleansing of the Victorian Capital*, Stroud: Sutton.

Halpern, A. L. (1992) 'The Insanity Verdict, the Psychopath, and Post-acquittal Confinement', *Psychiatric Quarterly*, 63: 209–43.

Ham, C. (2009) *Health Policy in Britain*, London: Palgrave Macmillan.

Hansen, B. G. (2011) 'Beyond the Boundary: Science, Industry, and Managing Symbiosis', *Bulletin of Science Technology and Society*, 31: 493–505.

Harden, V. (1986) *Inventing the NIH: Federal Biomedical Research Policy, 1887–1937*, Baltimore, MD and London: The Johns Hopkins University Press.

Harding, T. (1993) 'A Comparative Survey of Medico-legal Systems', in J. Gunn and P. J. Taylor (eds), *Forensic Psychiatry: Clinical, Legal and Ethical Issues*, Oxford: Butterworth-Heinemann, 118–66.

Hardy, A. and Tansey, E. M. (Tilli) (2006) 'Medical Enterprise and Global Response, 1945–2000', in W. F. Bynum, A. Hardy, S. Jacyna, C. Lawrence and E. M. (Tilli) Tansey (eds), *The Western Medical Tradition: 1800 to 2000*, Cambridge: Cambridge University Press.

Harker, R. (2012) *NHS Expenditure: Commons Library Standard Note*, London: House of Commons Library.

Harpuder, K. (1956) 'Basic Medical Principles in the Treatment of the Chronically Ill Patient', *Journal of Chronic Diseases*, 4: 170–6.

Harris, B. (2004) *The Origins of the British Welfare State: Social Welfare in England and Wales, 1800–1945*, Basingstoke: Palgrave.

Harris, J. (1977) *William Beveridge: A Biography*, Oxford: Clarendon Press.

——(1990) 'Enterprise and Welfare States: A Comparative Perspective', *Transactions of the Royal Historical Society*, 5th Series, 40: 175–95.

Harris, R. (1989) *Murders and Madness: Medicine, Law, and Society in the* fin de siècle, Oxford: Clarendon Press.

Harrison, M. (2012) *Contagion: How Commerce Has Spread Disease*, Oxford: Oxford University Press.

Harrison, S. and McDonald, R. (2008) *The Politics of Healthcare in Britain*, London: Sage.

Hassan, J. (1998) *A History of Water in Modern England and Wales*, Manchester: Manchester University Press.

Hațieganu, I. (1925) 'Rolul social al medicului în opera de consolidare a statului național', *Transilvania*, 54: 588.

Hayes, N. (2012) 'Did We Really Want a National Health Service? Hospitals, Patients and Public Opinions before 1948', *English Historical Review*, 127, 526: 660.

Hayes, P. (1987) *Industry and Ideology: IG Farben in the Nazi Era*, Cambridge: Cambridge University Press, 1987.

Head-König, A.-L. (2013) 'Citizens But Not Belonging: Migrants' Difficulties in Obtaining Entitlement to Relief in Switzerland from the 1550s to the Early Twentieth Century', in S. King and A. Winter (eds), *Migration, Settlement and Belonging in Europe 1500–1930s*, Oxford: Berghahn, 153–72.

Head-König, A.-L. and Schnegg, B. (eds) (1989) *Armut in der Schweiz, 17.-20. Jahrhundert*, Zurich: ZPD.

Healy, D. (1997) *The Antidepressant Era*, Cambridge, MA: Harvard University Press.

——(2004) *Let Them Eat Prozac: The Unhealthy Relationship between the Pharmaceutical Industry and Depression*, New York and London: New York University Press.

——(2009) *Bolshevik Sexual Forensics: Diagnosing Disorder in the Clinic and Courtroom, 1917–1939*, DeKalb: Northern Illinois University Press.

Healy, D. and Cattell, D. (2003) 'Interface between Authorship, Industry and Science in the Domain of Therapeutics', *British Journal of Psychiatry*, 183: 22–7.

Hekma, G. (1989) 'A History of Sexology: Social and Historical Aspects of Sexuality', in J. Bremmer (ed.), *From Sappho to De Sade: Moments in the History of Sexuality*, London and New York: Routledge, 173–93.

Henderson, R., Orsenigo, L. and Pisano, G. (1999) 'The Pharmaceutical Industry and the Revolution in Molecular Biology: Interactions among Scientific, Institutional and Organizational Change', in D. Mowery and R. Nelson (eds), *Sources of Industrial Leadership*, Cambridge: Cambridge University Press.

Hendrick, H. (1994) *Child Welfare: England, 1872–1989*, London and New York: Routledge.

——(2003) 'Children's Emotional Well-being and Mental Health in Early Post-Second World War Britain: The Case of Unrestricted Hospital Visiting', in Gijswijt-Hofstra and Marland, *Cultures of Child Health in Britain and the Netherlands in the Twentieth Century,* Amsterdam: Rodopi, 213–42.

Hennock, E. P. (1987) *British Social Reform and German Precedents: The Case of Social Insurance 1880–1914*, Oxford: Clarendon Press.

——(2007) *The Origins of the Welfare State in England and Germany, 1850–1914: Social Policies Compared*, Cambridge: Cambridge University Press.

Hering, S. and Waaldijk, B. (eds) (2006) *Guardians of the Poor – Custodians of the Public: Welfare History in Eastern Europe, 1900–1960*, Opladen: Barbara Budrich Publishers.

Herzberg, D. (2011) 'Blockbusters and Controlled Substances: Miltown, Quaalude, and Consumer Demand for Drugs in Postwar America', *Studies in History and Philosophy of Biological and Biomedical Sciences*, 42: 415–26.

Heywood, C. (1988) *Childhood in Nineteenth-Century France: Work, Health and Education among the 'classes populaires'*, Cambridge: Cambridge University Press, 183–214.

Hitchings, G. (1969) 'Chemotherapy and Comparative Biochemistry', G. H. A. Clowes Memorial Lecture, *Cancer Research*, 29: 1895–1903.

HMSO (1942) Cmd. 6404, *Social Insurance and Allied Services: Report*, London: HMSO.

Hobby, G. (1985) *Penicillin: Meeting the Challenge*, New Haven, NJ: Yale University Press.

Hoffman, B. (2012) *Health Care for Some: Rights and Rationing in the United States since 1930*, Chicago: Chicago University Press.

Hogg, C. (2008) *Citizens, Consumers and the NHS: Capturing Voices*, Basingstoke: Palgrave.

Homan, J. D. H. and Tepstra, J. (1984) 'Insulin', in M. J. Parnham and J. Bruinvels (eds), *Discoveries in Pharmacology, Volume 2: Haemodynamics, Hormones and Inflammation*, Amsterdam: Elsevier, 431–60.

Homburg, E. (1992) 'The Emergence of Research Laboratories in the Dyestuffs Industry, 1870–1900', *British Journal of the History of Science*, 25: 91–111.

Honigsbaum, F. (1989) *Health, Happiness and Security: The Creation of the National Health Service*, London: Routledge.

Horwitz, S. (2013) *Baragwanath Hospital, Soweto: A History of Medical Care 1941–1990*, Johannesburg: Wits University Press.

Howard, J. (1777) *The State of Prisons in England and Wales*, Warrington: William Eyres.

Howard-Jones, N. (1974) *The Scientific Background of the International Sanitary Conferences, 1851–1938*, Geneva: World Health Organization.

Howells, J. and Neary, I. (1988) *Intervention and Technological Innovation*, Basingstoke: Macmillan.

Howells, K., Day, A. and Thomas-Peter, B. (2004) 'Changing Violent Behaviour: Forensic Mental Health and Criminological Models Compared', *Journal of Forensic Psychiatry & Psychology*, 15: 391–406.

Hugo, J. (2005) 'Mid-level Health Workers in South Africa: Not an Easy Option', *South African Health Review*, Durban: Health Systems Trust, 148–59.

Huisman, F. (2010) 'Struggling for the Market: Strategies of Dutch Pharmaceutical Companies, 1880–1940', in V. Quirke and J. Slinn (eds), *Perspectives on Twentieth-Century Pharmaceuticals*, Oxford: Peter Lang, 63–89.

Hulverscheidt, M. (2010) 'The Scientist-Entrepreneur or Financing in Pharmaceutical Research: A Portrait of the Malariologist Werner Schulemann, 1888–1975', in V. Quirke and J. Slinn (eds), *Perspectives on Twentieth-Century Pharmaceuticals*, Oxford: Peter Lang, 121–48.

Humphrey, J. P. (1984) *Human Rights and the United Nations: A Great Adventure*, New York: Transnational Publishers.

Hüntelmann, A. (2013) 'Making Salvarsan: Experimental Therapy and the Development and Marketing of Salvarsan at the Crossroads of Science, Clinical Medicine, Industry and Public Health', in J.-P. Gaudillière and V. Hess (eds), *Ways of Regulating Drugs in the Nineteenth and Twentieth Centuries* (Houndmills, Basingstoke and New York: Palgrave Macmillan, 2013), 43–65.

Hunter, D. J. (1980) *Coping With Uncertainty: Policy and Politics in the National Health Service*, Chichester: Research Studies Press.

Hurd, H. M. (ed.) (1916) *The Institutional Care of the Insane in the United States and Canada*, Vol. 1, Baltimore, MD: The Johns Hopkins University Press.

Iftimovici, R. (2008) *Istoria universală a medicinii şi farmaciei*, Bucharest: Editura Academiei Române.

Iliffe, J. (1987) *The African Poor: A History*, Cambridge: Cambridge University Press, 158–61.

——(1995) *Africans: The History of a Continent*, Cambridge: Cambridge University Press.

Illich, I. (1974) *Medical Nemesis*, London: Calder & Boyars.

——(1975) 'The Medicalization of Life', *Journal of Medical Ethics*, 1 (2) (Jul.): 73–7.

Ingebrigtsen, E. (1964) *Private Conscience, Public Morality*, London: Andre Deutsch.

——(2010) '"National Models" and Reforms of Public Health in Interwar Hungary", in G. Péteri (ed.), *Imagining the West in Eastern Europe and the Soviet Union*, Pittsburgh, PA: Pittsburgh University Press, 36–58.

——(1965) *Drugs, Doctors and Disease: A Survey of the Pharmaceutical Industry*, London: Andre Deutsch.

Ionescu, T. (1999 [first published in 1906]) *Starea sanitară a României*, Bucharest: Ed. Viaţa Medicală Românească.

Israel, J. (1997) 'Dutch Influence on Urban Planning, Health Care and Poor Relief: The North Sea and Baltic Regions of Europe, 1567–1720', in O. Grell and A. Cunningham (eds), *Health Care and Poor Relief in Protestant Europe 1500–1700*, London: Routledge, 66–83.

Jackson, M. (2009) *Asthma: The Biography*, Oxford and New York: Oxford University Press.

Jahoda, M., Lazarsfeld, P. and Zeisel, H. (2002) *Marienthal: The Sociography of an Unemployed Community*, New Brunswick, NJ: Transaction Publishers.

James, D. V. (2010) 'Diversion of Mentally Disordered People from the Criminal Justice System in England and Wales: An Overview', *International Journal of Law and Psychiatry*, 33: 241–8.

Jeffreys, D. (2004) *The Remarkable Story of a Wonder Drug: Aspirin*, London: Bloomsbury.

Jeffreys, K. (1991) *The Churchill Coalition and Wartime Politics, 1940–1945*, Manchester: Manchester University Press.

Jewson, N. D. (1976) 'The Disappearance of the Sick Man from Medical Cosmology, 1770–1870', *Sociology*, 10: 225–44.

Jochelson, K. (2001) *The Colour of Disease: Syphilis and Racism in South Africa, 1880–1950*, London: Palgrave.

Johan, B. (1938) 'Public Health Services in Hungary', *The Hungarian Quarterly*, 4, 3: 427–33.

——(1939) *Rural Health Work in Hungary*, Budapest: The State Hygienic Institute.

John, H. (2013) 'Translating Leprosy: The Expert and the Public in Stanley Stein's Anti-stigmatization Campaigns, 1931–60', *Journal of the History of Medicine and Allied Sciences* 68: 659–87.

Johns, W. F. (1973) *Steroids*, London: Butterworths.

Johnson, R. and Khalid, A. (eds) (2011) *Public Health in the British Empire: Intermediaries, Subordinates, and Public Health Practice, 1850–1960*, London: Routledge.

Johnson, S. P. (1987) *World Population and the United Nations: Challenge and Response*, Cambridge: Cambridge University Press.

Johnston, N. (2006) *Forms of Constraint: A History of Prison Architecture*, Urbana: University of Illinois Press.

Jones, E. (2001) *The Business of Medicine*, London: Profile Books.

Jones, H. (1994) *Health and Society in Twentieth Century Britain*, London: Longmans.

Jones, T. (1991) 'The Value of Academia/Industry Links in R&D', in S. R. Walker (ed), *Creating the Right Environment for Drug Discovery*, Lancaster: Quay Publishing, 77–84.

Jordan, D. P. (1995) *Transforming Paris: The Life and Labors of Baron Haussmann*, New York: Simon & Schuster.

Jütte, R. (1994) *Poverty and Deviance in Early Modern Europe*, Cambridge: Cambridge University Press.

Kaartinen, M. (2013) 'Women Patients in the English Urban Medical Marketplace in the Long Eighteenth Century', in D. Simonton and A. Montenach (eds), *Female Agency in the Urban Economy: Gender in European Towns 1680–1830*, London: Routledge, 48–67.

Kaase, M. and Newton, K. (1998) 'What People Expect From the State: *plus ça change*', in R. Jowell, J. Curtice and A. Park (eds), *British – and European – Social Attitudes, the Fifteenth Report: How Britain Differs*, Aldershot: Ashgate, 39–54.

Kapronczay, K. and Kapronczay, K. (eds) (2005), *Az orvostörténelem Magyarországon*, Budapest: Semmelweis Orvostörténeti Múzeum.

Karakatsani, D. and Theodoru, V. (2010) *'Hygiene Imperatives': Medical Supervision and Child Welfare in Greece in the First Decades of the Twentieth Century*, Athens: Dionikos.

Karsh, J. and Heteny, G. (1997) 'A Historical Review of Rheumatoid Arthritis Treatment: 1948–1952', *Seminars in Rheumatism and Arthritis*, 27: 57–65.

Kaser, M. (1976) *Health Care in the Soviet Union and Eastern Europe*, Beckenham: Croom Helm.

Katz, E. (1994) *The White Death: Silicosis on the Witwatersrand Gold Mines*, Johannesburg: Witwatersrand University Press.

Kaufmann, D. (1993) 'Boundary Disputes: Criminal Justice and Psychiatry in Germany, 1760–1850', *Journal of Historical Sociology* 6: 276–87.

Keating, P. and Cambrosio, A. (2007) 'Cancer Clinical Trials: The Emergence and Development of a New Style of Practice', in David Cantor (ed.), 'Cancer in the Twentieth Century', *Bulletin for the History of Medicine*, 81: 197–223.

Kedrowski, K. M. and Sarow, M. S. (2007) *Cancer Activism: Gender, Media and Public Policy*, Urban and Chicago: University of Illinois Press, 2007.

Kennedy, C. (1986) *ICI: The Company That Changed Our Lives*, London: Hutchinson.

Kenny, S. (2010) '"A Dictate of Both Interest and Mercy"? Slave Hospitals in the Antebellum South', *Journal of the History of Medicine and Allied Sciences*, 65: 2–47.

Kilday, A.-M. (2013) *A History of Infanticide in Britain c. 1600 to the Present*, Basingstoke: Palgrave Macmillan.

King, C. R. (1993) *Children's Health in America: A History*, New York: Twayne Publishers.

King, M., Smith, G. and Bartlett, A. (2004) 'Treatments of Homosexuality in Britain since the 1950s – an Oral History: The Experience of Professionals', *British Medical Journal*, 328: 429–31.

King, S. (2007) 'Regional Patterns in the Experiences and Treatment of the Sick Poor, 1800–40: Rights, Obligations and Duties in the Rhetoric of Paupers', *Family and Community History* 10: 61–75.

King, S. and Winter, A. (eds) (2013), *Migration, Settlement and Belonging in Europe 1500–1930s*, Oxford: Berghahn.

Kipping, M. and Clark, T. (eds) (2013), *The Oxford Handbook of Management Consulting*, Oxford and New York: Oxford University Press.

Kipping, M. and Bjarnar, O. (eds) (2014), *The Americanisation of European Business: The Marshall Plan and the Transfer of US Management Models*, London and New York: Routledge.

Klein, R. (1995) *The New Politics of the NHS*, 3rd edn, London: Longman.

——(2000) 'The Crises of the Welfare States', in R. Cooter and J. Pickstone (eds), *Medicine in the Twentieth Century*, Abingdon: Harwood Academic Publishers.

——(2010) *The New Politics of the NHS: From Creation to Reinvention*, 6th edn, London: Radcliffe Publishing.

Knafla, L. A. (1996) 'Structure, Conjuncture, and Event in the Historiography of Modern Criminal Justice History', in C. Emsley and L. A. Knafla (eds), *Crime History and Histories of Crime: Studies in the Historiography of Crime and Criminal Justice in Modern History*, Westport, CT: Greenwood Press, 33–44.

Knoll, J. L. and Resnick, P. J. (2008) 'Insanity Defense Evaluations: Basic Procedure and Best Practices', *Psychiatric Times*, 1 Dec.

Kok, P. and Collinson, M. (2006) *Migration and Urbanisation in South Africa*, Pretoria: Statistics South Africa.

Konrad, N. and Völlm, B. (2014) 'Forensic Psychiatric Expert Witnessing within the Criminal Justice System in Germany', *International Journal of Law and Psychiatry*, 37: 149–54.

Kornberg, A. (1995) *The Golden Helix: Inside the Biotech Ventures*, Sausalito, CA: University Science Books.

Kott, S. and Joëlle Droux (eds) (2013), *Globalizing Social Rights: The ILO and beyond*, London: Palgrave Macmillan.

Kovács, M. M. (1994) *Liberal Professions & Illiberal Politics: Hungary from the Habsburgs to the Holocaust*, Washington, DC: Woodrow Wilson Center Press.

Koven, S. and Michel, S. (eds) (1993) *Mothers of a New World: Maternalist Policies and the Origins of Welfare States*, New York and London: Routledge.

Kragh, H. (1998) 'The Take-off Phase of Danish Chemical Industry, ca 1910–1940', in A. Travis, H. Schröter, E. Homburg and P. Morris (eds), *Determinants in the Evolution of the European Chemical Industry, 1900–1939: New Technologies, Political Frameworks, Markets and Companies*, Dordrecht: Kluwer Academic, 321–39.

Krementsov, N. *The Cure: A Story of Cancer and Politics from the Annals of the Cold War*, Chicago and London: University of Chicago Press, 2002.

Krementsov, N. and Solomon, S. (2001) 'Giving and Taking across Borders: The Rockefeller Foundation and Soviet Russia, 1919–1928', *Minerva*, 39: 265–98.

Kuehl, S. (2013) *For the Betterment of the Race: The Rise and Fall of the International Movement for Eugenics and Racial Hygiene*, Basingstoke: Palgrave.

Kutcher, G. (2009) *Contested Medicine: Cancer Research and the Military*, Chicago and London: University of Chicago Press.

Kynaston, D. (2007) *Austerity Britain, 1945–51*, pbk edn, London: Bloomsbury.

Labisch, A. and Sakai, S. (2009) *Transaction in Medicine and Heteronomous Modernization: Germany, Japan, Korea and Taiwan*, Tokyo: University of Tokyo Center for Philosophy.

Lambie, I. (2001) 'Mothers Who Kill: The Crime of Infanticide', *International Journal of Law and Psychiatry*, 24: 71–80.

Landau, R., Achilladelis, B. and Scriabine, A. (eds) (1999), *Pharmaceutical Innovation*, Philadelphia, PA: Chemical Heritage Press.

Landsman, S. (1995) 'Of Witches, Madmen, and Products Liability: A Historical Survey of the Use of Expert Testimony', *Behavioral Sciences and the Law*, 13: 131–57.

Laporte, D. (2000) *History of Shit*, Cambridge, MA: The MIT Press.

Largent, M. (2012) *Vaccine: The Debate in Modern America*, Baltimore, MD: The Johns Hopkins University Press.

Larson, F. (2009) *An Infinity of Things: How Sir Henry Wellcome Collected the World*, Oxford: Oxford University Press.

Law, J. (2006) *Big Pharma: How the World's Biggest Drug Companies Control Illness*, London: Constable, 2006.

Lawrence, C. (1997) 'Clinical Research', in J. Krige and D. Pestre (eds), *Science in the Twentieth Century*, Amsterdam: Harwood Academic, 439–60.

Lawson, N. (1992) *The View From No. 11: Memoirs of a Tory Radical*, London: Bantam.

Lawson, R. (1996) 'Germany: Maintaining the Middle Way', in V. George and P. Taylor-Gooby (eds), *European Welfare Policy: Squaring the Welfare Circle*, Basingstoke: Macmillan.

Lazell, H. G. (1975) *From Pills to Penicillin: The Beechams Story*, London: Heinemann.

Le Fanu, J. (2000) *The Rise and Fall of Modern Medicine*, London: Abacus.

Le Grand, J. (2007) *The Other Invisible Hand: Delivering Public Services through Choice and Competition*, Princeton: Princeton University Press.

League of Red Cross Societies (1919) *Proceedings of the Medical Conference Held at the Invitation of the Committee of Red Cross Societies Cannes, France April 1 to 11, 1919*, Geneva: LRCS.

Lees, A. (1985) *Cities Perceived: Urban Society in European and American Thought, 1820–1940*, Manchester: Manchester University Press.

Leimgruber, M. (2009) *Solidarity without the State? Business and the Shaping of the Swiss Welfare State, 1890–2000*, Cambridge: Cambridge University Press.

Leisering, L. (2003) 'Nation State and Welfare State: An Intellectual and Political History', *Journal of European Social Policy*, 13, 2: 175–85.

Lerner, B. (2001) *The Breast Cancer Wars: Fear, Hope and the Pursuit of a Cure in Twentieth-Century America* (Oxford and New York: Oxford University Press).

Lesch, J. (1999) 'Chemistry and Biomedicine in an Industrial Setting: The Invention of the Sulfa Drugs', in Seymour Mauskopf (ed.), *Chemical Sciences in the Modern World*, Philadelphia, PA: University of Pennsylvania Press, 158–215.

——(2007) *The First Miracle Drugs: How the Sulfa Drugs Transformed Medicine*, Oxford: Oxford University Press.

Levene, A., Powell, M. and Stewart, J. (2004) 'Patterns of Municipal Health Expenditure in Interwar England and Wales', *Bulletin of the History of Medicine*, 78, 3: 644–6.

Lewis, D. (1965) *From Newgate to Dannemora: The Rise of the Penitentiary in New York, 1796–1848*, Ithaca, NY: Cornell University Press.

Lewis, J. (1980) *The Politics of Motherhood: Child and Maternal Welfare in England, 1900–1939*, Beckenham: Croom Helm.

——(1992) *Women in Britain since 1945: Women, Family, Work and the State in the Post-war Years*, Oxford: Blackwell Publishing.

Lewis, J. and Brookes, B. (1983) 'A Reassessment of the Work of the Peckham Health Centre, 1926–1951', *Milbank Memorial Fund Quarterly: Health and Society*, 61, 2: 307–50.

Lewis, S. (1925) *Arrowsmith*, New York: Harcourt Brace.

Liebenau, J. (1984) 'Industrial R&D in Pharmaceutical Firms in the Early Twentieth Century', *Business History*, 26: 329–46.

——(1987) *Medical Science and Medical Industry: The Formation of the American Pharmaceutical Industry*, Baltimore, MD: The Johns Hopkins University Press.

——(1988) 'Ethical Business: The Formation of the Pharmaceutical Industry in Britain, Germany and the US before 1914', in Richard Davenport-Hines and Geoffrey Jones (eds), *The End of Insularity: Essays in Comparative Business History*, London: Cass, 117–29.

——(1989) 'The MRC and the Pharmaceutical Industry: The Model of Insulin', in J. Austoker and L. Bryder (eds), *Historical Perspectives on the Role of the Medical Research Council*, Oxford: Oxford University Press, 163–80.

——(1990) 'Paul Ehrlich as a Commercial Scientist and Research Administrator', *Medical History*, 34: 65–78.

Liebenau, J. and Robson, M. (1991) 'L'Institut Pasteur et l'industrie pharmaceutique', in M. Morange (ed.), *L'Institut Pasteur: Contributions à son histoire*, Paris: Presses Universitaires de France, 52–61.

Liebenau, J., Higby, G. and Stroud, E. (eds) (1990) *Pill Peddlers: Essays on the History of the Pharmaceutical Industry*, Madison, WI: American Institute of the History of Pharmacy.

Lind, J. (1762) *Essay on the Most Effectual Means of Preserving the Health of Seamen, in the Royal Navy*, London: D. Wilson.

Lindee, S. M. (1994) *Suffering Made Real: American Science and the Survivors at Hiroshima*, Chicago: University of Chicago Press.

Lindert, P. (2004) *Growing Public: Social Spending and Economic Growth since the Eighteenth Century, Volume 1*, Cambridge: Cambridge University Press.

Lloyd, M. G. and Bénézech, M. (1992) 'The French Mental Health Legislation of 1838 and Its Reform', *Journal of Forensic Psychiatry*, 3: 235–50.

Lomax, E. M. R. (1996) *Small and Special: The Development of Hospitals for Children in Victorian Britain*, London: Wellcome Institute for the History of Medicine.

Loudon, I., Horder, J. and Webster, C. (eds) (1998) *General Practice under the National Health Service, 1948–1997*, Oxford: Clarendon Press.

Loughlin, K. and Berridge, V. (eds) (2005) *Medicine, the Market and the Mass Media: Producing Health in the Twentieth Century*, London: Routledge.

Loughnan, A. (2012) 'The "Strange" Case of the Infanticide Doctrine', *Oxford Journal of Legal Studies*, 32: 685–711.

Loughnan, A. and Ward, T. (2014) 'Emergent Authority and Expert Knowledge: Psychiatry and Criminal Responsibility in the UK', *International Journal of Law and Psychiatry*, 37: 25–36.

Lowe, R. (1990) 'The Second World War, Consensus and the Foundation of the Welfare State', *Twentieth Century British History*, 1, 2: 152–82.

Löwy, I. (1992) 'The Strength of Loose Concepts: Boundary Objects, Federative Experimental Strategies and Discipline Growth: The Case of Immunology', *History of Science*, 30: 371–96.

Lundberg, A. (1999) *Care and Coercion: Medical Knowledge, Social Policy and Patients with Venereal Disease in Sweden, 1785–1903*, Umea: Umea Demographic Database Report 14.

MacDonald, G. (1994) *At the Back of the North Wind*, Ware: Wordsworth Editions.

Mackie, R. and Roberts, G. (2004) 'Career Patterns in the British Chemical Profession in the Twentieth Century', in D. Mitch, J. Brown and M. van Leeuwen (eds), *Origins of the Modern Career*, Aldershot: Ashgate, 317–36.

Macnicol, J. (1992) 'Welfare, Wages and the Family: Child Endowment in Comparative Perspective, 1900–50', in Cooter, R. (ed.), *In The Name of the Child: Health and Welfare, 1880–1940*, London and New York: Routledge, 244–76.

Mahoney, T. (1959) *The Merchants of Life: An Account of the American Pharmaceutical Industry*, New York: Harper.

Maja, P. 'A Painstaking Journey', *Mail & Guardian*, 14–20 December 2012.

Mander, M. (1998) *Marketing of Indigenous Medicinal Plants in South Africa – A Case Study in Kwazulu-Natal*, Rome: Food and Agriculture Organization of the United Nations.

Mander, M., Ntuli, L., Diederichs, N. and Mavundla, K. (2007) 'Economics of the Traditional Medicine Trade in South Africa', *South African Health Review*, Durban: Health Systems Trust, 189–99.

Manicatide, M. (1906) 'Pentru ce medical rural nu-şi poate face datoria', *Viaţa românească*, 1, 2: 315.

Marks, L. V. (2001) *Sexual Chemistry: A History of the Contraceptive Pill*, New Haven, NJ and London: Yale University Press.

Marks, S. (2001) *Divided Sisterhood: Race, Class and Gender in the South African Nursing Profession*, Johannesburg: University of Witwatersrand Press.

——(2002) 'An Epidemic Waiting to Happen?: The Spread of HIV/AIDS in South Africa in Social and Historical Perspective', *African Studies*, 61, 1: 13–26.

Marks, S., Weindling, P. and Wintour, L. (2011) *In Defence of Learning: The Plight, Persecution and Placement of Academic Refugees 1933–1980s*, Oxford: Oxford University Press for the British Academy.

Marland, H. (2004) *Dangerous Motherhood: Insanity and Childbirth in Victorian Britain*, Basingstoke: Palgrave Macmillan.

Marsa, L. (1997) *Prescription for Profit: How the Pharmaceutical Industry Bankrolled the Unlikely Marriage between Science and Business*, New York: Scribner.

Marshall, L. (1995) 'Gertrude Belle Elion, 1918– : American Biochemist', *Notable Twentieth Century Scientists*, Vol. 1, Detroit, MI: Gale Research, 583–4.

Marshall, T. H. (1950) *Citizenship and Social Class, and Other Essays*, Cambridge: Cambridge University Press.

Mass-Observation Papers (1943) 'A National Health Service', University of Sussex, File Report 1921, October.

——(1944) 'A National Health Service', University of Sussex, File Report 3140, January.

Matheson, A. (2008) 'Corporate Science and the Husbandry of Scientific and Medical Knowledge by the Pharmaceutical Industry', *Biosocieties*, 3: 355–82.

Mathias, P. (1975) 'Swords and Ploughshares: The Armed Forces, Medicine and Public Health in the Late Eighteenth Century', in J. M. Winter (ed.), *War and Economic Development: Essays in Memory of David Joslin*, Cambridge: Cambridge University Press, 73–90.

Mays, N., Dixon, A. and Jones, L. (2011) 'Return to the Market: Objectives and Evolution of New Labour's Market Reforms', in N. Mays, A. Dixon and L. Jones (eds), *Understanding New Labour's Market Reforms of the English NHS* (London: King's Fund, 2011).

Mazower, M. (2012) *Governing the World: The History of an Idea*, Harmondsworth: Penguin.

Mazumdar, P. (2003) 'In the Silence of the Laboratory: The League of Nations Standardises Syphilis Tests', *Social History of Medicine*, 16: 43–459.

Mazzucato, M. (2014) *The Entrepreneurial State: Debunking Public vs Private Sector Myths*, London, New York and Delhi: Anthem Press.

Mazzucato, M. and Dosi, G. (eds) (2006), *Knowledge Accumulation and Industry Evolution: The Case of Pharma Biotech*, Cambridge: Cambridge University Press.

McCulloch, J. (2002) *Asbestos Blues: Labour, Capital, Physicians and the State in South Africa*, James Currey: Oxford.

McDonald, D. (2013) *The Firm: The Inside Story of McKinsey, the World's Most Controversial Management Consultancy*, London: Simon & Schuster.

McHugh, T. (2007) *Hospital Politics in Seventeenth-Century France: The Crown, Urban Elites, and the Poor*, Farnham: Ashgate.

McKelvey, M. (1996) *Evolutionary Innovations: The Business of Biotechnology*, Oxford: Oxford University Press.

McKenna, C. (2006) *The World's Newest Profession: Management Consulting in the Twentieth Century*, Cambridge: Cambridge University Press.

McKeown, T. (1976) *The Modern Rise of Population*, London: Edward Arnold.

——(1976) *The Role of Medicine: Dream, Mirage or Nemesis?* London: Nuffield Trust.

Medawar, J. (2001) *Hitler's Gift: Scientists Who Fled Nazi Germany*, London: Piatkus, 2001.

Melosi, M. (2000) *The Sanitary City: Urban Infrastructure in America from Colonial Times to the Present*, Baltimore, MD: The Johns Hopkins University Press.

Messner, D. (2013) 'AZT and Drug Regulatory Reform in the Late Twentieth-Century US', in J.-P. Gaudillière and V. Hess (eds), *Ways of Regulating Drugs in the Nineteenth and Twentieth Centuries*, Houndmills, Basingstoke and New York: Palgrave Macmillan, 228–44.

Meyer-Thurow, G. (1982) 'The Industrialisation of Invention: A Case Study from the German Chemical Industry', *Isis*, 73: 363–81.

Michalik, K. (2006) 'The Development of the Discourse on Infanticide in the Late Eighteenth Century and the New Legal Standardization of the Offense in the Nineteenth Century', in U. Gleixner and M. W. Gray (eds), *Gender in Transition: Discourse and Practice in German-Speaking Europe, 1750–1830*, Ann Arbor: University of Michigan Press, 51–71.

Moberg, C. and Cohn, Z. (1990) *Launching the Antibiotic Era: Personal Accounts of the Discovery and Use of the First Antibiotics*, New York: Rockefeller University Press.

Mohan, J. (1995) *A National Health Service?: The Restructuring of Health Care in Britain since 1979*, New York: St. Martin's Press.

——(2002) *Planning, Markets and Hospitals*, London: Routledge.

Mohan, J. and Gorsky, M. (2001) *Don't Look Back? Voluntary and Charitable Finance of Hospital in Britain, Past and Present*, London: Office of Health Economics.

Mohr, J. C. (1993) *Doctors and the Law: Medical Jurisprudence in Nineteenth-Century America*, Baltimore, MD and London: The Johns Hopkins University Press.

Mold, A. (2010) 'Patient Groups and the Construction of the Patient-Consumer in Britain: An Historical Overview', *Journal of Social Policy*, 39, 4: 505–21.

——(2013) 'Repositioning the Patient: Patient Organisations, Consumerism and Autonomy in Britain during the 1960s and 1970s', *Bulletin of the History of Medicine*, 87: 225–49.

Mommsen, W. (ed.) (1981) *The Emergence of the Welfare State in Britain and Germany 1880–1950*, London: Croom Helm.

Moncrieff, J. (2009) *The Myth of the Chemical Cure: A Critique of Psychiatric Drug Treatment*, revised edn, Houndmills, Basingstoke and New York: Palgrave Macmillan.

Mooney, G. (2009) 'Diagnostic Spaces: Workhouse, Hospital and Home in Mid-Victorian London', *Social Science History*, 33: 357–90.

Moore, K. (1996) 'Organizing Integrity: American Science and the Creation of Public Interest Organizations', *American Journal of Sociology*, 101: 1592–1627.

Moorehead, C. (1998) *Dunant's Dream: War, Switzerland and the History of the Red Cross*, London: HarperCollins.

Moran, J. and Guerra, C. (2007) *Pill Pushers: A Big Pharma Battle for Market Share*, Charleston, SC: Booksurge.

Moran, R. (1981) *Knowing Right from Wrong: The Insanity Defense of Daniel McNaughtan*, New York: The Free Press.

——(1985) 'The Origin of Insanity as a Special Verdict: The Trial for Treason of James Hadfield (1800)', *Law and Society Review*, 19: 487–519.

Morgan, S., Lopert, R. and Greyson, D. (2008) 'Toward a Definition of Pharmaceutical Innovation', *Open Medicine*, 2: 4–7.

Morrell, D. (1998) 'Introduction and Overview', in I. Loudon, J. Horder and C. Webster (eds), *General Practice under the National Health Service, 1948–1997*, Oxford: Clarendon Press, 1–19.

Moscoso, J. (2012) *Pain: A Cultural History*, Basingstoke: Palgrave Macmillan.

Mukherjee, S. (2011) *The Emperor of All Maladies: A Biography of Cancer*, London: Fourth Estate.

Mulley, C. (2009) *The Woman Who Saved the Children: A Biography of Eglantyne Jebb*, London: Oneworld Publications.

Murray, J. (2007) *Origins of American Health Insurance: A History of Industrial Sickness Funds*, New Haven, CT: Yale University Press.

Needham, C. (2011) *Personalising Public Services: Understanding the Personalisation Narrative*, Bristol: Policy Press.

Newton, H. (2012) *The Sick Child in Early Modern England, 1580–1720*, Oxford: Oxford University Press.

Ngubane, H. (1992) 'The Predicament of the Sinister Healer', in S. Feierman and J. M. Janzen (eds), *The Social Basis of Health and Illness in Africa*, Berkeley: University of California Press.

Nilsson, R. and Sjöström, H. (1972) *Thalidomide and the Power of the Drug Companies*, Harmondsworth: Penguin.

Niquette, M. and Buxton, W. (2010) 'Relieving Twentieth-Century Excesses: The Socialization of Antacid and Laxative Uses through Advertising', in V. Quirke and

J. Slinn (eds), *Perspectives on Twentieth-Century Pharmaceuticals*, Oxford: Peter Lang, 257–81.

No author (1881) 'Birmingham Sewage Works: Discussion', *Proceedings of the Association of Municipal Sanitary Engineers and Surveyors: Volume VII, 1880–81*, London: E. & F. N. Spon, 89.

No author (1890) 'The "Hercules" Street-Cleansing Machine', *The Builder*, 58: 179.

No author (1891) 'A Modern Police Station', *Public Health (Supplement to the International Congress of Hygiene and Demography)*: 53.

No author (1974) 'Editorial', *South African Medical Journal*, 48: 45.

No author (1988) 'Editorial', *South African Health Review*, Durban: Health Systems Trust, 1.

No author (1997) 'Editorial', *South African Health Review*, Durban: Health Systems Trust, 1

Nottingham, C. and De Rooy, P. (2007) 'The Peculiarities of the Dutch: Social Security in the Netherlands', in S. King and J. Stewart (eds), *Welfare Peripheries*, Oxford: Peter Lang, 39–66.

Oberman, M. (2002) 'Understanding Infanticide in Context: Mothers Who Kill, 1870–1930 and Today', *Journal of Criminal Law and Criminology*, 92: 707–37.

——(2003) 'Mothers Who Kill: Cross-cultural Patterns in and Perspectives on Contemporary Maternal Filicide', *International Journal of Law and Psychiatry*, 26: 493–514.

O'Dowd, A. (2012) 'The "Self-Funding" NHS Patient: Thin End of the Wedge?', *British Medical Journal*, 345: e5128.

Ogle, M. (1996) *All the Modern Conveniences: American Household Plumbing, 1840–1890*, Baltimore, MD: The Johns Hopkins University Press.

Ogle, R. and Maier-Katkin, D. (1993) 'A Rationale for Infanticide Laws', *Criminal Law Review* (Dec.): 903–14.

O'Hara, G. (2007) *From Dreams to Disillusionment: Economic and Social Planning in 1960s Britain*, Basingstoke: Palgrave Macmillan.

——(2013) 'The Complexities of "Consumerism": Choice, Collectivism and Participation within Britain's National Health Service, c. 1961–c. 1979', *Social History of Medicine*, 26, 2: 12–13.

Oikonomou, H. and Spyridakis, M. (eds) (2012), *Anthropological and Sociological Perspectives on Health*, Athens: I. Sideris.

Omran, A. R. (2008[1971]) 'The Epidemiologic Transition: A Theory of the Epidemiology of Population Change', *Milbank Memorial Fund Quarterly*, 49, 1: 1–42.

Oosterhuis, H. (1999) 'Medical Science and the Modernisation of Sexuality', in F. X. Eder, L. A. Hall and G. Hekma (eds), *Sexual Cultures in Europe: National Histories*, Manchester: Manchester University Press, 221–41.

——(2000) *Stepchildren of Nature: Krafft-Ebing, Psychiatry, and the Making of Sexual Identity*, Chicago: University of Chicago Press.

Oosterhuis, H. and Loughnan, A. (eds) (2014) 'Historical Perspectives on Forensic Psychiatry', *International Journal of Law and Psychiatry*, 37: 1–134.

Oppenheimer, H. (1909) *The Criminal Responsibility of Lunatics: A Study in Comparative Law*, London: Sweet & Maxwell.

Oppenheimer, M. (2011) 'Beveridge in the Antipodes: The 1948 Tour', in M. Oppenheimer and N. Deakin (eds), *Beveridge and Voluntary Action in Britain and the Wider British World*, Manchester: Manchester University Press.

Orsenigo, L. (1989) *The Emergence of Biotechnology: Institutions and Markets in Industrial Innovation*, London: Pinter.

Oudshoorn, N. (1993) 'United We Stand: The Pharmaceutical Industry, Laboratory and Clinic in the Development of Sex Hormones into Scientific Drugs, 1920–1940', *Science, Technology and Human Values*, 18: 5–24.

Oudshoorn, N. and Pinch, T. (eds) (2003) *How Users Matter: The Co-construction of Users and Technologies*, Cambridge, MA and London: MIT Press.

Owen, D. (1964) *English Philanthropy 1660–1960*, Cambridge: Belknap Press.

Packard, R. M. (1989) *White Plague, Black Labor: Tuberculosis and the Political Economy of Health and Disease in South Africa*, Durban: University of Natal Press.

Palló, G. (2002) 'Make a Peak on the Plain: The Rockefeller Foundation's Szeged Project', in W. H. Schneider (ed.), *Rockefeller Philanthropy and Modern Medicine: International Initiatives from World War I to the Cold War*, Bloomington: Indiana University Press, 2002, 87–105.

Parascandola, J. (1981) 'The Theoretical Basis of Paul Ehrlich's Chemotherapy', *Journal of the History of Medicine*, 36: 19–43.

——(2008) *Sex, Sin and Science: A History of Syphilis in America*, Westport: Kreager.

Parkes, E. A. (1966) *A Manual of Practical Hygiene, Prepared Especially for Use in the Medical Service of the Army*, 2nd edn, London: John Churchill & Sons.

Pater, J. (1981) *The Making of the National Health Service*, London: King's Fund.

Patron, C. (1999) 'New Labour's Health Policy: The New Healthcare State', in Martin Powell (ed.), *New Labour, New Welfare State?* Bristol: Policy Press.

Patterson, J. (1987) *The Dread Disease: Cancer and Modern American Culture*, Harvard, MA and London: Harvard University Press.

Pelling, M. (2002) 'Public and Private Dilemmas: The College of Physicians in Early Modern London', in S. Sturdy (ed.), *Medicine, Health and the Public Sphere in Britain, 1600–2000*, London and New York: Routledge.

Petermann, L. (2007) 'From a Cough to a Coffin: The Child's Medical Encounter in England and France, 1762–1888', unpublished PhD thesis, University of Warwick.

Phillips, H. (2012) *Plague, Pox and Pandemics*, Auckland Park: Jacana.

Pick, D. (1989) *Faces of Degeneration: A European Disorder, c. 1848–c. 1918*, Cambridge: Cambridge University Press.

Pickstone, J. (ed.) (1993) *Medical Innovations in Historical Perspective*, Basingstoke: Macmillan.

Pieters, T. (2005) *Interferon: The Science and Selling of a Miracle Drug*, Abingdon and New York: Routledge.

Pieters, T. and Majerus, B. (2011) 'The Introduction of Chlorpromazine in Belgium and the Netherlands (1951–1968): Tango between Old and New Treatment Features', *Studies in History and Philosophy of Biological and Biomedical Science*, 42: 443–52.

Pisano, G. (2006) *Science Business: The Promise, the Reality, and the Future of Biotech*, Boston, MA: Harvard Business School Press.

Pohl, L. M. (2012) 'African American Southerners and White Physicians: Medical Care at the Turn of the Twentieth Century', *Bulletin of the History of Medicine*, 86: 178–205.

Porter, D. (ed.) (1994) *The History of Public Health and the Modern State*, Amsterdam: Rodopi.

——(1995) 'The Mission of Social History of Medicine: An Historical View', *Social History of Medicine*, 8, 345–59.

——(1999) *Health, Civilization and the State: A History of Public Health from Ancient to Modern Times*, London: Routledge.

Porter, D. and Porter, R. (1988) 'The Politics of Prevention: Anti-vaccinationism and Public Health in Nineteenth-Century England', *Medical History*, 32: 231–52.

Porter, R. (1985) 'The Patient's View: Doing Medical History from Below', *Theory and Society*, 14: 175–98.

——(1999) *The Greatest Benefit to Mankind: A Medical History of Humanity from Antiquity to the Present*, London: Fontana.

Porter, R. and Porter, D. (1989) *Patient's Progress: Doctors and Doctoring in Eighteenth-Century England*, Cambridge: Polity Press.

Power, S. (2002) *A Problem from Hell: America and the Age of Genocide*, New York: Basic Books.

Pretorius, E. (1999) 'Traditional Healers', *South African Health Review*, Durban: Health Systems Trust, 249–56.

Price, K. (2013) '"Where is the Fault?" The Starvation of Edward Cooper at the Isle of Wight Workhouse in 1877', *Social History of Medicine*, 26: 21–37.

Price, M. (1987) 'Health Care beyond Apartheid: Economic Issues in the Reorganisation of South Africa's Health Services', *Critical Health*, March.

Pringle, J. (1753) *Observations on the Diseases of the Army, in Camp and Garrison*, 2nd edn, London: A. Millar, D. Wilson and T. Durham, 1753.

Prior, P. M. (2008) *Madness and Murder: Gender, Crime and Mental Disorder in Nineteenth-Century Ireland*, Dublin: Irish Academic Press.

Promitzer, C. (2011) 'Typhus, Turks, and Roma: Hygiene and Ethnic Difference in Bulgaria, 1912–1944', in C. Promitzer, S. Trubeta and M. Turda (eds), *Health, Hygiene and Eugenics in Southeast Europe to 1945*, Budapest: CEU Press, 87–125.

Promitzer, C., Trubeta, S. and Turda M. (eds) (2011) *Health, Hygiene and Eugenics in Southeast Europe to 1945*, Budapest: CEU Press.

*Propositions and Resolutions of the Association of Medical Superintendents of American Institutions for the Insane* (Philadelphia: The Association, 1876), 20–21.

Protais, C. (2014) 'Psychiatric Care or Social Defense?: The Origins of a Controversy over the Responsibility of the Mentally Ill in French Forensic Psychiatry', *International Journal of Law and Psychiatry*, 37: 17–24.

Prüll, C.-R. (2003) 'Part of a Scientific Master Plan? Paul Ehrlich and the Origins of His Receptor Concept', *Medical History*, 47: 332–56.

——(2010) 'Scientists, Doctors and Drug Development: The History of Raymond P. Ahlquist's Receptor Theory, 1948–1988', in V. Quirke and J. Slinn (eds), *Perspectives on Twentieth-Century Pharmaceuticals*, Oxford: Peter Lang, 149–84.

Quirke, V. (2004) 'War and Change in the Pharmaceutical Industry: A Comparative Study of Britain and France in the Twentieth Century', in Sophie Chauveau (ed.), 'Industries du médicament et du vivant', *Enterprises et Histoire*, 36: 64–83.

——(2005) 'From Evidence to Market: Alfred Spinks's 1953 Survey of New Fields for Pharmacological Research, and the Origins of ICI's Cardiovascular Research Programme', in K. Loughlin and V. Berridge (eds), *Medicine, the Market and the Mass Media: Producing Health in the Twentieth Century*, London: Routledge, 146–71.

——(2005) 'Making *British* Cortisone: Glaxo and the Development of Corticosteroid Drugs in the UK in the 1950s and 1960s', *Studies in History and Philosophy of Biology and Biomedical Sciences*, 36: 645–74.

——(2006) 'Putting Theory into Practice: James Black, Receptor Theory, and the Development of the Beta-blockers at ICI', *Medical History*, 50: 69–92.

——(2008) *Collaboration in the Pharmaceutical Industry: Changing Relationships in Britain and France*, Abingdon and New York: Routledge.

——(ed.) (2008) 'Pharmaceutical Styles of Thinking and Doing: French and British Spheres of Influence in the Nineteenth and Early-Twentieth Centuries', *Pharmacy in History*, 52: 134–47.

——(2009) 'Anglo–American Relations and the Co-production of American "Hegemony" in Pharmaceuticals', in H. Bonin and F. de Goey (eds), *American Firms in Europe*, Geneva: Droz, 363–84.

——(2009) 'Standardizing R&D in the Second Half of the Twentieth Century: ICI's Nolvadex Development Programme in Historical and Comparative Perspective', in C. Bonah, C. Masutti, A. Ramusse and J. Simon (eds), *Harmonizing Drugs: Standards in Twentieth-Century Pharmaceutical History*, Paris: Eds Glyphe, 105–32.

——(2010) 'Foreign Influences, National Styles, and the Creation of a Modern Pharmaceutical Industry in Britain and France', in V. Quirke (ed.), 'Pharmaceutical Styles of Thinking and Doing: French and British Spheres of Influence in the Nineteenth and Early-Twentieth Centuries', *Pharmacy in History*, 52: 134–47.

——(2013) 'Thalidomide, Drug Safety Regulation and the British Pharmaceutical Industry: The Case of Imperial Chemical Industries', in J.-P. Gaudillière and V. Hess (eds), *Ways of Regulating Drugs in the Nineteenth and Twentieth Centuries*, Houndmills, Basingstoke and New York: Palgrave Macmillan, 151–180.

——(forthcoming) 'Targeting the American Market for Medicines: ICI and Rhône-Poulenc Compared, *c*. 1950s–1970s', *The Bulletin for the History of Medicine*.

Quirke, V. and Gaudillière, J.-P. (2008) 'The Era of Biomedicine: Science, Medicine and Health in Britain and France, ca 1945–65', in V. Quirke and J.-P. Gaudillière (eds), special issue of *Medical History*, 52: 441–52.

Quirke, V. and Slinn, J. (eds) (2010) *Perspectives on Twentieth-Century Pharmaceuticals*, Oxford: Peter Lang.

Rafter, N. (2004) 'The Unrepentant Horse-slasher: Moral Insanity and the Origins of Criminological Thought', *Criminology*, 42: 979–1008.

——(2005) 'The Murderous Dutch Fiddler: Criminology, History and the Problem of Phrenology', *Theoretical Criminology*, 9: 65–96.

Rama, P. and McLeod, H. (2001) *An Historical Study of Trends in Medical Schemes in South Africa: 1974–1999*, Cape Town: Centre for Actuarial Research, University of Cape Town.

Râmneanţu, P. (1945) 'Fundaţia Rockefeller', *Buletin eugenic şi biopolitic*, 16, 1–12: 120–43.

Ramsey, M. (1994) 'Public Health in France', in D. Porter (ed.), *The History of Public Health and the Modern State*, Amsterdam: Rodopi, 95–98.

Rasmussen, N. (2002) 'Steroids in Arms: Science, Government, Industry and the Hormones of the Adrenal Cortex in the United States, 1930–1950', *Medical History*, 46: 299–324.

——(2004) 'The Moral Economy of the Drug Company–Medical Scientist Collaboration in Interwar America', *Social Studies of Science*, 34: 161–85.

——(2008) *On Speed: The Many Lives of Amphetamine*, New York and London: New York University Press.

Rawcliffe, C. (2013) *Urban Bodies: Communal Health in Late Medieval English Towns and Cities*, Woodbridge: Boydell & Brewer.

Ray, I. (1839) *Treatise on the Medical Jurisprudence of Insanity*, London: G. Henderson.

Reader, W. (1975) *Imperial Chemical Industries: A History, Volume 2: The First Quarter-Century, 1926–52*, London: Oxford University Press.

Redmayne, M. (2001) *Expert Evidence and Criminal Justice*. Oxford: Oxford University Press.

Regidor, E., Pascual, C., Martínez, D., Calle, M. E., Ortega, P. and Astasio, P. (2001) 'The Role of Political and Welfare State Characteristics in Infant Mortality: A Comparative Study in Wealthy Countries since the Late Nineteenth Century', *International Journal of Epidemiology*, 40, 5: 1187–95.

Reinisch, J. (2008) '"We Shall Rebuild Anew a Powerful Nation": UNRRA, Internationalism and National Reconstruction in Poland', *Journal of Contemporary History*, 43: 451–476.

——(2013) 'Auntie UNRRA at the Crossroads', in R. Mitter and M. Hilton (eds), 'Transnationalism and Contemporary Global History', *Past and Present Supplement*, 218, 8: 70–97.

Renner, A. and Kreuder-Sonnen, K. (2013) focuses on 'Öffentliche Hygiene in Osteuropa/Public Hygiene in Eastern Europe', *Jahrbücher für Geschichte Osteuropas*, 61, 4.

Reverby, S. M. (2009) *Examining Tuskegee: The Infamous Syphilis Study and Its Legacy*, Chapel Hill: University of North Carolina Press.

Reynolds, S. (1909) *A Poor Man's House*, London: John Lane.

Richardson, B. W. (1876) 'Address on Health', *Transactions of the National Association for the Promotion of Social Science: 1875*, Longmans, Green, & Co.: London, 100–20.

Richardson, H. (ed.) (1998) *English Hospitals, 1660–1948: A Study of Their Architecture and Design*, Swindon: Royal Commission on the Historical Monuments of England.

Richardson, R. (1988) *Death, Dissection and the Destitute*, London: Routledge.

Richter, J. S. (1998) 'Infanticide, Child Abandonment, and Abortion in Imperial Germany', *Journal of Interdisciplinary History*, 28: 511–51.

Riedl, R. (1990) 'A Brief History of the Pharmaceutical Industry in Basel', in J. Liebenau, G. Higby and E. Stroud (eds), *Pill Peddlers: Essays on the History of the Pharmaceutical Industry*, Madison, WI: American Institute of the History of Pharmacy, 49–72.

Rivett, G. (1997) *From Cradle to Grave: Fifty Years of the NHS*, London: King's Fund.

Roberts, G. (1997) 'Dealing with Issues at the Academic–Industry Interface in Interwar Britain: UCL and ICI', *Science and Public Policy*, 24: 29–35.

Roberts, R. (1976) *A Ragged Schooling: Growing up in the Classic Slum*, Manchester: Mandolin.

Rodger, R. (1995) *Housing in Urban Britain, 1780–1914*, Cambridge: Cambridge University Press.

Rodwin, M. (2011) *Conflicts of Interest and the Future of Medicine: The United States, France, and Japan*, Oxford and New York: Oxford University Press.

Roemer, M. (ed.) (1960), *Henry E. Sigerist on the Sociology of Medicine*, New York: MD Publications.

Rose, W. and Carless, A. (1902) *A Manual of Surgery for Students and Practitioners*, 5th edn, New York: William Wood & Company.

Rosen, G. (1993) *A History of Public Health*, Baltimore, MD: The Johns Hopkins University Press.

Rosenbaum, S. and Burke, T. (2003) 'Lawrence v. Texas: Implications for Public Health Policy and Practice', *Public Health Reports*, 118: 559–61.

Rosenberg, C. E. (1977) 'The Therapeutic Revolution: Medicine, Meaning and Social Change in Nineteenth-Century America', *Perspectives in Biology and Medicine*, 20: 485–506.

——(1978) 'Social Class and Medical Care in Nineteenth-Century America: The Rise and Fall of the Dispensary', in J. W. Leavitt and R. L. Numbers (eds), *Sickness and Health in America: Readings in the History of Medicine and Public Health*, Madison: University of Wisconsin Press, 157–71.

Rosental, P.-A. (2011) 'Migrations, souveraineté, droits sociaux. Protéger et expulser les étrangers en Europe du 19e siècle à nos jours', *Annales HSS*, 66: 335–73.

Ross, J. S., Hill, K., Egilman, D. and Krumholz, H. (2008) 'Guest Authorship and Ghostwriting in Publications Related to Rofecoxib: A Case Study of Industry Documents from Rofecoxib Litigation', *Journal of the American Medical Association*, 299: 1800–12.

Ruffat, M. (1996) *175 Ans d'industrie pharmaceutique française: Histoire de Synhélabo*, Paris: La Découverte.

Ryan, C. S. and Sandes, J. (1897) *Under the Red Crescent. Adventures of an English Surgeon with the Turkish Army at Plevna and Erzeroum, 1877–1878*, New York: Charles Scribner's Sons.

Saives, A.-L., Ebrahimi, M. and Desmarteau, R. H. with Garnier, C. (2010) 'Knowledge Creation Dynamics and the Growth of Biotech Firms in Quebec', in V. Quirke and J. Slinn (eds), *Perspectives on Twentieth-Century Pharmaceuticals*, Oxford: Peter Lang, 435–66.

Santesmases, M. J. (2010) 'Distributing Penicillin: The Clinic, the Hero and Industrial Production in Spain, 1943–1952', in V. Quirke and J. Slinn (eds), *Perspectives on Twentieth-Century Pharmaceuticals*, Oxford: Peter Lang, 90–117.

Savitt, T. (2007) *Race and Medicine in Nineteenth- and Early-Twentieth-Century America*, Kent, OH: Kent State University Press.

Savoja, V., Godet, P. F. and Dubuis, J. (2008–9) 'Compulsory Treatments in France', *International Journal of Mental Health*, 37: 17–32.

Schneider, W. H. (2003) 'The Model American Foundation Officer: Alan Gregg and the Rockefeller Foundation Medical Divisions', *Minerva*, 41: 155–66.

Schroeder-Gudehus, B. (1978) *Les scientifiques et la paix*, Montreal: Presses de l'Université de Montreal.

Schwartz, L. L. and Isser, N. K. (2007) *Child Homicide: Parents Who Kill*, Boca Raton, FL: CRC Press.

Schwartzman, D. (1976) *Innovation in the Pharmaceutical Industry*, Baltimore, MD: The Johns Hopkins University Press.

Sechel, D. T. (ed.) (2011) *Medicine within and between the Habsburg and Ottoman Empires, Eighteenth–Nineteenth Centuries*, Bochum: Winkler Verlag.

——(2013) 'Networks of Medical Knowledge in Central and Eastern Europe', *East-Central Europe,* 40, 1.

——(2013) 'The Politics of Medical Translations and Its Impact upon Medical Knowledge in the Habsburg Monarchy, 1770–1830', *East Central Europe*, 40, 3: 296–318.

Sennett, R. (1994) *Flesh and Stone: The Body and the City in Western Civilization*, London: Faber & Faber.

Shapin, S. (1992) 'Discipline and Bounding', *History of Science*, 30: 33–69.

Shapiro, A. L. (1985) *Housing the Poor of Paris, 1850–1902*, Madison: University of Wisconsin Press.

Shapiro, J. (2010) 'The NHS: The Story So Far', *Clinical Medicine*, 10, 3: 336–8.

Shapiro, K. (1987) 'Doctors or Medical Aids – The Debate over the Training of Black Medical Personnel for the Black Rural Population in South Africa in the 1920s and 1930s', *Journal of Southern African Studies*, 13: 234–55.

Shaw, E. (2007) *Losing Labour's Soul?: New Labour and the Blair Government 1997–2007*, London: Routledge.

Sheard, S. and Gorsky, M. (eds) (2007) *Financing Medicine: The British Experience since 1750*, London: Routledge.

Shelton, J. L. E., Muirhead, Y. and Canning, K. E. (2010) 'Ambivalence toward Mothers Who Kill: An Examination of 45 US Cases of Maternal Neonaticide', *Behavioral Sciences and the Law*, 28: 812–31.

Shinn, T. (1980) 'The Triple Helix and the New Production of Knowledge', *Social Science Information*, 19: 607–40.

Siddiqi, J. (1995) *World Health and World Politics: The World Health Organisation and the UN System*, London: Hurst.

Siena, K. (2004) *Venereal Disease, Hospitals and the Urban Poor: London's Foul Wards 1600–1800*, Rochester: University of Rochester Press.

Sigerist, H. E. (1939) 'Yugoslavia and the Eleventh International Congress of the History of Medicine', *Bulletin of the History of Medicine*, 7: 99–147.

——(1940) 'The Social History of Medicine', *The Western Journal of Surgery, Obstetrics and Gynaecology*, 48: 715–22.

Silverstein, A. (2002) *Paul Ehrlich's Receptor Immunology: The Magnificent Obsession*, San Diego and London: Academic Press.

Simon, J. and Hüntelmann, A. (2010) 'Two Models of Production and Regulation: The Diphtheria Serum in Germany and France', in V. Quirke and J. Slinn (eds), *Perspectives on Twentieth-Century Pharmaceuticals*, Oxford: Peter Lang, 37–61.

Sinding, C. (2002) 'Making the Unit of Insulin: Standards, Clinical Work, and Industry, 1920–1925', *Bulletin of the History of Medicine*, 76: 231–70.

Sismondo, S. (2009) 'Ghosts in the Machine: Publication Planning in the Medical Sciences', *Social Studies of Science*, 39: 171–98.

Slack, P. (1985) *The Impact of Plague in Tudor and Stuart England*, Oxford: Clarendon Press.

Slater, L. (2000) 'Industry and Academy: The Synthesis of Steroids', *Historical Studies in the Physical and Biological Sciences*, 30: 443–79.

Slinn, J. (1984) *A History of May & Baker, 1834–1984*, Cambridge: Hobsons.

——(1996) 'Research and Development in the UK Pharmaceutical Industry from the Nineteenth Century to the 1960s', in M. Teich and R. Porter (eds), *Drugs and Narcotics in History*, Cambridge: Cambridge University Press, 168–86.

Sloan, F. and Hsieh, C.-R. (eds) (2007), *Pharmaceutical Innovation: Incentives, Competition, and Cost-Benefit Analysis in International Perspective*, Cambridge: Cambridge University Press.

Smith, G., Bartlett, A. and King, M. (2004) 'Treatments of Homosexuality in Britain since the 1950s – an Oral History: The Experience of Patients', *British Medical Journal*, 328: 427–31.

Smith, R. (1981) *Trial by Medicine: Insanity and Responsibility in Victorian Trials*, Edinburgh: Edinburgh University Press.

Smith, T. (2003) *Creating the Welfare State in France, 1880–1940*, Montreal: McGill-Queen's University Press.

Smith, V. (2007) *Clean: A History of Personal Hygiene and Purity*, Oxford: Oxford University Press.

Sneader, W. (1985) *Drug Discovery: The Evolution of Modern Medicines*, Chichester: John Wiley & Sons.

Solomon, S. (2000) 'Through a Glass Darkly: The Rockefeller Foundation's International Health Board and Soviet Public Health', *Studies in the History and Philosophy of the Biomedical Sciences*, 31: 409–18.

Solomon, S. G., Murard, L. and Zylberman, P. (eds) (2008), *Shifting Boundaries of Public Health: Europe in the Twentieth Century*, Rochester, NY: University of Rochester Press.

Soper, G. A. (1909) *Modern Methods of Street Cleaning*, New York: The Engineering News Publishing Company.

Sparr, L. F. (2009) 'Personality Disorders and Criminal Law: An International Perspective', *Journal of the American Academy of Psychiatry and Law*, 37: 168–81.

Spitzer, R. L. (1981) 'The Diagnostic Status of Homosexuality in DSM-III: A Reformulation of the Issues', *American Journal of Psychiatry*, 138: 210–15.

Spree, R. (1988) *Health and Social Class in Imperial Germany: A Social History of Mortality, Morbidity and Inequality*, Oxford: Berg.

Štampar, A. (1938) *Public Health in Jugoslavia*, London: School of Slavonic and East European Studies.

Star, S. and Griesemer, J. (1989) 'Institutional Ecology, "Translations", and Boundary Objects: Amateurs and Professionals in Berkeley's Museum of Vertebrate Zoology, 1907–1939', *Social Studies of Science*, 19: 387–420.

Starr, P. (1982) *The Social Transformation of American Medicine: The Rise of a Sovereign Profession and the Making of a Vast Industry*, New York: Basic Books.

Steadman, H. J., Redlich, A. D., Griffin, P., Petrila, J. and Monahan, J. (2005) 'From Referral to Disposition: Case Processing in Seven Mental Health Courts', *Behavioral Sciences and the Law*, 23: 215–26.

Steffen, K. (2013) 'Experts and the Modernization of the Nation: The Arena of Public Health in Poland in the First Half of the Twentieth Century', *Jahrbücher für Geschichte Osteuropas*, 61, 4: 574–90.

Stevens, A. (2004) 'The Enactment of Bay-Dohle', *Journal of Technology Transfer*, 29: 93–9.

Stevens, M. (2013) *Broadmoor Revealed: Victorian Crime and the Lunatic Asylum*, Barnsley: Pen & Sword Social History.

Stevens, R. (1999) *In Sickness and in Wealth: American Hospitals in the Twentieth Century*, Baltimore, MD: The Johns Hopkins University Press.

Stevenson, J. and Cook, C. (2013) *The Slump: Britain in the Great Depression*, 3rd edn, Abingdon: Pearson Education.

Stewart, J. (1999) *The Battle for Health: A Political History of the Socialist Medical Association, 1930–51*, Aldershot: Ashgate.

——(2008) 'The Political Economy of the British National Health Service, 1945–1975: Opportunities and Constraints?', *Medical History*, 52, 4: 453–70.

Stewart, J. and Bryder, L. (forthcoming) '"Some Abstract Socialistic Ideal or Principle": British Reactions to New Zealand's 1938 Social Security Act', *Historical Research*.

Steyn, L. 'Measuring the Waves of Migration', *Mail & Guardian Business*, 11–17 January 2013.

Sturdy, S. (1993) 'Medical Chemistry and Clinical Medicine: Academics and the Scientisation of Medical Practice in Britain, 1900–1925', in I. Löwy (ed.), *Medicine and*

*Change: Historical and Sociological Studies of Medical Innovation*, Montrouge: John Libbey Eurotext, and Paris: INSERM, 371–93.

——(ed.) (2002) *Medicine, Health and the Public Sphere in Britain, 1600–2000*, London and New York: Routledge.

——(2011) 'Looking for Trouble: Medical Science and Clinical Practice in the Historiography of Modern Medicine', *Social History of Medicine*, 24: 739–57.

Sturdy, S., Freeman, R. and Smith-Merry, J. (2013) 'Making Knowledge for International Policy: WHO Europe and Mental Health Policy, 1970–2008', *Social History of Medicine*, 26, 3: 532–54.

Svobodný, P. and Hlaváčková, L. (2004) *Dějiny lékařství v českých zemích*, Prague: Triton.

Swann, J. (1988) *Academic Scientists and the Pharmaceutical Industry: Cooperative Research in Twentieth-Century America*, Baltimore, MD: The Johns Hopkins University Press.

——(2005) 'Pharmaceutical Regulation before and after the Food and Drug Cosmetic Act', in I. R. Berry (ed.), *The Pharmaceutical Regulatory Process*, New York: Marcel Dekker, 1–46.

Swanson, M. W. (1977) 'The Sanitation Syndrome: Bubonic Plague and Urban Native Policy in the Cape Colony, 1900–1909', *Journal of African History*, 18: 387–410.

Swart, H. 'Class Action for Silicosis Payout Tarnishes Gold Industry', Mail & Guardian, 26–31 January 2013.

Swazey, J. (1974) *Chlorpromazine in Psychiatry: A Study of Therapeutic Innovation*, Cambridge, MA: MIT Press.

Symonds, R. and Carder, M. (1973) *The United Nations and the Population Question 1945–1970*, London: Chatto & Windus for Sussex University Press.

Szpilfogel, S. A. (1984) 'Adrenalcortical Steroids and Their Synthetic Analogues', in M. J. Parnham and J. Bruinvels (eds), *Discoveries in Pharmacology*, Vol. 2, Amsterdam: Elsevier, 253–84.

Tabili, L. (2011) *Global Migrants, Local Culture: Narratives and Newcomers in Provincial England 1840–1939*, Basingstoke: Palgrave Macmillan.

Tanner, A. (2007) 'Choice and the Children's Hospital: Great Ormond Street Hospital Patients and Their Families, 1855–1900', in A. Borsay and P. Shapely (eds), *Medicine, Charity and Mutual Aid: The Consumption of Health and Welfare in Britain, c. 1550–1950*, Aldershot: Ashgate, 135–161.

Tansey, E. M. (Tilli) (1988) '"They Used to Call it Psychiatry": Aspects of the Development and Impact of Psychopharmacology', in M. Gijswijt-Hofstra and R. Porter (eds), *Cultures of Psychiatry and Mental Health Care in Postwar Britain and the Netherlands*, Amsterdam: Rodopi, 79–101.

Tansey, E. M. (Tilli) and Lois Reynolds (eds), (2000) *Wellcome Witnesses to Twentieth Century Medicine: Volume 6, Post Penicillin Antibiotics: From Acceptance to Resistance?* London: Wellcome Trust.

Taylor, C. (2007) *A Secular Age*, Cambridge, MA: Belknap Press.

Taylor, M. L. (1993) '"My Work Came out of Agony and Grief": Mothers and the Making of the Sheppard-Towner Act', in S. Koven and S. Michel (eds), *Mothers of a New World: Maternalist Policies and the Origins of Welfare States*, New York and London: Routledge, 321–42.

Teich, M. and Porter, R. (eds) (1996) *Drugs and Narcotics in History*, Cambridge: Cambridge University Press.

Terreblanche, S. (2002) *A History of Inequality in South Africa 1652–2002*, Pietermaritzburg: University of Natal Press.

Terry, J. (1999) *An American Obsession: Science, Medicine, and Homosexuality in Modern Society*, Chicago: University of Chicago Press.

Thackray, A. (ed.) (1998) *Private Science: Biotechnology and the Rise of the Molecular Sciences*, Philadelphia: University of Pennsylvania Press.

Theodoru, V. and Karakatsani, D. (2008) 'Health Policy in Interwar Greece: The Intervention by the League of Nations Health Organisations', *Dynamis*, 28: 53–75.

Thompson, J. D. and Goldin, G. (1975) *The Hospital: A Social and Architectural History*, New Haven, CT: Yale University Press.

Thorne, B. (2011) 'Assimilation, Invisibility, and the Eugenic Turn in the "Gypsy Question" in Romanian Society, 1938–1942', *Romani Studies*, 21, 2: 177–205.

Timmins, N. (2001) *The Five Giants: A Biography of the Welfare State*, new edn, London: HarperCollins.

——'How New Labour Succeeded with NHS Policy', *The Financial Times*, 13 March 2010.

Tinková, D. (2005) 'Protéger ou punir? Les voies de la décriminalisation de l'infanticide en France et dans le domaine des Habsbourg (XVIIIe–XIXe siècles)', *Crime, History & Societies*, 9: 43–72.

Titmuss, R. M. (1950) *Problems of Social Policy*, London: HMSO, 1950.

——(1963) *Essays on 'The Welfare State'*, London: Unwin University Books.

Tobbell, D. (2008) 'Allied against Reform: Pharmaceutical Industry–Academic Physician Relations in the United States, 1945–1970', *Bulletin of the History of Medicine*, 82: 878–912.

——(2010). 'Charitable Innovations: The Political Economy of Thalassemia Research and Drug Development in the United States, 1960–2000', in V. Quirke and J. Slinn (eds), *Perspectives on Twentieth-Century Pharmaceuticals*, Oxford: Peter Lang, 302–37.

Tomes, N. (1998) *The Gospel of Germs: Men, Women and the Microbe in American Life*, Cambridge, MA: Harvard University Press.

Tomkins, A. (2008) '"The Excellent Examples of the Working Class": Medical Welfare, Contributory Funding and the North Staffordshire Infirmary from 1815', *Social History of Medicine*, 21: 13–30.

Tone, A. (2007) 'Tranquilizers on Trial: Psychopharmacology in the Age of Anxiety', in A. Tone and E. S. Watkins (eds), *Medicating Modern America: Prescription Drugs in History*, New York and London: New York University Press, 156–79.

——(2009) *The Age of Anxiety: A History of America's Turbulent Affair with Tranquilizers*, New York: Basic Books.

Toole, C. J. (2012) 'Medical Diagnosis of Legal Culpability: The Impact of Early Psychiatric Testimony in the Nineteenth Century English Criminal Trial', *International Journal of Law and Psychiatry*, 35: 82–7.

Trubeta, S. (2013) *Physical Anthropology, Race and Eugenics in Greece 1880s–1970s*, Leiden: Brill.

Turda, M. (2008) *Eugenism şi antropologie rasială în România*, Bucharest: Cuvântul.

——(2008) 'Focus on Social History of Medicine in Central and Eastern Europe', *Social History of Medicine*, 21, 2: 395–401.

——(2010) 'Focus on Austria and Germany', *Social History of Medicine* 23, 2: 408–12.

——(2011) 'Controlling the National Body: Ideas of Racial Purification in Romania, 1918–1944', in C. Promitzer, S. Trubeta and M. Turda (eds), *Health, Hygiene and Eugenics in Southeastern Europe* (Budapest: Central European University Press), 325–50.

——(2011) 'History of Medicine in Eastern Europe, Including Russia', in M. Jackson (ed.), *The Oxford Handbook of the History of Medicine*, Oxford: Oxford University Press, 208–24.

——(ed.) (2012) 'Private and Public Medical Traditions in Greece and the Balkans', *Deltos: Journal of the History of Hellenic Medicine*, 33–6.

——(2013) 'Crafting a Healthy Nation: European Eugenics in Historical Context', in Marius Turda (ed.), *Crafting Humans: From Genesis and Genetics and Beyond*, Göttingen: V&R Unipress, 109–26.

——(2013) 'In Pursuit of Greater Hungary: Eugenic Ideas of Social and Biological Improvement, 1940–1941', *The Journal of Modern History*, 85, 3: 558–91.

——(2014) *Eugenics and Nation in Early Twentieth Century Hungary*, Basingstoke: Palgrave Macmillan.

——(forthcoming, 2015) *The History of Eugenics in East Central Europe, 1900–1945: Sources and Commentaries*, Bloomsbury.

Turda, M. and Weindling, P. J. (eds) (2007) *Eugenics and Racial Nationalism in Central and Southeast Europe, 1900–1940*, Budapest: CEU Press.

Turda, M. and King, S. (2011) 'Journeying Across Empires: An Agenda for Future Research in Central and Southeastern European History of Medicine', in T. D. Sechel (ed.), *Medicine within and between the Habsburg and Ottoman Empires, Eighteenth–Nineteenth Centuries*, Bochum: Winkler, 235–42.

Turkowska, J. A. (2013) 'Im Namen der "großen Kolonisationsaufgaben": Das Hygiene Institut in Posen (1899–1920) und die preußische Hegemonialpolitik in der Ostmark', *Jahrbücher für Geschichte Osteuropas*, 61, 4: 552–73.

Tweedale, G. (1990) *At the Sign of the Plough: 275 Years of Allen & Hanburys and the British Pharmaceutical Industry, 1715–1990*, London: Murray.

van Leeuwen, M. (1994) 'Logic of Charity: Poor Relief in Pre-industrial Europe', *Journal of Interdisciplinary History*, 24: 589–613.

Vernon, J. (2007) *Hunger: A Modern History*, Cambridge, Mass.: Harvard University Press.

Versteeg, M. (2011) 'The State of the Right to Health in Rural South Africa', *South African Health Review*, Durban: Health Systems Trust: Durban, 100–6.

Veyne, P. (ed.) (1992) *A History of Private Life: From Pagan Rome to Byzantium*, Cambridge, MA: Harvard University Press.

Vigarello, G. (1988) *Concepts of Cleanliness: Changing Attitudes in France since the Middle Ages*, Cambridge: Cambridge University Press.

Vogel, M. J. (1996) 'The Transformation of the American Hospital', in Norbert Finzsch and Robert Jütte (eds), *Institutions of Confinement: Hospitals, Asylums and Prisons in Western Europe and North America, 1500–1950*, Cambridge: Cambridge University Press.

von Krafft-Ebing, R. (1965) *Psychopathia Sexualis, with Especial Reference to the Anti-pathetic Sexual Instinct: A Medico-forensic Study*, 12th edn, London: Staples Press.

Waksman, S. (1964) *The Conquest of Tuberculosis*, London: Cambridge University Press.

Walker, N. (1968) *Crime and Insanity in England, Vol. 1: The Historical Perspective*, Edinburgh: Edinburgh University Press.

Waller, R. D. (2003) 'Witchcraft and Colonial Law in Kenya', *Past and Present*, 180: 241–76.

Ward, T (1999) 'The Sad Subject of Infanticide: Law, Medicine and Child Murder, 1860–1938', *Social & Legal Studies*, 8: 163–80.

Warsh, C. K. (2010) *Prescribed Norms: Women and Health in Canada and the United States since 1800*, Toronto: Toronto University Press.

Warsh, C. K. and Strong-Boag, V. (eds) (2005) *Children's Health Issues in Historical Perspective*, Waterloo, ON: Wilfrid Laurier University Press.

Watkin, B. (1978) *The National Health Service: The First Phase, 1948–1974 and after*, London: Allen and Unwin, 1978.

Watkins, E. (1998) *On the Pill: A Social History of Contraceptives, 1950–1970*, Baltimore, MD: The Johns Hopkins University Press, 1998.

Watson, K. D. (2011) *Forensic Medicine in Western Society: A History*, Abingdon: Routledge.

Webster, C. (1979) *Health, Medicine, and Mortality in the Sixteenth Century*, Cambridge: Cambridge University Press.

——(1982) 'Healthy or Hungry Thirties?', *History Workshop Journal*, 13: 110–29.

——(1988) *Problems of Health Care: The National Health Service before 1957*, London: HMSO.

——(1988) *The health services since the war; Vol.1, Problems of health care: the national health service before 1957*, London: HMSO.

——(1996) *The Health Services since the War, Vol. 2, Government and Health Care: The National Health Service 1958–1979*, London: TSO.

——(2002) *The National Health Service: A Political History*, Oxford: Oxford University Press.

——(2008) *Paracelsus: Medicine, Magic, and Mission at the End of Time*, New Haven, NJ: Yale University Press.

Weiden, D. L. 'Comparing Judicial Institutions: Using an Inquisitorial Trial Simulation to Facilitate Student Understanding of International Legal Traditions', *PS: Political Science and Politics*, 42 (2009): 759–63.

Weindling, P. J. (1989) *Health, Race and German Politics between National Unification and Nazism*, Cambridge: Cambridge University Press.

——(1992) 'Children's Hospitals and Diphtheria Wards in *fin de siècle* Paris, London and Berlin', in Roger Cooter (ed.), *In the Name of the Child*, London and New York: Routledge, 124–45.

——(1992) 'From Infectious to Chronic Diseases: Changing Patterns of Sickness in the Nineteenth and Twentieth Centuries', in A. Wear (ed.), *Medicine in Society*, Cambridge: Cambridge University Press, 303–16.

——(1992) 'From Medical Research to Clinical Practice: Serum Therapy for Diphtheria in the 1890s', in J. Pickstone (ed.), *Medical Innovations in Historical Perspective*, London and Basingstoke: Macmillan, 72–83.

——(1992) 'Scientific Elites and Laboratory Organization in *fin de siècle* Paris and Berlin: The Pasteur Institute and Robert Koch's Institute for Infectious Diseases Compared', in A. Cunningham and P. Williams (eds), *The Laboratory Revolution in Medicine*, Cambridge: Cambridge University Press, 170–88.

——(1993) 'The Politics of International Co-ordination to Combat Sexually Transmitted Diseases, 1900–1980s', in V. Berridge and P. Strong (eds), *AIDS and Contemporary History*, Cambridge: Cambridge University Press, 93–107.

——(1993) 'Public Health and Political Stabilisation: Rockefeller Funding in Interwar Central/Eastern Europe', *Minerva*, 31: 253–67.

——(ed.) (1995) *International Health Organisations and Movements 1918–1939*, Cambridge: Cambridge University Press.

——(ed.) (1995), 'Social Medicine at the League of Nations Health Organisation and International Labour Office Compared', *International Health Organisations*, Cambridge: Cambridge University Press, 134–53.

——(2000) *Epidemics and Genocide in Eastern Europe, 1890–1945*, Oxford: Oxford University Press.

——(2002) 'From Moral Exhortation to Socialised Primary Care: The New Public Health and the Healthy Life, 1918–45', in E. Rodriguez Ocana (ed.), *The Politics of the Healthy Life: An International Perspective*, Sheffield: European Association for the History of Medicine and Health, 113–30.

——(2009) 'A City Regenerated: Eugenics, Race and Welfare in Interwar Vienna', in D. Holmes and L. Silverman (eds), *Interwar Vienna: Culture between Tradition and Modernity*, Rochester, NY: Camden House, 81–113.

——(2010) *John W. Thompson, Psychiatrist in the Shadow of the Holocaust*, Rochester, NY: Rochester University Press.

——(2012) 'From Disease Prevention to Population Control: The Realignment of Rockefeller Foundation Policies 1920s–1950s', in H. Rausch and J. Krige (eds), *American Foundations and the Coproduction of World Order in the Twentieth Century*, Göttingen: Vandenhoeck & Ruprecht, 125–45.

——(2014) *Victims and Survivors of Nazi Human Experiments: Science and Suffering in the Holocaust*, London: Bloomsbury.

Weintraub, J. A. and Kumar, K. (eds) (1997) *Public and Private in Thought and Practice: Perspectives on a Grand Dichotomy*, Chicago: Chicago University Press.

Weissmann, B. M. (1974) *Herbert Hoover and Famine Relief to Soviet Russia 1921–23*, Stanford, CA: Hoover Press.

Weiss-Wendt, A. and Yeomans, R. (eds) (2013) *Racial Science in Hitler's New Europe, 1938–1945*, Lincoln: University of Nebraska Press.

Weisz, G. (2014) *Chronic Disease in the Twentieth Century*, Baltimore: The Johns Hopkins University Press.

Wells, N. E. J. (1983) *Pharmaceutical Innovation: Recent Trends, Future Prospects*, London: Office of Health Economics.

Whipple, A. C. (2010) '"Into Every Home, into Every Body": Organicism and Anti-statism in the British Anti-fluoridation Movement, 1952–1960', *Twentieth Century British History*, 21, 3: 330–49.

White, P. D. (1920) 'Public Health in Eastern Macedonia', *American Journal of Public Health*, 19, 1: 14.

White, S. (1985) 'The Insanity Defense in England and Wales Since 1843', *Annals of the American Academy of Political and Social Science*, 477: 43–57.

Wilde, S. (2009) 'Truth, Trust, and Confidence in Surgery, 1890–1910: Patient Autonomy, Communication and Consent', *Bulletin of the History of Medicine*, 83: 302–30.

Wilkinson, L. (1997) 'Sir Austin Bradford Hill: Medical Statistics and the Quantitative Approach to Disease', *Addiction*, 92: 657–66.

Williams, M. T. (1991) *Washing 'the Great Unwashed': Public Baths in Urban America, 1840–1920*, Columbus: Ohio State University Press.

Williamson, J. G. (1990) *Coping with City Growth during the British Industrial Revolution*, Cambridge: Cambridge University Press.

Wilson, L. G. (1993) 'Fevers', in W. F. Bynum and R. Porter (eds), *Companion Encyclopaedia of the History of Medicine*, London: Routledge, 382–411.

World Health Organization (1958) *The First Ten Years of the World Health Organization*, Geneva: WHO.

——(1968) *The Second Ten Years of the World Health Organization 1958–1967*, Geneva: WHO.

——(1988) *Four Decades of Achievement: Highlights of the Work of the WHO* (1988) Geneva: WHO.

Wreford, J. (2010) 'Loosening the Bonds of Historical Prejudice: Traditional Practitioners as Agents of Reconciliation and Change in Contemporary South Africa', in A. Digby, W. Ernst and P. Mukharji (eds), *Crossing Colonial Historiographies: Histories of Colonial and Indigenous Medicines in Transnational Perspective*, Newcastle upon Tyne: Cambridge Scholars Publishing, 220–42.

Wulf, S. (1994) *Das Hamburger Tropeninstitut 1919 bis 1945. Auswärtige Kulturpolitik und Kolonialrevisionismus nach Versailles*, Berlin: Dietrich Reimer Verlag.

Yasigawa, Y. (1980) 'Early History of Antibiotics in Japan', in J. Parascandola (ed.), *The History of Antibiotics: A Symposium*, Madison, WI: American Institute of the History of Pharmacy, 69–90.

Yoshioka, A. (1998) 'Use of Randomisation in the Medical Research Council's Clinical Trial of Streptomycin in Pulmonary Tuberculosis in the 1940s', *British Medical Journal*, 317: 1220–3.

——(2002) 'Streptomycin in Postwar Britain: A Cultural History of a Miracle Drug', in M. Gijswijt-Hofstra, G. van Heteren and E. M. (Tilli) Tansey (eds), *Biographies of Remedies: Drugs, Medicines and Contraceptives in Dutch and Anglo-American Healing Cultures*, Amsterdam: Rodopi, 203–27.

Young, J. (1883–4) 'The Scavenging of Towns', *Transactions of the Sanitary Institute*, 5: 248.

Zelizer, V. (1981) *Pricing the Priceless Child: The Changing Social Value of Children*, New York: Basic Books.

Zimmermann, S. (2011) *Divide, Provide and Rule: An Integrative History of Poverty Policy, Social Policy, and Social Reform in Hungary under the Habsburg Monarchy*, Budapest: CEU Press.

Zukulu, S., Dold, T., Abbott, T. and Raimondo, D. (2012) *Medicinal and Charm Plants of Pondoland*, Pretoria: South African National Biodiversity Institute.

Zylberman, P. (2004) 'Fewer Parallels than Antitheses: René Sand and Andrija Štampar on Social Medicine, 1919–1955', *Social History of Medicine*, 17, 1: 77–92.

——(2005) 'Mosquitos and the Komitadjis: Malaria and Borders in Macedonia (1919–1938)', in I. Borowy and W. D. Gruner (eds), *Facing Illness in Troubled Times: Health in Europe in the Interwar Years, 1918–1939*, Bern: Peter Lang, 305–43.

# Index

Wellcome, Henry 202; Burroughs
  Wellcome 164, 173, 175, 177, 191
Western Cape 150
Western medicine 11, 142-4, 147f
Westphal, Carl 67
White, Paul Dudley 104
WHO *see* World Health Organization
Willink, Henry 133
Wilson, Woodrow 202
Witwatersrand 149, 151
WMA *see* World Medical Association
World Health Organization (WHO) 7,
  21, 143, 155, 207–10

World Medical Association 208

Yugoslavia 102f, 107–14, 117, 204, 208;
  Central Institute for Hygiene in
  Belgrade 111; Institute of Hygiene and
  School of Public Health in Sofia 111;
  Ministerial Commission for
  Epidemiology 111; National Popular
  Health Education Act 111

Zambia 143
Zelizer, Viviane 37
Zimbabwe 143